Electrocardiography of Arrhythmias

A COMPREHENSIVE REVIEW

Electrocardiography of Arrhythmias

A COMPREHENSIVE REVIEW

A COMPANION TO CARDIAC ELECTROPHYSIOLOGY: FROM CELL TO BEDSIDE

SECOND EDITION

MITHILESH K. DAS, MD

Professor of Clinical Medicine
Director, Electrophysiology Service
Cardiovascular Institute
Indiana University Health
Indianapolis, Indiana

DOUGLAS P. ZIPES, MD

Distinguished Professor
Professor Emeritus of Medicine, Pharmacology,
and Toxicology
Director Emeritus, Division of Cardiology and
the Krannert Institute of Cardiology
Indiana University School of Medicine
Editor, Practice Update Cardiology and Trends in
Cardiovascular Medicine
Indianapolis, Indiana

ELSEVIER

ELSEVIER
1600 John F. Kennedy Blvd.
Ste 1800
Philadelphia, PA 19103-2899

ELECTROCARDIOGRAPHY OF ARRHYTHMIAS:
A COMPREHENSIVE REVIEW, SECOND EDITION

ISBN: 9780323680509

Notice

Previous editions copyrighted 2012.

Library of Congress Control Number: 2020945514

Content Strategist: Robin Carter
Content Development Manager: Meghan Andress
Content Development Specialist: Angie Breckon
Publishing Services Manager: Shereen Jameel
Senior Project Manager: Karthikeyan Murthy
Design Direction: Renee Duenow

Printed in the United States of America.

Last digit is the print number: 9 8 7 6 5 4 3 2 1

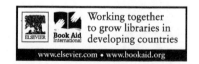

To our wives and families,
without whose support we could not have accomplished
a fraction of what we have achieved

To my parents, Ganpati Lal Das and Bimla Das; my wife, Rekha;
and my children, Awaneesh, Ruchi, Mohineesh, Kriti, and Avyukt

—MKD

To my wife, Joan,
and my children, Debra, Jeffrey, and David

—DPZ

Clinical cardiac electrophysiology continues to play a critically important role in the care of patients of all ages. Being able to interpret the electrocardiogram (ECG) accurately is vital for their evaluation and treatment. As more people live to older ages, arrhythmias become an ever-increasing component to their health and well-being. We have thoroughly revised and updated this second edition to facilitate learning the fundamental aspects of arrhythmia interpretation. Similar to the first edition, we have designed the book for learners at all levels of training, including internists with an interest in cardiology, trainees in cardiology and electrophysiology, and experienced cardiologists. This volume also continues as a companion to the well-known text, *Cardiac Electrophysiology: From Cell to Bedside*, soon in its eighth edition. We hope you find it a useful addition to help with your ECG reading skills.

Mithilesh K. Das, MD
Douglas P. Zipes, MD

CONTENTS

1 **Important Concepts,** 1

2 **Sinus Node Dysfunction,** 37

3 **Atrioventricular Conduction Abnormalities,** 61

4 **Junctional Rhythm,** 99

5 **Atrioventricular Nodal Reentrant Tachycardia,** 125

6 **Atrioventricular Reentrant Tachycardias,** 151

7 **Atrial Tachycardia,** 179

8 **Atrial Flutter,** 223

9 **Atrial Fibrillation,** 273

10 **Wide Complex Tachycardia,** 297

11 **Ventricular Tachycardia in the Absence of Structural Heart Disease,** 329

12 **Ventricular Tachycardia in Structural Heart Disease,** 361

13 **Polymorphic Ventricular Tachycardia and Ventricular Fibrillation in the Absence of Structural Heart Disease,** 411

Index, 463

1

Important Concepts

A normal 12-lead electrocardiogram (ECG) includes P, QRS, T, and sometimes the U waves (Fig. 1.1). The P wave is generated by activation of the atria, the P-R segment represents the duration of atrioventricular (AV) conduction, the QRS complex is produced by the activation of the two ventricles, and the ST-T wave reflects ventricular recovery. Normal values for the various intervals and waveforms of the ECG are shown in Table 1.1. The range of normal values of these measurements reflects the substantial interindividual variability related to (among other factors) differences in age, sex, body habitus, heart orientation, and physiology. In addition, significant differences in electrocardiographic patterns can occur in an individual's ECGs recorded days, hours, or even minutes apart. These intraindividual variations may be caused by technical issues (e.g., changes in electrode position) or the biologic effects of changes in posture, temperature, autonomics, or eating habits, and may be sufficiently large to alter diagnostic evidence for conditions, such as chamber hypertrophy.

P WAVE

Normal P waves (duration equal to <110 ms and amplitude <0.25 mV) are generated in the sinus node, which depolarizes in the direction from right to left atria and superior to inferior. P wave patterns in the precordial leads correspond to the direction of atrial activation wave fronts in the horizontal plane. Atrial activation early in the P wave is over the right atrium and is oriented primarily anteriorly; later, it shifts posteriorly as activation proceeds over the left atrium. Therefore P waves are positive in lead I and inferior in leads. The P wave in the right precordial leads (V1 and, occasionally, V2) is upright or, often, biphasic, with an initial positive deflection followed by a later negative deflection. In the more lateral leads, the P wave is upright and reflects continual right to left spread of the activation fronts. Variations in this pattern may reflect differences in pathways of interatrial conduction.

P waves with prolonged duration usually denote atrial conduction abnormalities and occur in atrial enlargement or myopathy, which can be a substrate for reentrant atrial tachycardia (Fig. 1.2 and Table 1.2). Negative P waves in lead I represent lead arm reversal or dextrocardia (Fig. 1.3). Isolated dextrocardia is not a precursor for arrhythmias, but when dextrocardia is associated with congenital heart disease, atrial arrhythmias caused by atrial myopathy or scarring related to cardiac surgery can occur. An abnormal P wave axis denotes an ectopic atrial rhythm, and intermittently changing P wave morphology from sinus to nonsinus represents wandering atrial pacemakers (Fig. 1.4). Frequent premature atrial complexes can provoke atrial tachyarrhythmia (atrial tachycardia, atrial fibrillation, and atrial flutter). Paroxysmal atrial fibrillation often is triggered by premature atrial complexes generated in the muscle sleeves of one or more pulmonary veins. Electrical isolation of these veins prevents the recurrence of atrial fibrillation (Fig. 1.5). P waves can enlarge in right and left atrial hypertrophy or enlargement.

Sinus P waves have prolonged duration and generally have a low amplitude after a maze surgery for atrial fibrillation (Fig. 1.6).

P-R INTERVAL AND P-R SEGMENT

The P-R segment is usually the isoelectric region beginning with the end of the P wave to the onset of the QRS complex. The P-R interval is measured from the onset of the P wave to the onset of the QRS complex. The P-R interval represents the initiation of atrial depolarization to the initiation of ventricular depolarization. It is the time taken by the sinus impulse to travel to the ventricles by way of the atrium, AV node, bundle of His, and bundle branches. A delay in any part of the conduction will prolong the P-R interval. Prolonged P-R interval results mostly from AV nodal disease and His-Purkinje disease but can occur due to atrial myopathy causing prolonged intra- or interatrial conduction. His-Purkinje disease is almost always associated with a bundle branch block (BBB). PR prolongation (>200 ms) caused by AV nodal disease or severe His-Purkinje disease represents a potential substrate for various degrees of heart block (see Chapter 3). A short P-R interval (<120 ms) can result from enhanced AV nodal conduction (Fig. 1.7), ventricular preexcitation (Fig. 1.8), or an atrial rhythm. Isorhythmic AV dissociation can also falsely appear as short P-R interval (Fig. 1.9).

QRS WAVE

Normal QRS complexes represent the depolarization of both ventricles (normal QRS duration = 60–120 ms). This is represented by the beginning of the Q wave and end of the S wave. Ventricular depolarization begins at the left side of the interventricular septum near the AV junction and progresses across the interventricular septum from left to right. The impulse then travels simultaneously to both the ventricles endocardially by way of the right and left bundle branches. It also progresses from the endocardial surface through the ventricular wall to the epicardial surface. The normal Q wave is the first negative deflection of the QRS, which is not preceded by any R wave and represents interventricular depolarization. The R wave is the first positive deflection in the QRS complex. Subsequent positive deflection in the QRS above the baseline represents a bundle branch delay or bundle branch block (BBB) called R′ (R prime). The S wave is the first negative deflection (below the baseline) after an R wave. The QS wave is a QRS complex that is entirely a negative wave without any positive deflection (R wave) above the baseline. The larger waves that form a major deflection in QRS complexes are usually identified by uppercase letters (QS, R, S), whereas smaller waves with amplitude less than the half of the major positive (R wave) or negative (S wave) deflection are denoted by lowercase letters (q, r, s). Therefore notches in R, S, or QS waves can be defined as qR, Rs, RSR, QrS, or rS patterns. The QRS morphology on a particular ECG lead depends on the sum vector of depolarization toward or away from that

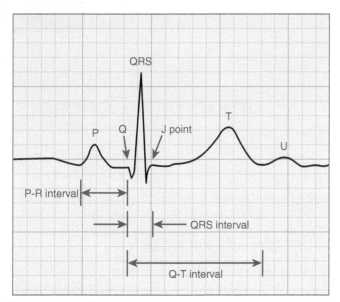

Fig. 1.1 Normal QRS waves and baseline intervals.

TABLE 1.1   Normal Electrocardiogram Parameters

Electrocardiogram Waves or Intervals	Duration in MS
P wave duration	<110
P-R interval	120 to <200 ms
QRS duration	<100 ms
QTc (corrected Q-T interval)[a]	≤460 for men and ≤470 for women
U wave[b]	N/A

N/A, Not applicable.

[a]The QTc is traditionally reported in units of ms; however, the units of the QTc will vary with the formula used for the rate correction. The commonly applied Bazett formula is a ratio of Q-T interval in ms to the square root of R-R interval in seconds. Fridericia formula: $QTc = QT/\sqrt[3]{RR}$.

[b]U waves may normally be present in midprecordial leads in a few individuals. The normal range of amplitude and duration is not well defined.

lead. Usually, the R waves are upright in limb leads and augmented limb leads except for lead aVR. A QS pattern in lead V1-V2 may represent normal myocardial depolarization, but a Q wave in lead V3 represents myocardial scarring, usually caused by a septal myocardial infarction. QRS transition is seen in lead V3-V4 with R wave amplitude larger than S wave amplitude. R waves are upright in lead V5-V6 because of a positive net vector toward these precordial leads. Poor progression of R wave amplitude across the precordial leads represents severe myocardial disease. It is seen in severe nonischemic and ischemic cardiomyopathy with severely reduced left ventricular ejection fraction.

Q WAVES

The normal Q wave duration is less than 40 ms with amplitude less than one-fourth of the amplitude of the succeeding R wave. Q waves in the baseline ECG of a patient with palpitations can be a clue to reentrant ventricular arrhythmias. Q waves more than 40 ms may be due to scarring from a myocardial infarction. Noninfarction Q waves (pseudoinfarction pattern) are also encountered in ventricular hypertrophy, fascicular blocks, preexcitation, cardiomyopathy, pneumothorax, pulmonary embolus, amyloid heart disease, primary and metastatic tumors of the heart, traumatic heart disease, intracranial hemorrhage, hyperkalemia, pericarditis, early repolarization, and cardiac sarcoidosis.

INTRAVENTRICULAR CONDUCTION ABNORMALITIES

QRS prolongation can be because of the conduction system abnormality resulting from a right bundle branch block (RBBB) or a left bundle branch block (LBBB). When the QRS duration is prolonged, often called *wide* (> 120 ms), and its morphology does not qualify for a BBB, then it is called an *interventricular conduction defect* (IVCD). IVCD can result from myocardial disease, such as coronary artery disease or cardiomyopathy. IVCD can also result from electrolyte abnormalities, such as hypokalemia or antiarrhythmic drug therapy, mainly with the use of class I drugs (sodium channel blockers), which prolong the conduction velocity of the myocardial depolarizing waves (Fig. 1.10). IVCD can represent a substrate for ventricular arrhythmias. Other causes of a wide QRS include premature ventricular complexes, ventricular preexcitation, or a paced ventricular rhythm.

FRAGMENTED QRS COMPLEXES

Fragmented QRS is defined as the presence of one or more notches in the R wave or S wave without any BBB in two contiguous leads. *Fragmented wide QRS* is defined as QRS duration greater than 120 ms with 2 or more notches in the R wave or the S wave in two contiguous leads. QRS fragmentation and Q waves represent myocardial infarction scarring and can indicate a substrate for reentrant ventricular arrhythmias (Figs. 1.11–1.14).

BUNDLE BRANCH BLOCK AND FASCICULAR BLOCKS

Conduction block or delay in one of the bundle branches results in the depolarization of the corresponding ventricle by way of the contralateral bundle (Table 1.3). The RBBB has rSR′ pattern in lead V1-V2, whereas LBBB has rSR′ pattern in lead V6 and lead I (Figs. 1.15–1.17). The QRS duration between 100 ms and less than 120 ms is called *incomplete BBB*, and greater than 120 ms is called a *complete BBB*. Narrow QRS at baseline and a physiologic delay in one of the bundle branches at higher heart rates can cause BBB and is called *ventricular aberrancy* (see Chapter 6). A wide complex tachycardia is more commonly a ventricular tachycardia but can also be a supraventricular tachycardia with BBB or ventricular aberrancy.

MULTIFASCICULAR BLOCK

Conduction delay in any two fascicles is called a *bifascicular block*, and delay in all three fascicles is termed a *trifascicular block* (Table 1.4). The term *bilateral bundle branch block* has been used to refer to concomitant conduction abnormalities in both the left and right bundle branch systems. Trifascicular block involves conduction delay in the right bundle branch plus delay in the main left bundle branch or in both the left anterior and the left posterior fascicles.

Rate-dependent conduction block or ventricular aberrancy, BBB, fascicular block, or IVCD can occur with changes in the heart rate.

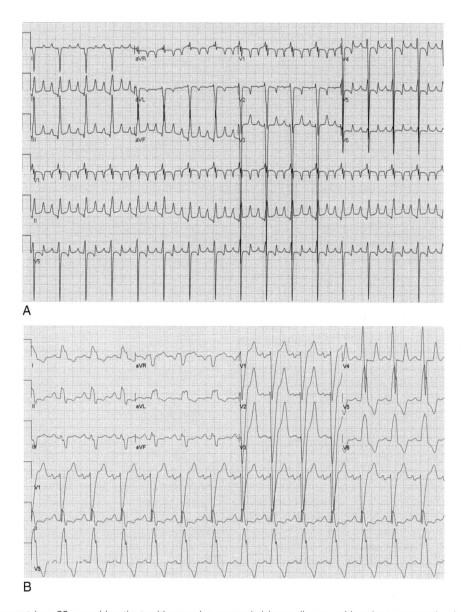

Fig. 1.2 Biatrial enlargement in a 32-year-old patient with complex congenital heart disease with pulmonary atresia, double inlet ventricle, and multiple cardiac shunts (A). Lead II shows tall P waves greater than 0.25 mV, and lead V1 shows deep inverted T waves. The patient suffered from atrial arrhythmias. (B) Biatrial enlargement with left bundle branch block in a patient with nonischemic dilated cardiomyopathy with severely reduced left ventricular systolic function.

TABLE 1.2 **Right and Left Atrial Enlargement**	
Left Atrial Abnormality	**Right Atrial Abnormality**
P wave duration >120 ms in lead II	Peaked P waves with amplitudes in lead II >0.25 mV (P pulmonale)
Prominent notching of P wave, usually most obvious in lead II, with interval between notches of 0.40 ms (P mitrale)	Prominent initial positivity in lead V_1 or V_2 >0.15 mV
Ratio between the duration of the P wave in lead II and duration of the PR segment >1.6	Increased area under initial positive portion of the P wave in lead V_1 to >0.06 mm-sec
Increased duration and depth of terminal-negative portion of P wave in lead V_1 (P terminal force) so that area subtended by >0.04 mm-sec	Rightward shift of mean P wave axis to more than +75°
Leftward shift of mean P wave axis to between −30° and −45°	

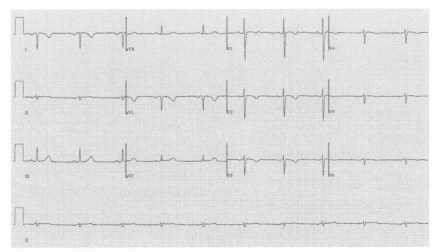

Fig. 1.3 Electrocardiogram showing inverted P and QRS waves in lead I along with poor progression of R wave. This is due to dextrocardia. The arm lead reversal is also associated with similar P and QRS axis in lead I, but the QRS progression in precordial leads is unaffected.

1. Ashman phenomenon: The duration of the refractory period of the ventricular myocardium is a function primarily of the immediately preceding cycle length(s). If the preceding cycle length is long, the refractory period of the subsequent QRS complex is long and may conduct with BBB aberrancy (Ashman phenomenon) as part of a long cycle—short cycle sequence, often when there is an abrupt prolongation of the immediately preceding cycle. The RBBB aberrancy is more common than LBBB aberrancy because the refractory period of the right bundle is usually longer than that of the left bundle at slower heart rates (Fig. 1.18).
2. Acceleration (tachycardia)-dependent block or conduction delay: It is manifest as either RBBB or LBBB, which occurs when the heart rate exceeds a critical value. At the cellular level, this aberration is the result of encroachment of the impulse on the relative refractory period (sometime during phase 3 of the action potential) of the preceding impulse, which results in slower conduction (Figs. 1.19–1.23).
3. Deceleration (bradycardia)-dependent block or conduction delay: It occurs when the heart rate falls below a critical level. It is thought to be due to abnormal phase 4 depolarization of cells so that activation occurs at reduced resting potentials. Deceleration-dependent block is less common than acceleration-dependent block and usually occurs in the setting of a significant conduction system disease (Fig. 1.23).

FASCICULAR BLOCK

Fascicular block is an abnormal delay or conduction block in one of the fascicles of the LBBB. This alters ventricular activation, and therefore the axis of the QRS is altered. Isolated fascicular block (without any BBB) does not prolong the QRS significantly. Left anterior fascicular block is associated with qR pattern in lead aVL, QRS axis between −45° and −90°, and the time to peak R wave in aVL 45 ms or more. Left posterior fascicular block is associated with a qR pattern in lead III and aVF, rS pattern in lead I and aVL, and QRS axis between +90° and +180°. Other causes of QRS wave changes similar to that of left posterior fascicular block include right ventricular hypertrophy and lateral wall myocardial infarction.

J POINT AND J WAVE

The J point is the junction between the end of QRS and initiation of the ST segment. A J wave is a dome- or hump-shaped wave caused by J point elevation. The amplitude of the normal J point and ST segment varies with race, sex, autonomic input, and age. The upper limits of J point elevation in leads V2 and V3 are 0.2 mV for men older than 40 years, 0.25 mV for men younger than 40 years, and 0.15 mV for women. In other leads the accepted upper limit is 0.1 mV.

The J wave can be prominent as a normal variant called *early repolarization* (Figs. 1.24 and 1.25). However, the incidence of early repolarization abnormality in the inferolateral leads is higher in patients who were resuscitated after sudden cardiac death, and therefore it may not always be benign, as was previously believed. In addition, the J wave can be seen in systemic hypothermia (Osborn wave), Brugada pattern, coronary artery disease, and electrolyte abnormalities and during vagal stimulation. Its origin has been related to a prominent notch (phase 1) of the action potentials on the epicardium but not on the endocardium (Figs. 1.26–1.28).

U WAVE

In some patients the T wave can be followed by an additional low-amplitude wave known as the *U wave*. This wave, usually less than 0.1 mV in amplitude, normally has the same polarity as the preceding T wave and is best seen in anterior precordial leads. It is most often seen at slow heart rates. Its electrophysiologic basis is uncertain; it may be caused by the late repolarization of the Purkinje fibers, by the long action potential of midmyocardial M cells, or by delayed repolarization in areas of the ventricle that undergo late mechanical relaxation. Prominent U waves can be seen in hypokalemia (discussed later). Inverted U waves are a sign of coronary ischemia.

ST-T WAVES

Normal ST segment is almost always isoelectric to the PR and TP segments. ST segment elevation can be defined morphologically as coving, concavity upward, or downsloping. ST horizontal or coving segment elevation occurs in acute myocardial infarction, coronary vasospasm, and left ventricular aneurysm (Box 1.1). ST segment elevation with concavity upward is seen in acute pericarditis. Coved or saddleback ST segment elevation with incomplete RBBB is called a Brugada pattern ECG. Persistence of juvenile pattern of T wave inversion in precordial adults is encountered in 1% to 3% of the population.

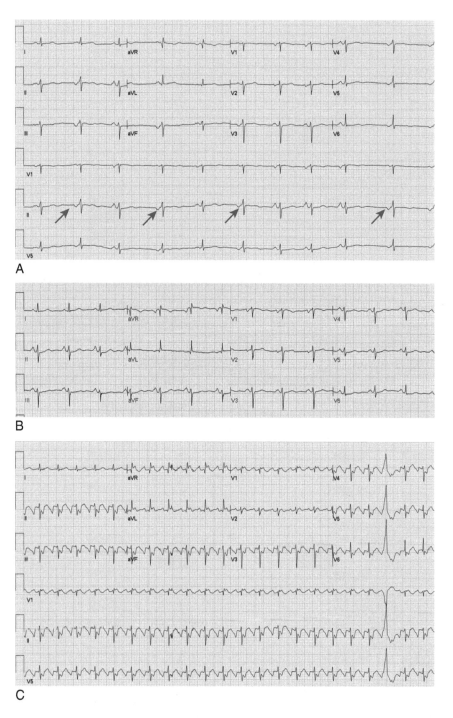

Fig. 1.4 Wandering atrial pacemaker. (A) Electrocardiogram depicts intermittent change in P wave morphology from sinus rhythm to low atrial rhythm (inverted P waves in lead II, *arrows*). (B) Electrocardiogram shows P wave morphology and axis during sinus rhythm. Wandering atrial pacemaker usually does not denote atrial pathology, however, this patient later developed atrial flutter with 2:1 atrioventricular block (C).

When ST segment or T wave changes (or both) occur without any cardiac pathology or abnormal physiologic state, they are called *nonspecific ST-T changes*. This includes slight ST depression or T wave inversion or T wave flattening.

Q-T INTERVAL

The Q-T interval extends from the onset of the QRS complex to the end of the T wave. Thus it includes the total duration of ventricular depolarization and repolarization. Ventricular depolarization, and therefore repolarization, does not occur instantaneously. Electrophysiologically, the Q-T interval is therefore a summation of action potentials in both ventricles. It is measured from the onset of the QRS to the end of the T wave. The Q-T interval duration will vary from lead to lead in a normal ECG by as much as 50 to 60 ms. The difference between the longest and shortest Q-T interval is called *Q-T dispersion*. Accurately measuring the Q-T interval is challenging for several reasons, including identifying the beginning of the QRS

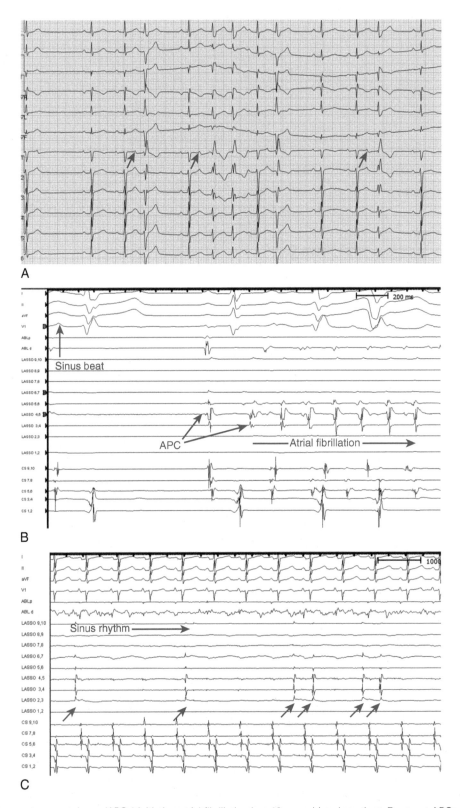

Fig. 1.5 Frequent atrial premature complexes (APCs) initiating atrial fibrillation in a 40-year-old male patient. Frequent APCs, mostly originating from pulmonary veins, can trigger focal atrial fibrillation. (A) Electrocardiogram shows frequent monomorphic APCs with right bundle branch block aberrancy initiating a short run of atrial tachycardia. The APC was mapped to be originating from the right superior pulmonary vein. (B) APC was mapped by a circular decapolar catheter (Lasso 1,2 to Lasso 9,10) and an ablation catheter (Abl D and Abl P) placed at the ostium of the pulmonary vein. (C) These APCs repeatedly initiated atrial fibrillation. All these rapid focal discharges in the right pulmonary veins do not reach the left atrium, as shown by the coronary sinus recording (CS 1,2 [distal] to CS 9,10 [proximal]). Electrical isolation of the right superior pulmonary vein during catheter ablation is confirmed because these focal discharges are still present in the pulmonary vein during the sinus rhythm but do not reach the left atrium; therefore the initiation atrial fibrillation is prevented. Arrows indicate atrial premature complexes.

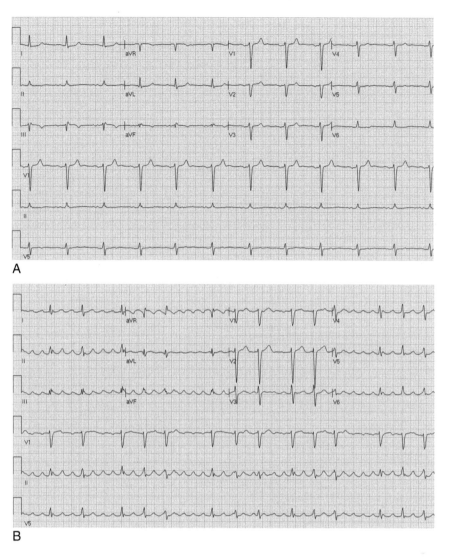

Fig. 1.6 Low voltage and prolonged P waves in a patient with a history of maze procedure for atrial fibrillation (A). (B) Patient developed atrial flutter 2 years after the procedure. Flutter waves are positive in inferior leads, negative in lead aVR and aVL, and isoelectric/negative in V1. Flutter circuit was mapped at the right superior pulmonary vein ostium during electrophysiology study.

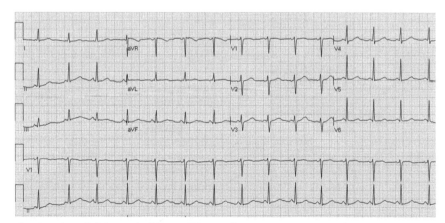

Fig. 1.7 Electrocardiogram showing short P-R interval with no evidence of preexcitation. This is called *enhanced atrioventricular nodal conduction* because of the minimum normal delay at the atrioventricular nodal level for the atrial impulse to reach the ventricle by way of the His-Purkinje system. This is not a precursor of arrhythmia but can conduct impulses rapidly from the atria to the ventricles during an atrial arrhythmia.

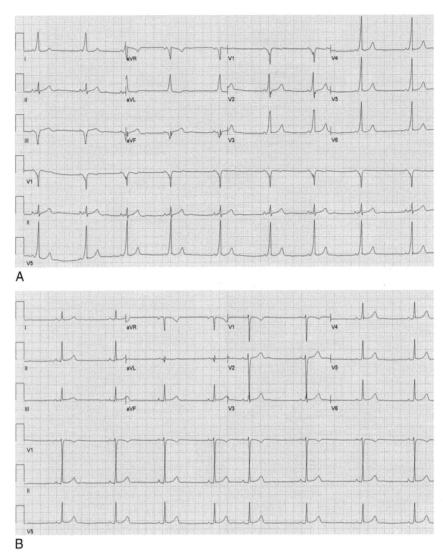

Fig. 1.8 Short P-R interval caused by preexcitation in a 19-year-old female patient. Electrocardiogram shows a short P-R interval of 80 ms resulting from preexcitation (negative delta waves in lead V1 and inferior leads and positive delta waves in lead I and aVL) over a right posteroseptal accessory pathway (A) that was successfully ablated. The P-R interval normalized after the ablation (B).

complex and end of the T wave; determining which lead(s) to use; and adjusting the measured interval for rate, QRS duration, and sex. The presence of U waves also complicates the measurement. Q-T interval should be measured in the lead at which it is longest, and without a prominent U wave. In automated electrocardiographic systems, the interval is typically measured from a composite of all leads, with the interval beginning with the earliest onset of the QRS in any lead and ending with the latest end of the T wave in any lead.

The Q-T interval changes with heart rates, shorter at faster heart rates and longer at slower ones. Therefore numerous formulas have been proposed to correct the measured Q-T interval for this rate effect to a rate of 60 bpm. The Bazett formula is commonly used in the clinical practice. The corrected Q-T interval (QTc) is measured by the ratio of Q-T interval in seconds and the root square of the R-R interval in seconds (QTc [ms] = Q-T/ $\sqrt{RR}$ [sec]).

Because the Bazett correction exaggerates the correction at faster heart rates and undercorrects at slower heart rates, the Fridericia correction is often preferred. It uses cube root of R-R interval instead of square root of R-R interval used in Bazett formula (QTc = Q-T/ $\sqrt[3]{RR}$).

LEFT AND RIGHT VENTRICULAR HYPERTROPHY

ECG manifestation of left ventricular hypertrophy (LVH) includes increased amplitude of the QRS complex. R waves in lateral leads (I, aVL, V_5, and V_6) and S waves in right precordial leads are increased in LVH, whereas ST-T segment changes in LVH are varied. The common findings are downsloping ST segment from a depressed J point and asymmetrically inverted T waves. Apart from QRS wave changes, ventricular hypertrophy is also associated with atrial abnormalities (Table 1.5 and Box 1.2).

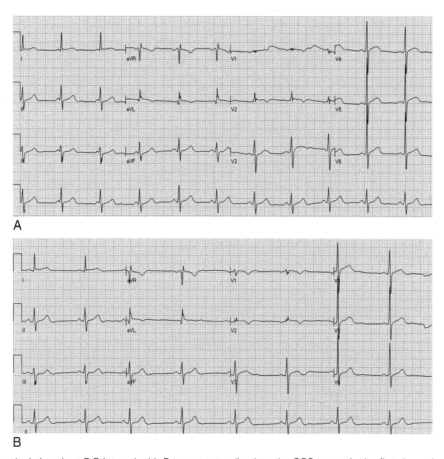

Fig. 1.9 Electrocardiogram depicting short P-R interval with P waves extending into the QRS waves in the first three sinus complexes followed by short P-R interval (A). It is an isorhythmic atrioventricular dissociation. (B) Electrocardiogram showing normal sinus rhythm of the same patient with a normal P-R interval of 164 ms.

RIGHT-SIDED PRECORDIAL LEAD PLACEMENT

Right-sided lead placement is needed when dextrocardia or right ventricular infarction is suspected. In acute right ventricular infarction, V_{4R} shows ST elevation. Dextrocardia and arm reversal is suspected when the P wave is negative in lead I. However, in dextrocardia, the QRS morphology of the precordial leads shows poor progression of R waves, whereas in arm lead reversal precordial progression of R wave is unchanged. In dextrocardia, ECG placement can be corrected when the left arm lead is placed on the right arm, the right arm lead is placed on the left arm, and the V1 through V6 leads are placed in the V1, V2, and V3R through V6R positions. When Brugada syndrome is suspected and the typical coving pattern of ST-T segment is present but J point elevation is less than 2 mm in a routine ECG, precordial leads V1 and V2 can be placed in third or second intercostal spaces, which may elicit typical Brugada pattern with more than 2 mm J point elevation and coved pattern spontaneously or with the use of a class I antiarrhythmic drug.

GENERALIZED LOW VOLTAGE

Generalized low voltage is defined when the amplitude of the QRS complexes in precordial leads is less than 1 mV and in the limb leads are <0.5 mV. This is commonly present in obesity, pericardial effusion,

chronic obstructive lung disease, and severe myopathy, such as cardiac amyloidosis. Cardiac amyloidosis is a substrate for conduction block or ventricular arrhythmias.

CORONARY ARTERY DISEASE

Coronary artery disease is the second most common cause of conduction system disease and the most common cause of ventricular arrhythmias. The ECG plays a major role in the diagnosis of acute and chronic coronary artery disease. ECG changes result from depolarization or repolarization abnormalities (or both). Acute ST elevation myocardial infarction (STEMI) may be associated with serial changes: transient hyperacute (tall) T waves, ST elevation in two contiguous leads, and later abnormal Q waves in two contiguous leads. Non-ST elevation myocardial infarction (NSTEMI) is more difficult to diagnose, and the diagnosis depends on the elevation of cardiac biomarkers. ECG signs of NSTEMI include T wave inversion, ST depression, and fragmentation of the QRS waves in two contiguous leads. Atrial arrhythmias, such as atrial fibrillation, can occur during an acute myocardial infarction (MI). Bifascicular block, when it occurs with anterior MI, carries a poor prognosis. Complete heart block during anterior MI also carries a poor prognosis because it represents a large infarction with an extensive involvement of His-Purkinje system. AV block with an inferior MI usually results

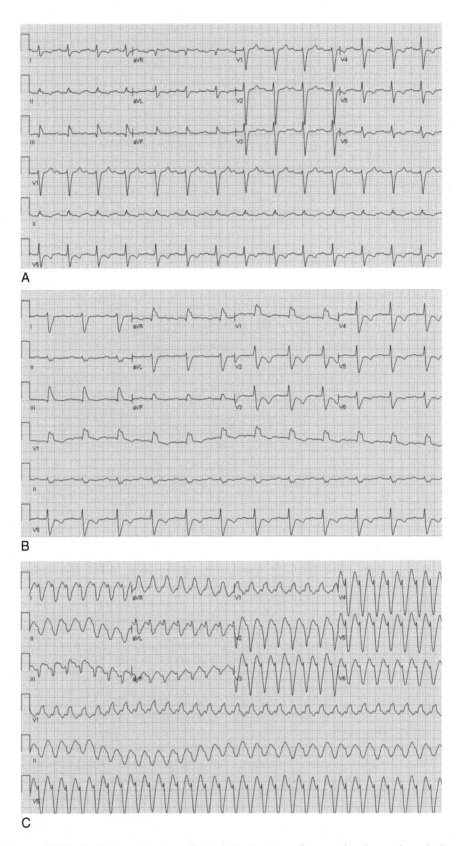

Fig. 1.10 (A) Electrocardiogram (ECG) of a 59-year-old male patient with ischemic cardiomyopathy shows sinus rhythm with a long P-R interval (270 ms) and intraventricular conduction delay (QRS duration = 156 ms). (B) ECG of the same patient after 3 months shows long P-R interval, left bundle branch block, and right axis deviation suggestive of a multifascicular block. (C) ECG showing wide complex tachycardia that is an atrial tachycardia left bundle branch block with further prolongation of QRS waves.

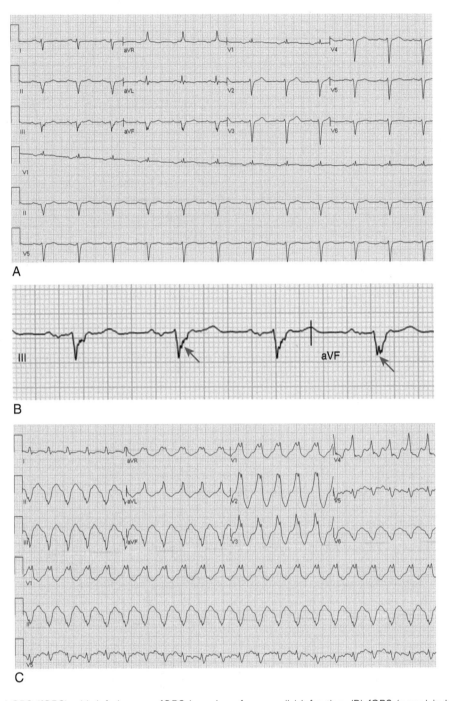

Fig. 1.11 (A) Fragmented QRS (fQRS) with inferior scar. fQRS is a sign of myocardial infarction. (B) fQRS (*arrow*) in lead III, and aVF signifies inferior myocardial scar. (C) Electrocardiogram of the same patient shows a wide complex tachycardia, which is a ventricular tachycardia arising from the inferoposterior wall of the left ventricle.

from a high vagal tone or ischemia to the AV nodal artery and generally carries a good prognosis (Fig. 1.29). Polymorphic ventricular tachycardia and ventricular fibrillation can also be the presenting manifestation of an acute MI (Fig. 1.30). Repetitive monomorphic idioventricular rhythm is encountered during the reperfusion phase of MI (reperfusion arrhythmia) (Fig. 1.31). Sinus node dysfunction and AV block can occur within the first few months of MI. Patients with a remote MI are at a risk for scar-related monomorphic, polymorphic VT, and ventricular fibrillation (Fig. 1.32A). Fig. 1.32B

shows the baseline ECG showing fragmented QRS inferior leads, which represents myocardial scar.

QRS ALTERNANS AND T WAVE ALTERNANS

Beat-to-beat variation of QRS or T wave amplitude are called *QRS* and *T wave alternans*, respectively. QRS alternans can occur in pericardial tamponade, in severe myocardial disease, or during a supraventricular or ventricular tachycardia (Figs. 1.33 and 1.34). Macroscopic T wave

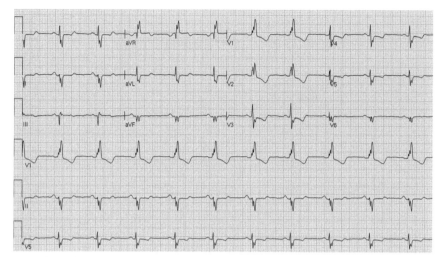

Fig. 1.12 Electrocardiogram depicting sinus rhythm with right bundle branch block pattern in lead V1-V2, which has three notches, and therefore is defined as fragmented right bundle branch block. The patient had inferior myocardial scar. The patient developed scar-related ventricular tachycardia originating near the mitral annulus.

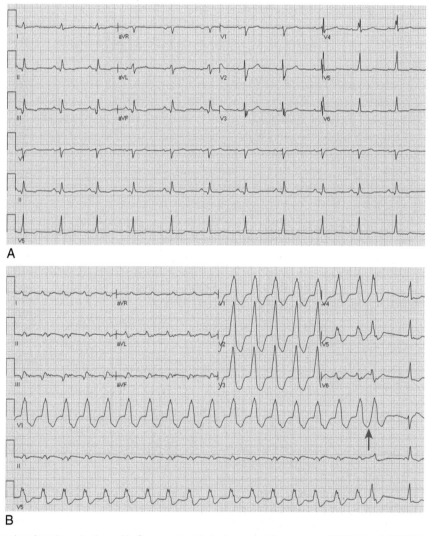

Fig. 1.13 Electrocardiogram showing sinus rhythm with Q waves in inferior leads and fragmented QRS in leads V2-V4 in a 64-year-old male patient with anteroseptal and inferoposterior scar (A). Patient presented with a ventricular tachycardia (B) that terminated spontaneously after a premature ventricular contraction (*arrow*).

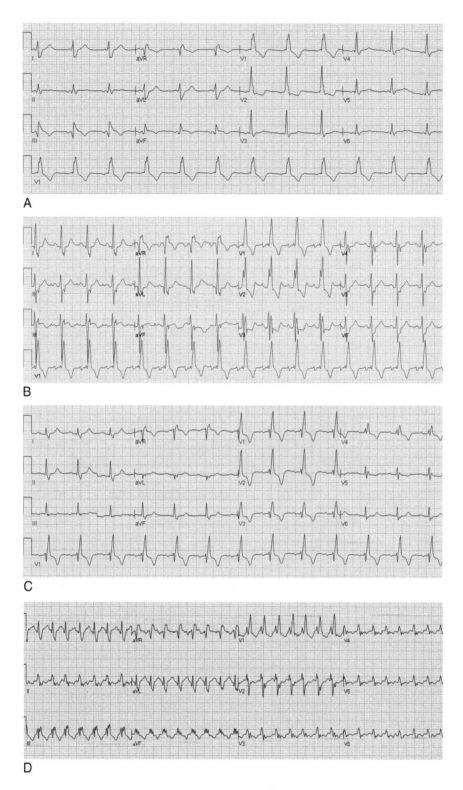

Fig. 1.14 Electrocardiogram showing typical right bundle branch block with RsR′ (A), rsR′ (B), rSR′ (C), and rsR′ (D) pattern in lead V1, and wide and slurred S wave in lead V5.

alternans is uncommon and is reported in long QT syndrome preceding an episode of torsades de pointes.

ELECTROLYTE IMBALANCE

Electrolyte imbalance, such as hypokalemia, hyperkalemia, hypocalcemia, and hypercalcemia, can cause various ECG changes. Isolated hypernatremia or hyponatremia does not produce consistent effects on the ECG. Metabolic acidosis and alkalosis, which are often associated with hyperkalemia and hypokalemia, respectively, can provoke arrhythmias. Severe hypermagnesemia can cause AV and intraventricular conduction disturbances, including complete heart block. Hypomagnesemia is usually associated with hypocalcemia or hypokalemia. Hypomagnesemia and hypokalemia can potentiate certain

TABLE 1.3 Electrocardiogram Criteria for Bundle Branch Block and Fascicular Block

Block	Electrocardiogram Signs
Complete RBBB	QRS duration ≥ 120 ms
	Broad, notched secondary R waves (rsr, rsR, or rSR patterns) in right precordial leads (V1 and V2)
	Wide, deep S waves (qRS pattern) in left precordial leads (V5 and V6)
	Delayed intrinsicoid deflection (> 50 ms) in right precordial leads
Complete LBBB	QRS duration ≥ 120 ms
	Broad, notched, monophasic R waves in V5 and V6, and usually in leads I and aVL
	Small or absent initial r waves in V1 and V2, followed by deep S waves (rS or QS patterns)
	Absent septal q waves in left-sided leads (leads I, V5, and V6)
	Delayed intrinsicoid deflection (> 60 ms) in V5 and V6
	ST segment and T wave directed opposite to the predominant deflection of the QRS complex
LAFB	Frontal plane mean QRS axis of −45° to −90°
	rS patterns in leads II, III, and aVF (the S wave in lead III is deeper than lead II)
	qR pattern in aVL
	Delayed intrinsicoid deflection in aVL
	QRS duration <120 ms
LPFB	Frontal plane of mean QRS axis ≥ 100°
	rS pattern in leads I and aVL, and qR patterns in leads II, III, and aVF (S1-Q3 pattern)
	QRS duration <110 ms
	Exclusion of other factors causing right axis deviation (right ventricular overload patterns, lateral MI)
	Delayed intrinsicoid deflection in aVF

LAFB, Left anterior fascicular block; *LBBB*, left bundle branch block; *LPFB*, left posterior fascicular block; *MI*, myocardial infarction; *RBBB*, right bundle branch block.

digitalis toxic arrhythmias. ECG signs of electrolyte imbalance may be lacking even in severe imbalance and may not correlate with the levels of the electrolyte.

Hypokalemia

ECG manifestations of hypokalemia include ST depression with flattened T waves and increased U wave prominence (Fig. 1.35). The U waves can exceed the amplitude of T waves. Clinically, distinguishing T waves from U waves can be difficult or impossible from the 12-lead ECG. The prolongation of repolarization with hypokalemia, as part of an acquired long QT(U) syndrome, predisposes to torsades de pointes.

Hyperkalemia

Mild hyperkalemia is associated with narrowing and peaking (tenting) of the T wave (Fig. 1.36). With the progressive increase in potassium level, the P wave decreases in amplitude and the QRS begins to widen. P-R interval prolongation can occur. It may be followed by AV block. Sinus activity is suppressed, P waves may disappear, and junctional escape rhythm, or so-called sinoventricular rhythm, may appear. The putative sinoventricular rhythm is explained by persisting sinus rhythm with conduction between the sinus and AV nodes, without producing an overt P wave. Experimental evidence of this phenomenon is lacking, and it most likely results from very-low-amplitude P waves. Moderate to severe hyperkalemia occasionally induces ST elevation in the right precordial leads (V1 and V2) and simulates an ischemic current of injury or Brugada-type patterns. Very marked hyperkalemia leads to eventual asystole, sometimes preceded by a slow undulatory ("sine-wave") ventricular flutter-like pattern.

HYPOCALCEMIA AND HYPERCALCEMIA

Changes in serum calcium levels predominantly alter the myocardial action potential duration. Hypercalcemia shortens the ventricular action potential duration by shortening phase 2 of the action potential, thereby shortening the ST segment, which results in shortening of the Q-T interval. In contrast, hypocalcemia prolongs phase 2 of the action potential and prolongs the ST segment, and therefore the Q-T interval (Figs. 1.37−1.39).

GAP PHENOMENON

The gap phenomenon is an unexpected sequence of AV nodal or bundle branch conduction in which a late premature atrial beat fails to conduct the ventricles or one of the bundle branches, but the conduction resumes when a premature atrial beat occurs earlier (shorter R-P′ interval) (Fig. 1.39). The physiologic basis of the gap phenomenon depends on a distal area with a long refractory period and a proximal site with a shorter refractory period. During the gap phenomenon, initial block occurs distally. With earlier impulses, proximal conduction delay is encountered, which allows the distal site of early block to recover excitability and resume conduction. Therefore, proximal delay in conduction allows distal recovery of refractoriness.

PARASYSTOLE

Parasystole is due to the function of a secondary pacemaker in the heart (Figs. 1.40−1.42) and requires not only "focal" impulse formation but also an area that protects (shields) the "focus" from discharge of the rest of the myocardium. Generally, the protected "focus" of automaticity of this type can fire at its own intrinsic frequency. The three classical criteria are (1) varying coupling intervals, (2) mathematically related interectopic intervals, and (3) presence of fusion beats. Pure ventricular parasystole is usually classified as continuous, but without exit block; continuous with exit block; or intermittent. Frequently, however, modulated parasystole occurs in which the normal QRS complex modulates the timing of the parasystolic focus.

CONCEALED CONDUCTION

Concealed conduction is defined as the propagation of an impulse within the specialized conduction system (AV node and His-Purkinje system), which cannot be recognized on surface ECG because of its low amplitude. This impulse travels only a limited distance within the conduction tissue with incomplete anterograde or retrograde penetration.

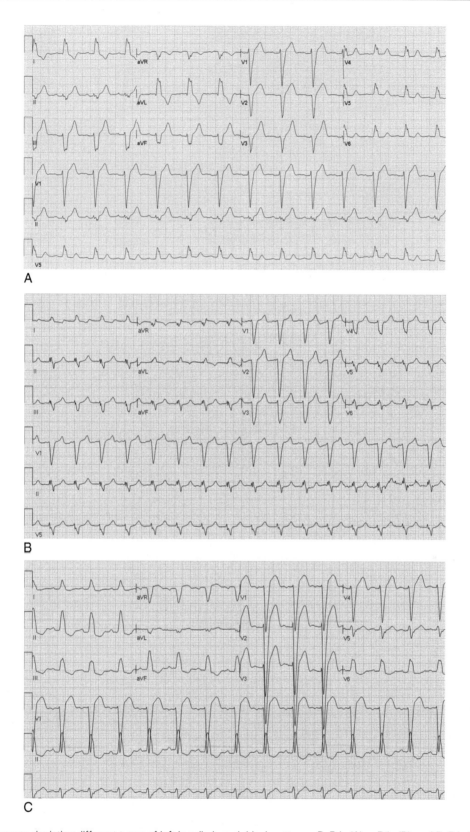

Fig. 1.15 Electrocardiograms depicting different types of left bundle branch block patterns: RsR in (A), rsR in (B), and RsR in lead V6 in (C).

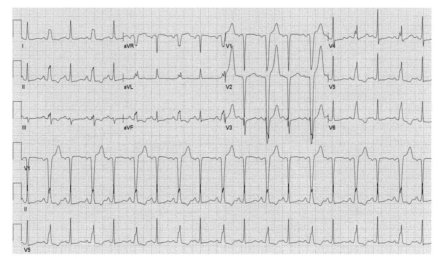

Fig. 1.16 Electrocardiogram showing sinus rhythm with left bundle branch block in alternate QRS complexes.

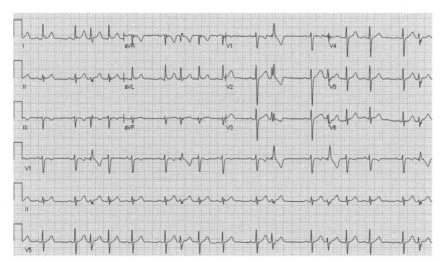

Fig. 1.17 Electrocardiogram showing sinus rhythm with frequent premature atrial contractions initiating short, long-short cycles conducting to the ventricles with right bundle branch block aberrancy (Ashman phenomenon).

TABLE 1.4	**Electrocardiographic Manifestations of Multifasciular Block**	
Type of Block	**Cause**	**Electrocardiogram Manifestations**
Bifascicular block	RBBB + LAFB	RBBB with left axis deviation beyond −45°
	RBBB + LPFB	RBBB with a mean QRS axis deviation to the right of +120°
	LAFB + LPFB	LBBB alone that may be caused by delay in both the anterior and posterior fascicles.[a]
Trifascicular block	RBBB + LAFB + LPFB	PR >200 ms + RBBB + LAD
	RBBB + LBBB	Alternate RBBB and LBBB

LAD, Left axis deviation; *LAFB*, left anterior fascicular block; *LBBB*, left bundle branch block; *LPFB*, left posterior fascicular block; *RBBB*, right bundle branch block.

[a]This form of LBBB represents one of the inadequacies of current electrocardiographic terminology and the simplification inherent in the trifascicular schema of the conduction system.

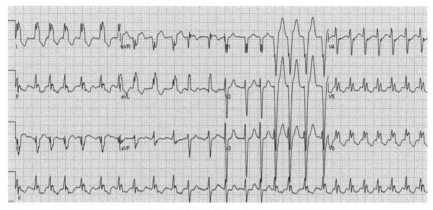

Fig. 1.18 Electrocardiogram showing atrial fibrillation with intermittent left bundle branch block aberrancy.

Therefore it can interfere with the formation or propagation of subsequent supraventricular or ventricular impulse. It can be recognized on the ECG by a change in subsequent interval or cycle length.

Concealment at the Atrioventricular Nodal Level

The commonest example of concealment is seen at the AV nodal level. During atrial fibrillation a slow ventricular rate is due to repeated concealed conduction with varying degrees of penetration and block into the AV node. This is an example of anterograde concealment of AV node. Prolongation of the P-R interval or AV nodal block after a non-conducted premature depolarization of any origin (ventricle or His bundle) can also occur. When premature ventricular complexes or a junctional complex incompletely penetrates the AV node, it resets its refractoriness and can make it fully or partially refractory in the face of the next sinus impulse. Therefore the next sinus impulse can be blocked or can conduct with a longer P-R interval. Typically, it occurs with interpolated premature ventricular complex with retrograde concealment in the AV node resulting in a longer P-R interval in the subsequent cycle (Figs. 1.43 and 1.44; see also Chapter 4).

CONCEALED CONDUCTION AT THE HIS-PURKINJE LEVEL

Concealment of conduction at the His-Purkinje level occurs as a result of perpetuation of aberrant conduction during supraventricular tachycardia with a BBB aberrancy. The perpetuation of aberrant conduction results from retrograde penetration of the BBB subsequent to transseptal conduction. Perpetuation of aberrant ventricular conduction (functional BBB) is induced by a sudden increase in the

ventricular rate. Often, the aberrancy shows hysteresis and persists even after the ventricular rate slows to rates less than the rate that initiated the functional BBB. This phenomenon can be explained by transseptal activation of the aberrant bundle from the contralateral bundle branch. Alternatively, a premature ventricular complex from the left ventricle during a supraventricular tachycardia can activate the left bundle branch early and then conduct transseptally and later penetrate the right bundle branch retrogradely. Subsequently, the left bundle branch recovers in time for the next supraventricular impulse, whereas the right remains refractory. Therefore the next supraventricular tachycardia impulse travels to the left ventricle over the left bundle branch (with an RBBB pattern). Conduction subsequently propagates from the left ventricle across the septum to the right ventricle. By this time the distal right bundle branch has recovered, allowing for retrograde penetration of the right bundle branch by the transseptal wavefront, thereby rendering the right bundle branch refractory to each subsequent supraventricular tachycardia impulse. This scenario is repeated, and RBBB continues until another, well-timed premature ventricular complex preexcites the right bundle branch (and either peels back or shortens its refractoriness), so that the next impulse from above finds the right bundle branch fully recovered and conducts without aberration (Figs. 1.45 and 1.46).

UNEXPECTED FACILITATION OF CONDUCTION

Mechanistically, when a premature impulse penetrates the conduction system, it can result in facilitation of AV conduction and normalization of a previously present AV block or BBB. For example, sometimes a premature ventricular complex abruptly normalizes the aberrancy by retrograde concealment into the AV node or the bundle branch tissue.

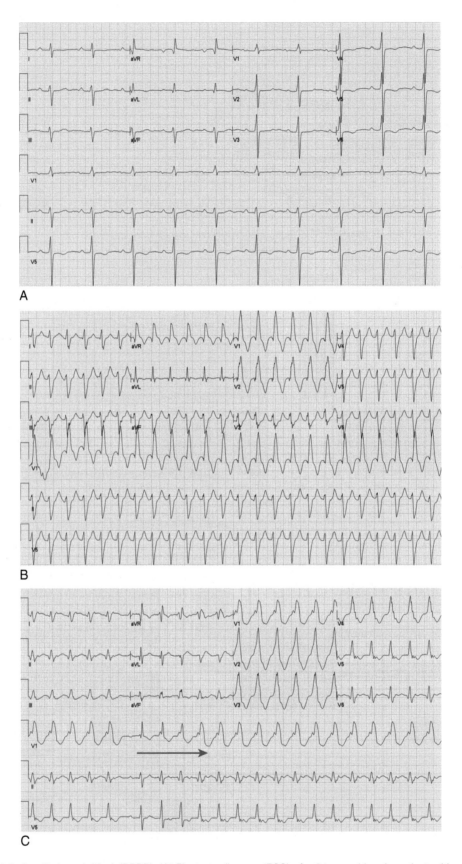

Fig. 1.19 Rate-related right bundle branch block (RBBB). (A) Electrocardiogram (ECG) of a 34-year-old male patient with congenital heart disease shows sinus rhythm, right axis deviation, and poor progression of R waves in the precordial leads. (B) ECG depicting RBBB aberrancy with right axis deviation during atrial tachycardia. (C) ECG showing RBBB aberrancy with a progressive widening of the QRS complexes for few complexes (*arrow*) followed by a wide QRS tachycardia during the same atrial tachycardia. The QRS morphology is wider in ECG because of amiodarone therapy, which was initiated for ventricular tachycardia.

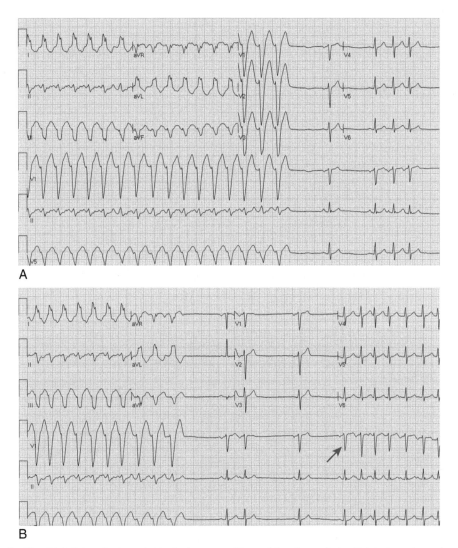

Fig. 1.20 Atrial tachycardia (A) with left bundle branch block aberrancy. The atrial tachycardia is slightly irregular and terminates spontaneously followed by three sinus beats and a three-beat run of atrial tachycardia without aberrancy. (B) Similar aberrancy pattern during the atrial tachycardia, which terminates spontaneously. The atrial tachycardia reinitiates (*arrow*), but this time there is no aberrancy, although the cycle length of the atrial tachycardia is similar to that associated with the aberrancy.

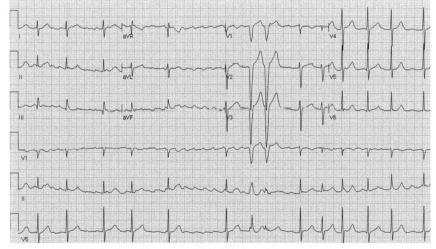

Fig. 1.21 Electrocardiogram depicting atrial fibrillation with narrow QRS complexes. There are two successive left bundle branch block morphology QRS complexes after a short-long-short sequence. This is most likely a left bundle branch block aberrancy, although a ventricular couplet cannot be ruled out.

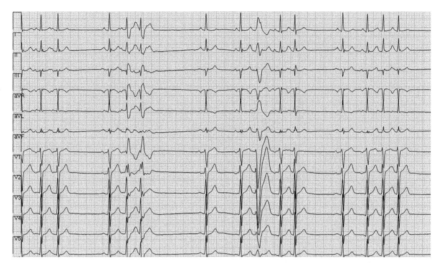

Fig. 1.22 Electrocardiogram showing sinus rhythm with frequent premature atrial complexes. QRS morphology varies between narrow QRS complex similar to that during the sinus rhythm, and right bundle branch block aberrancy and a QSR complex with left bundle branch block aberrancy.

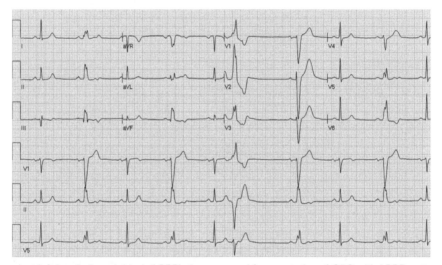

Fig. 1.23 Bradycardia-dependent left bundle branch block (LBBB) aberrancy and fragmentation of QRS with LBBB pattern and fragmentation of the premature ventricular complex. Electrocardiogram shows sinus rhythm with LBBB in alternate QRS complexes. R-R interval preceding the aberrant complexes is longer than R-R interval preceding the narrow QRS complexes. A premature ventricular complex is followed by a compensatory pause that is significantly longer than sinus R-R interval; still, the QRS complex followed by the long pause has LBBB aberrancy. This is an example of bradycardia-dependent (phase IV) BBB. There is fragmentation of the QRS with LBBB pattern in lead I and aVL (>2 notches) and fragmentation of the premature ventricular complex (notches are >40 ms apart).

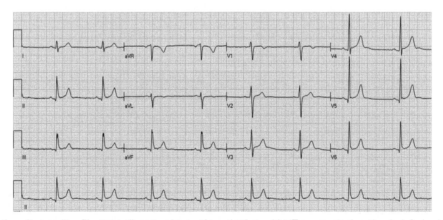

Fig. 1.24 Early repolarization abnormality. Electrocardiogram shows sinus rhythm with JT segment elevation in inferior leads and leads V5 and V6 in a patient without structural heart disease.

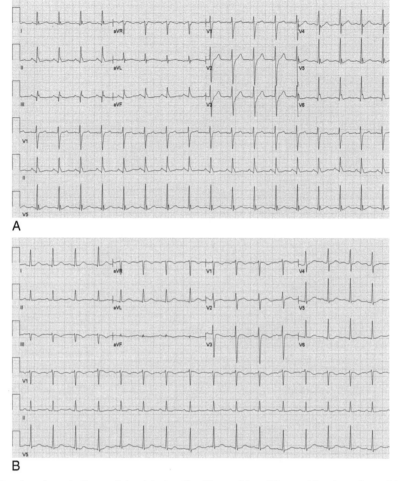

A

B

Fig. 1.25 Electrocardiogram showing sinus rhythm and J point elevation (J wave) in a 32-year-old male patient with methadone overdose (A) and severe acidosis (arterial pH = 7.1) (B). The electrocardiogram normalized after the correction of acidosis.

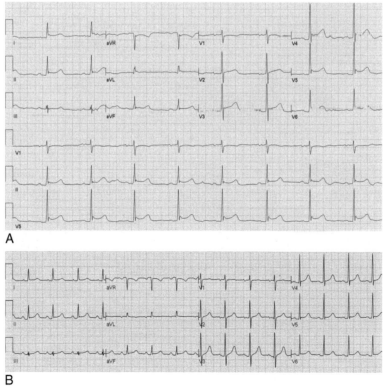

A

B

Fig. 1.26 (A) Electrocardiogram with prominent J waves (Osborn wave) in inferolateral leads and leads V2 to V4 in a patient who suffered from hypothermia. (B) Electrocardiogram depicts resolution of Osborn wave after correction of hypothermia.

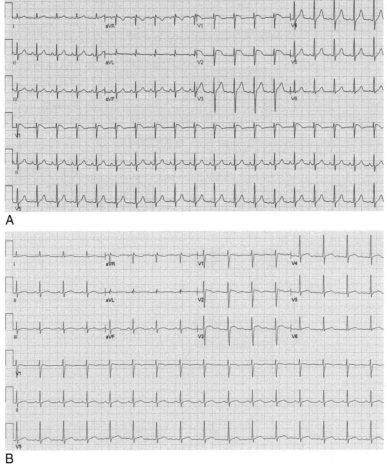

Fig. 1.27 (A) Incomplete right bundle branch block pattern caused by J point elevation and downsloping (coved) ST segment in lead V1–V2. It is called *Brugada pattern electrocardiogram*. ST-T waves can vary day by day, probably as a result of autonomic tone (vagal stimulation increases the J wave elevation) and can even normalize at times. (B) Electrocardiogram of the same patient shows no right bundle branch pattern but J point elevation and mild concavity upward (saddleback) in ST segment in lead V2.

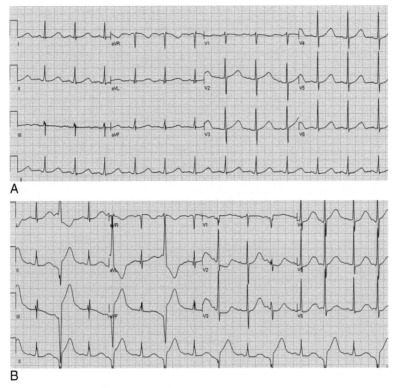

Fig. 1.28 (A) Electrocardiogram of a 55-year-old male patient with long QT syndrome type 1. The sinus rate is 80 bpm, the Q-T interval is 525, and corrected Q-T interval by Bazett formula is 581 ms. (B) Electrocardiogram of the same patient depicts frequent premature ventricular complexes in a bigeminal pattern. Premature ventricular complexes with a shorter coupling interval in this patient would be on the T wave and could trigger torsades de pointes.

BOX 1.1 Occurrence of ST horizontal or covering segment elevation

Myocardial ischemia or infarction

Noninfarction, transmural ischemia (e.g., Prinzmetal angina pattern, takotsubo syndrome)

Postmyocardial infarction (ventricular aneurysm pattern)

Acute pericarditis

Normal variants (including the classic early repolarization pattern)

LVH, LBBB (V_1-V_2 or V_3 only)

Other (rarer)

    Acute pulmonary embolism (right midchest leads)

    Hypothermia (J wave, Osborn wave)

    Myocardial injury

Myocarditis (may resemble myocardial infarction or pericarditis)

Tumor invading the left ventricle

Hypothermia (J wave, Osborn wave)

DC cardioversion (just following)

Intracranial hemorrhage

Hyperkalemia[a]

Brugada pattern (RBBB-like pattern and ST-segment elevations in right precordial leads)[a]

Type 1C antiarrhythmic drugs[a]

Hypercalcemia[a]

[a] Usually most apparent in V1 to V2.

DC, Direct current; *LBBB,* left bundle branch block; *LVH,* left ventricular hypertrophy; *RBBB,* right bundle branch block.

Modified from Goldberger AL. *Clinical Electrocardiography: A Simplified Approach.* 7th ed. St. Louis, MO: Mosby; 2017.

TABLE 1.5 Left Ventricular Hypertrophy

Measurements	Criteria
Sokolow-Lyon voltages	SV1 + RV5 >3.5 mV (35 mm) or
	RaVL >1.1 mV (11 mm)
Romhilt-Estes point score system[a]	Any limb lead R wave or S wave >2.0 mV (3 points)
	or SV1 or SV2 ≥3.0 mV (3 points)
	or RV5 to RV6 ≥3.0 mV (3 points)
	ST-T wave abnormality, no digitalis therapy (3 points)
	ST-T wave abnormality, digitalis therapy (1 point)
	Left atrial abnormality (3 points)
	Left axis deviation −30° or more (2 points)
	QRS duration ≥90 ms (1 point)
	Intrinsicoid deflection in V5 or V6 ≥50 ms (1 point)
Cornell voltage criteria	SV3 + RaVL ≥2.8 mV (for men)
	SV3 + RaVL >2.0 mV (for women)

[a] Probable left ventricular hypertrophy (LVH) is diagnosed if four points are present, and definite LVH is diagnosed if five or more points are present.

BOX 1.2 Right ventricular hypertrophy

R in V_1 ≥0.7 mV

QR in V_1

R/S in V_1 >1 with R >0.5 mV

R/S in V_5 or V_6 <1

S in V_5 or V_6 >0.7 mV

R in V_5 or V_6 ≥0.4 mV with S in V_1 ≤0.2 mV

Right axis deviation (>90°)

S_1Q_3 pattern

$S_1S_2S_3$ pattern

P pulmonale

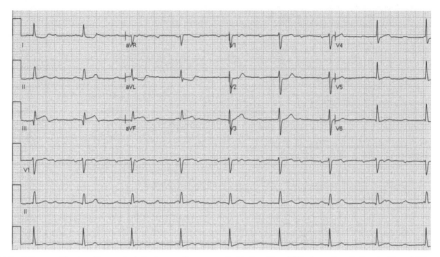

Fig. 1.29 Complete heart block in a patient with acute inferior wall myocardial infarction (ST elevation in leads II and III and aVF).

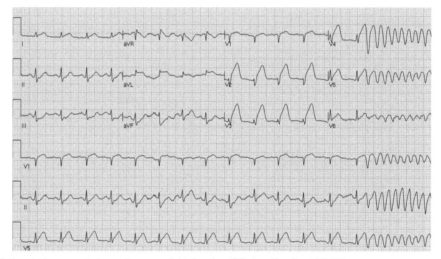

Fig. 1.30 Ventricular fibrillation during an anterior wall myocardial infarction (ST elevation from V1-V5).

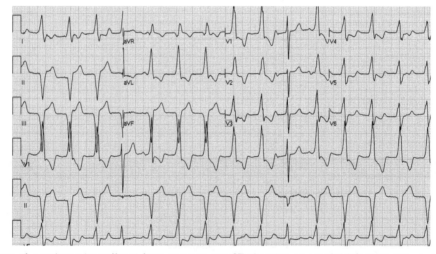

Fig. 1.31 Electrocardiogram of a patient who suffered from an acute non-ST elevation myocardial infarction shows sinus rhythm with salvos of idioventricular rhythm after percutaneous intervention. This is a reperfusion arrhythmia.

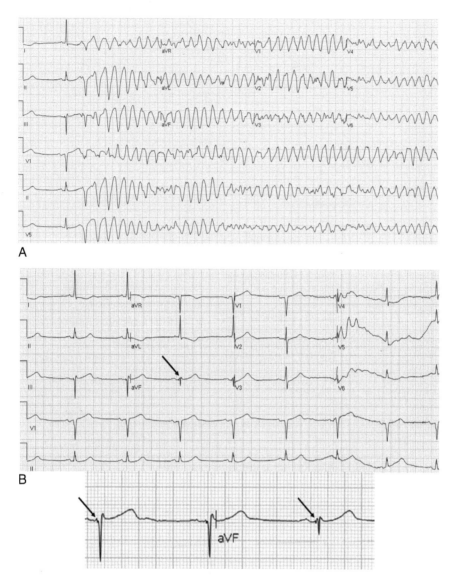

Fig. 1.32 Ventricular fibrillation in a patient with remote myocardial infarction. (A) Electrocardiogram showing polymorphic ventricular tachycardia initiated by an R on T phenomenon that degenerates into ventricular fibrillation. (B) Electrocardiogram depicting fragmented QRS in inferior leads (*arrow*) and no Q waves are present. The position emission tomography computed tomography scan confirmed inferior myocardial scar.

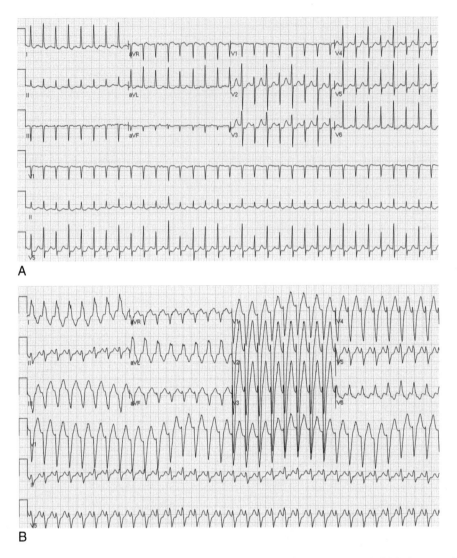

Fig. 1.33 (A) Electrocardiogram (ECG) showing a long RP' tachycardia with narrow QRS complexes with QRS alternans. ECG of the same patient depicting same tachycardia with the same rate as ECG (B). This is an example of atrial tachycardia with left bundle branch aberrancy.

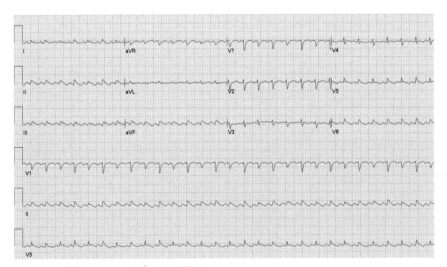

Fig. 1.34 Electrocardiogram showing QRS alternans during atrial flutter.

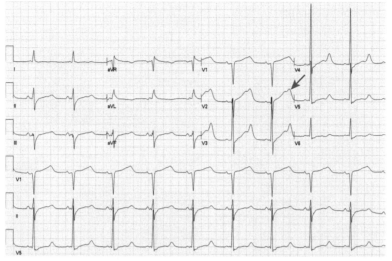

Fig. 1.35 Electrocardiogram depicting sinus rhythm at 57 bpm with prolonged QT-U interval (638 ms) in a 56-year-old female patient in the setting of hypokalemia. There are prominent U waves in inferior leads and leads V2 to V5 (*arrow*).

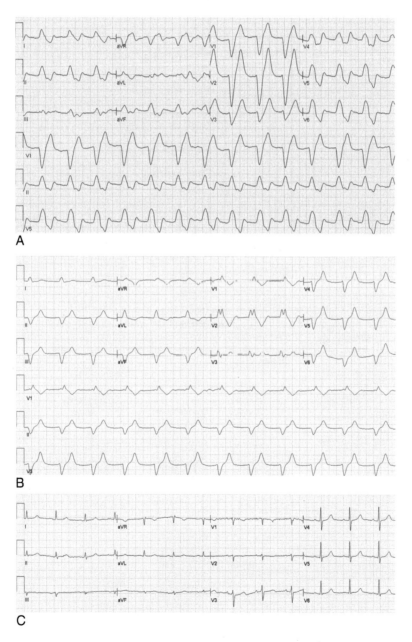

A

B

C

Fig. 1.36 (A) Electrocardiogram of a 58-year-old male patient with renal failure and K + level of 8.1 mEq/L shows no P waves and a wide QRS (A and B). The baseline electrocardiogram (C) of the same patient shows sinus rhythm with a normal P-R interval and narrow QRS and T waves after correction of hyperkalemia.

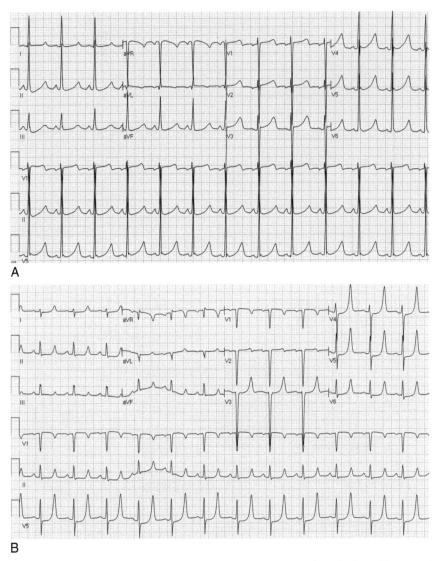

Fig. 1.37 Electrocardiogram of a 58-year-old female patient with chronic renal failure shows sinus rhythm with a prominent T wave (hyperkalemia) in leads V3 to V5 and a prolonged QTc interval of 516 ms. (A) The prolongation of Q-T interval is mainly due to prolongation of JT segment caused by associated hypocalcemia. (B) A peaked T wave (from hyperkalemia), Q-T prolongation (from hypocalcemia), and left ventricular hypertrophy (from hypertension) on an electrocardiogram is strongly suggestive of chronic renal failure in another patient.

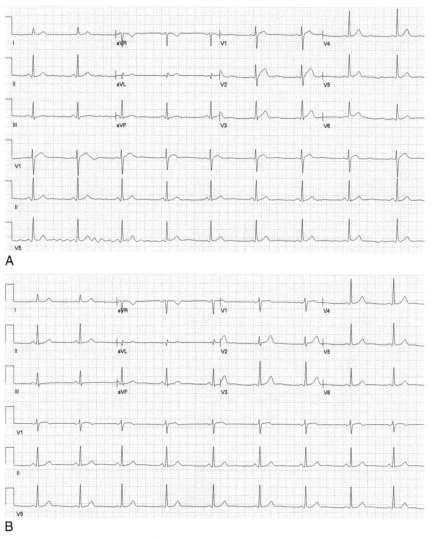

Fig. 1.38 (A) Electrocardiogram of a 58-year-old female patient with hyperparathyroidism and a serum calcium level of 13.2 mEq/L shows sinus rhythm at 54 bpm with a short corrected Q-T interval of 358 ms. (B) The QTc interval normalized to 400 ms with a calcium level of 9.4 mEq/L after parathyroidectomy in the same patient.

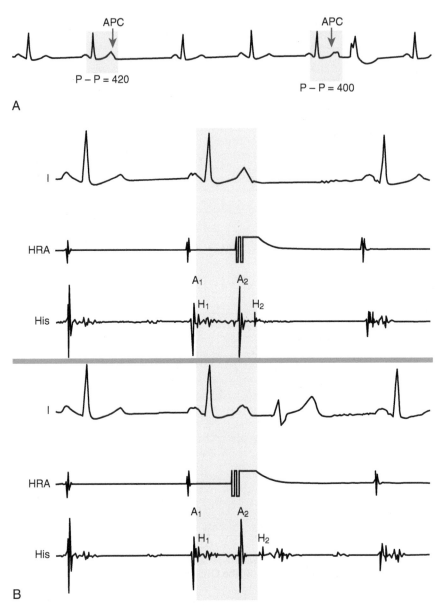

Fig. 1.39 Gap phenomenon of atrioventricular (AV) nodal conduction. Rhythm strip (A) shows sinus rhythm followed by blocked premature atrial complexes (premature atrial complexes do not conduct to the ventricles). The second premature atrial complex has a shorter coupling interval (in ms) but conducts to the ventricle with right bundle branch block aberrancy. (B) Anterograde AV gap phenomenon demonstrated during the electrophysiology study. Atrial extrastimulus (A2) (*upper panel*) conducting with modest delay through the AV node finds the His bundle still refractory, causing AV block. Earlier atrial extrastimulus (*lower panel*) results in further prolongation of the A2-H2 interval and the subsequent H1-H2 interval (*shaded area*). The longer H1-H2 interval now exceeds the refractory period of the His bundle, and by the time the impulse traverses the atrioventricular node the His bundle has completed its effective refractory period and conduction resumes; however, the conducted QRS has a left bundle branch block, morphology, and a longer HV interval because the left bundle is still refractory. (From Issa ZF, Miller JM, Zipes DP, eds. *Clinical Arrhythmology and Electrophysiology: A Companion to Braunwald's Heart Disease.* 1st ed. Philadelphia, PA: WB Saunders; 2019.)

Continuous tracings

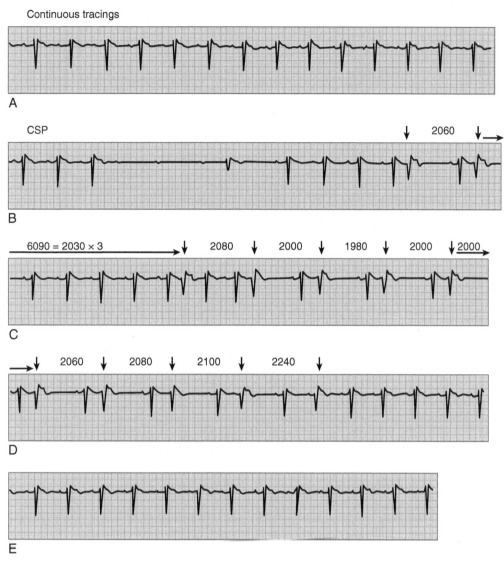

Fig. 1.40 Intermittent ventricular parasystole. (A) Continuous rhythm shows sinus rhythm. Note that the ventricular parasystole appears unexpectedly (B) at a cycle length (2060 ms) that is shorter than the immediately preceding ventricular pause elicited by carotid sinus pressure (CSP). After "warming up" to 1980 ms (C), the parasystole gradually "cools off" to 2240 ms (D) before it disappears (E). Although several other mechanisms have been shown in other figures, variants of this type of parasystole constitutes the one most frequently found when the diagnosis is made from Holter recordings. (*Arrows* indicate manifest parasystolic beats.) (From Zipes DP, Jalife J, eds. *Cardiac Electrophysiology: From Cell to Bedside.* 5th ed. St. Louis, MO: WB Saunders; 2018.)

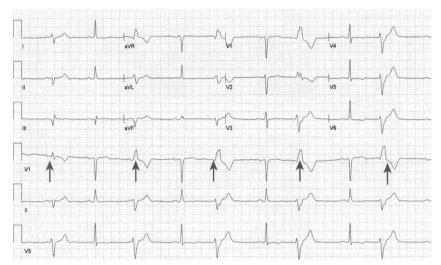

Fig. 1.41 Ventricular parasystole. Electrocardiogram shows sinus rhythm with premature ventricular contractions occurring at a regular interval (*blue arrow*). First and third wide complexes are fusion beats between the sinus complex and premature ventricular contraction (*red arrow*).

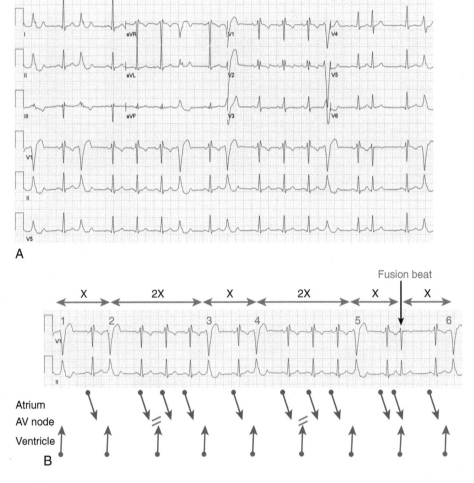

Fig. 1.42 (A) Intermittent ventricular parasystole with exit block. The rhythm strip (B) of the same electrocardiogram shows that the interval between the PVC2 and PVC3 is double the interval between PVC1 and PVC2 and between PVC3 and PVC4. Between PVC5 and PVC6 is the fusion beat following a premature atrial complex that conducts with a narrow QRS. Because the baseline QRS has incomplete right bundle branch block but the PVC originates from the right ventricle (left bundle branch block morphology), the fusion beat normalizes the QRS. Blue arrows depict impulses originating from the sinus node and the red arrows depict impulses originating from the ventricle. *AV*, atrioventricular.

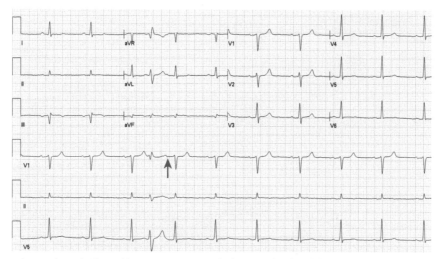

Fig. 1.43 Electrocardiogram shows sinus rhythm with a premature ventricular complex that does not change the next sinus cycle length; however, the P-R interval prolongs after the next P wave (*arrow*) because of a retrograde concealment of the ventricular impulse generated by the premature ventricular contraction in the atrioventricular node.

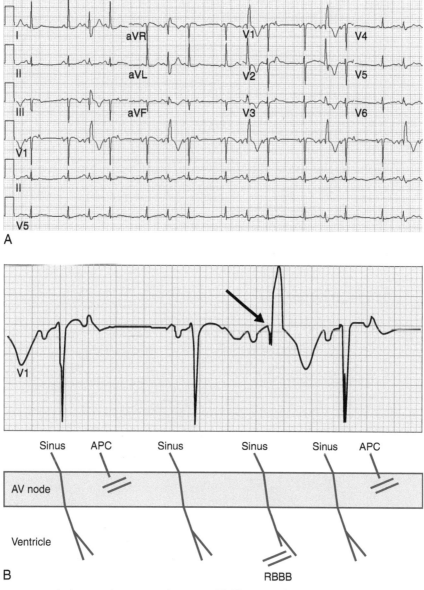

Fig. 1.44 Interpolated premature ventricular complex versus aberrancy. (A) Electrocardiogram showing sinus rhythm with a right bundle branch block (RBBB) morphology QRS between the alternate narrow QRS complexes. On close observation (B) the RBBB pattern QRS complexes are aberrantly conducted (*arrow*), and the QRS following that has a normal duration, which may be a result of a supernormal conduction via the RBBB. The P wave next to it is an atrial premature contraction and does not penetrate the atrioventricular node (blocked atrial premature contraction). Red double lines show the sites of block of supraventricular impulses. *APC*, atrial premature complexes; *AV*, atrioventricular.

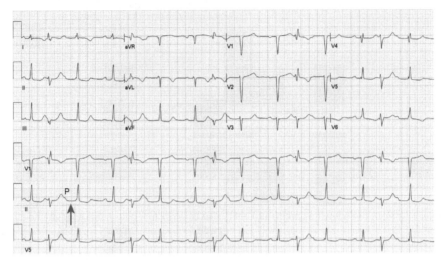

Fig. 1.45 Electrocardiogram depicting sinus rhythm with frequent interpolated premature ventricular contractions. The P-R interval (*arrow*) after these premature ventricular contractions is longer compared with the baseline P-R interval. This is because of retrograde concealment into the atrioventricular node of ventricular impulse generated by the premature ventricular contraction.

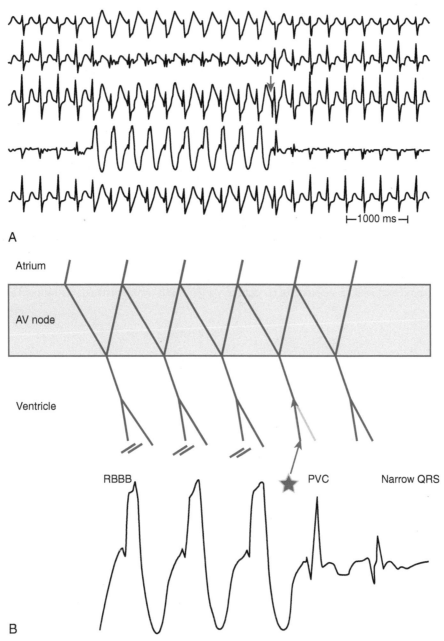

Fig. 1.46 Supraventricular tachycardia with tachycardia-dependent (phase 3) right bundle branch block. Electrocardiogram (A) depicts a short RP′ tachycardia with narrow QRS tachycardia. The tachycardia spontaneously changes to a wide complex tachycardia with the same tachycardia cycle length. This is an example of right bundle branch block aberrancy. An extrastimulus (premature ventricular contraction) delivered during the wide complex tachycardia changes the QRS duration to a narrow complex tachycardia. Delivery of a late ventricular extrastimulus (*arrow*) during the supraventricular tachycardia (B) preexcites the right bundle branch (and either peels back or shortens its refractoriness) and restores normal conduction. *PVC*, premature ventricular impulse. (From Issa ZF, Miller JM, Zipes DP, eds. *Clinical Arrhythmology and Electrophysiology: A Companion to Braunwald's Heart Disease.* 1st ed. Philadelphia, PA: Saunders; 2019.)

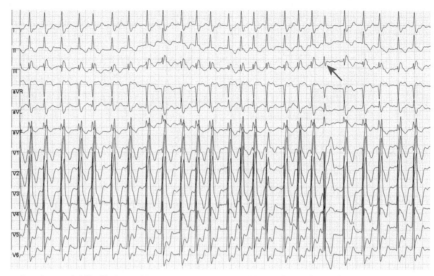

Fig. 1.47 Electrocardiogram showing atrial fibrillation with right bundle branch block. One of the QRS complexes is narrow without any signs of bundle branch block. This can be explained as supernormal conduction via the RBBB, which resulted in a narrow QRS. Narrow QRS complex is marked by an arrow.

SUPERNORMAL CONDUCTION

Supernormal conduction implies conduction that is better than anticipated or conduction that occurs when block is expected. At the AV nodal level, intermittent AV conduction can occur during periods of high-degree AV block. At the His-Purkinje level, supernormal conduction can occur with a paradoxical normalization of bundle branch conduction at an R-R interval shorter than that with BBB. This can also occur with an atrial premature complex conducting with a narrow QRS during baseline sinus rhythm with BBB, or with acceleration-dependent BBB that normalizes at even faster rates (Fig. 1.47).

BIBLIOGRAPHY

Goldberger AL. *Clinical Electrocardiography: A Simplified Approach.* 7th ed. St. Louis, MO: Mosby; 2006.

Issa ZF, Miller JM, Zipes DP, eds. *Clinical Arrhythmology and Electrophysiology: A Companion to Braunwald's Heart Disease.* 1st ed. Philadelphia, PA: WB Saunders; 2019.

Zipes DP, Jalife J, eds. *Cardiac Electrophysiology: From Cell to Bedside.* 5th ed. St. Louis, MO: WB Saunders; 2018.

2

Sinus Node Dysfunction

The normal sinoatrial node (SAN) is capable of generating impulses at a rate that meets metabolic demands at rest and during increased requirements, such as during exercise. The symptoms reported by patients with sinus node disease include palpitations, dizzy spells, presyncope, and syncope. These symptoms can be persistent or intermittent. More than half of the patients affected are aged older than 50 years. The normal heart rate for an adult is 60 to 100 bpm. Sinus node dysfunction (SND) includes symptomatic sinus bradycardia, sinus pauses, sinus arrest, tachycardia-bradycardia syndrome, and symptomatic chronotropic incompetence (Table 2.1). Patients with sinus bradycardia or chronotropic incompetence can present with decreased exercise capacity or fatigue. Sinus bradycardia may be physiologic in well-trained athletes because of high vagal tone (Fig. 2.1). Marked sinus bradycardia (40 bpm) can result in emergence of a junctional rhythm at 30 to 40 beats (Figs. 2.2 and 2.3). SND can occur in the setting of intrinsic sinus node disease (e.g., primary conduction system disease, coronary artery disease, cardiomyopathy, heart failure) or as a result of extrinsic factors. such as autonomic imbalance (neurocardiogenic syncope, carotid sinus hypersensitivity, autonomic neuropathy), cardiac surgery (maze surgery, mitral valve surgery) electrolyte imbalance (hyperkalemia), or drug therapy (e.g., antiarrhythmic drugs, clonidine, lithium) (Figs. 2.4 through 2.8). Usually an electrocardiogram confirms persistent sinus node abnormalities in symptomatic patients. However, intermittent arrhythmia with frequent symptoms requires 24- or 48-hour ambulatory Holter monitoring. Less frequent arrhythmias require cardiac event monitoring or implantable loop recorders for diagnosis. Wearable technology, such as smart watches and phones, can be useful to document SND in some patients. Invasive electrophysiology testing can be performed in symptomatic patients in whom SND is suspected but cannot be documented in association with symptoms. Electrophysiology study can be of value in evaluation of other potential causes for symptoms of syncope and palpitations, such as atrioventricular (AV) node disease or ventricular tachycardia. Head-up tilt test is also helpful in patients with neurocardiogenic syncope (bradycardia, hypotension, or both during upright posture) and postural orthostatic tachycardia syndrome (POTS).

SINUS ARRHYTHMIA

Sinus arrhythmia is usually a normal physiologic response to respiration or vagal stimulation. In sinus arrhythmia, P wave morphology is consistent with sinus rhythm, and the P-P intervals vary by more than 160 ms (Figs. 2.9 through 2.12). In respiratory sinus arrhythmia, the sinus rate increases with inspiration and decreases with expiration. A respiratory variation in the sinus P wave contour can be seen in the inferior leads. It is most commonly seen in young healthy subjects. Nonrespiratory sinus arrhythmia of unknown mechanisms can occur during digitalis and morphine administration.

VENTRICULOPHASIC SINUS ARRHYTHMIA

Ventriculophasic sinus arrhythmia is a nonpathological arrhythmia that occurs during sinus rhythm with high-grade or complete AV block. Electrographic recording shows shorter P-P intervals when they enclose QRS complexes and longer P-P intervals when no QRS complexes are enclosed (Fig. 2.13). The mechanism of this arrhythmia is not known but may be related to the effects of the mechanical ventricular systole, which increases the blood supply to the sinus node, thereby transiently increasing its firing rate. Alternatively, it could be carotid sinus stimulation with a larger stroke volume leading to reflex slowing of the sinus node in the next P-P cycle.

SINOATRIAL EXIT BLOCK

Sinoatrial exit block results when the sinus impulse fails to conduct to the atria because of delay in conduction or block within the sinus node area or perinodal tissue. Sinoatrial exit block produces a pause that is a multiple of the P-P interval unless there is type 1 second-degree sinoatrial block or sinus arrhythmia because the normal impulse is formed on time and just cannot exit. These pauses are eventually terminated by a delayed sinus beat or subsidiary escape beats from the atrium, His bundle, or ventricle. Like AV node block, sinoatrial block is classified into three types (Table 2.2).

CHRONOTROPIC INCOMPETENCE

Chronotropic incompetence is defined as the inability to accelerate the sinus rate appropriately to the level needed by the body's metabolism, usually during exercise. This definition includes the inability to reach the 80th percentile of maximum predicted heart rate, delayed peak of heart rate (heart rate peaks during recovery period after the exercise), early peaking of heart rate (before the peak exercise), fluctuations of heart rate during exercise, or the inability to reach a heart rate of 100 to 120 bpm. However, this definition of chronotropic incompetence is not universally agreed upon. The heart rate response to exercise also depends on several factors, such as deconditioning, drug therapy, and comorbidities.

TABLE 2.1   Sinus Node Dysfunction (with Accompanying Symptoms)

- Sinus bradycardia: Sinus rate <50 bpm.
- Ectopic atrial bradycardia: Atrial depolarization attributable to an atrial pacemaker other than the sinus node with a rate <50 bpm.
- Sinoatrial exit block: Evidence that blocked conduction between the sinus node and adjacent atrial tissue is present. Multiple electrocardiographic manifestations including "group beating" of atrial depolarization and sinus pauses.
- Sinus pause: Sinus node depolarizes >3 s after the last atrial depolarization.
- Sinus node arrest: No evidence of sinus node depolarization.
- Tachycardia-bradycardia ("tachy-brady") syndrome: Sinus bradycardia, ectopic atrial bradycardia, or sinus pause alternating with periods of abnormal atrial tachycardia, atrial flutter, or atrial fibrillation (S2.1-1). The tachycardia may be associated with suppression of sinus node automaticity and a sinus pause of variable duration when the tachycardia terminates.
- Chronotropic incompetence: Broadly defined as the inability of the heart to increase its rate commensurate with increased activity or demand, in many studies translates to failure to attain 80% of expected heart rate reserve during exercise.
- Isorhythmic dissociation: Atrial depolarization (from either the sinus node or ectopic atrial site) is slower than ventricular depolarization (from an atrioventricular nodal, His bundle, or ventricular site).
- Sinus node arrest: No evidence of sinus node depolarization.
- Tachycardia-bradycardia ("tachy-brady") syndrome: Sinus bradycardia, ectopic atrial bradycardia, or sinus pause alternating with periods of abnormal atrial tachycardia, atrial flutter, or atrial fibrillation. The tachycardia may be associated with suppression of sinus node automaticity and a sinus pause of variable duration when the tachycardia terminates.

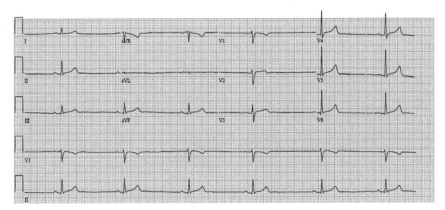

Fig. 2.1 Sinus bradycardia at 36 bpm in a professional athlete.

SINUS TACHYCARDIA

Sinus tachycardia (heart rate >100 bpm) is a normal physiologic response to meet the metabolic demand of the body. It is commonly encountered during exercise. It can be a manifestation of hyperadrenergic/hypovagotonic state (anxiety, stress, hyperthyroidism), physiologic stress (heart failure, pain, surgery, sepsis), hypovolemia (shock), or drug therapy (antianxiety medications, adrenergic drugs) (Fig. 2.24). Rarely, it may occur without any discernible cause (syndrome of inappropriate sinus tachycardia) or can occur during orthostatic stress (e.g., POTS) (Figs. 2.25 and 2.26).

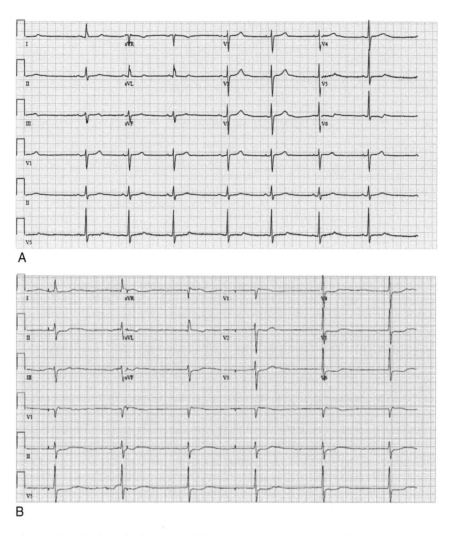

Fig. 2.2 Electrocardiogram shows sinus bradycardia (heart rate, 50 bpm) and sinus arrhythmia (A). A few hours later, sinus node dysfunction progressed and the junctional rhythm at 37 bpm appeared (B).

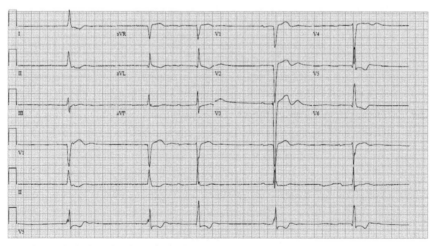

Fig. 2.3 Electrocardiogram reveals marked sinus bradycardia and junctional escape at 33 bpm. The third QRS complex is probably a conducted sinus beat with a long PR interval.

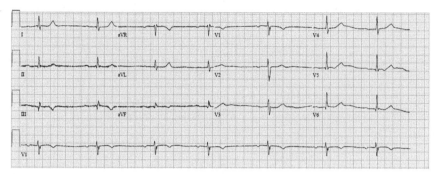

Fig. 2.4 Sinus bradycardia after mitral valve replacement was most likely caused by injury to the sinus node artery during surgery.

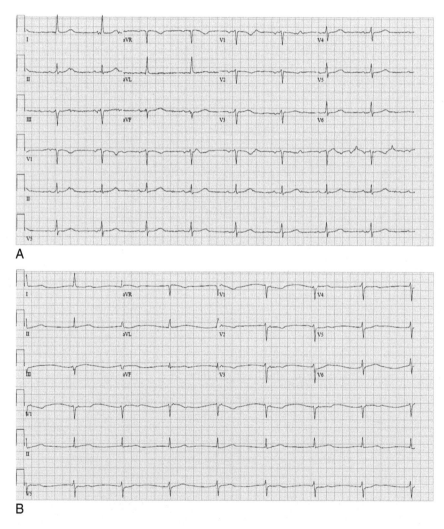

A

B

Fig. 2.5 Sinus bradycardia at 52 bpm (A) and with intermittent junctional rhythm with retrograde atrial capture at 48 bpm (B).

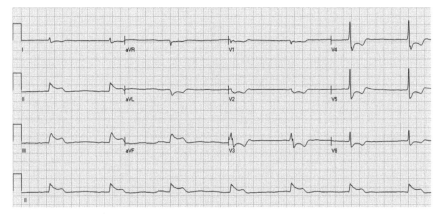

Fig. 2.6 Marked sinus bradycardia with ST elevation caused by right coronary artery occlusion producing inferior myocardial infarction.

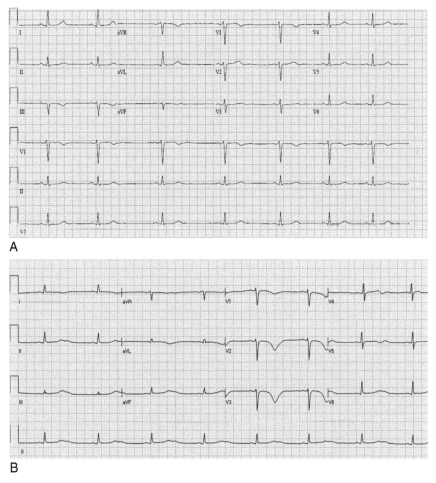

A

B

Fig. 2.7 Sinus bradycardia due to drug therapy. (A) A sinus bradycardia at 47 bpm due to lithium therapy. (B) Sinus bradycardia with prolonged QTc of 612 ms caused by amiodarone therapy.

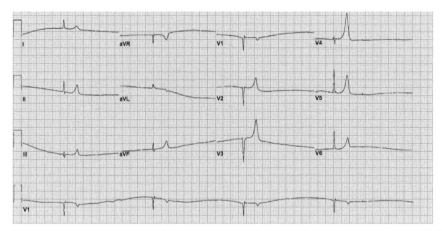

Fig. 2.8 Junctional escape rhythm in a patient with sinus node dysfunction associated with hyperkalemia (K + 8.2 mMol/L).

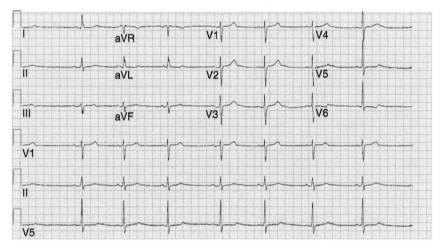

Fig. 2.9 Electrocardiogram shows sinus arrhythmia with P wave morphology consistent with sinus rhythm. The P-P intervals vary by more than 160 ms or 10% of the cycle length.

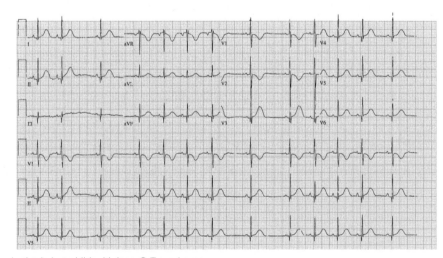

Fig. 2.10 Marked sinus arrhythmia in a child with long Q-T syndrome.

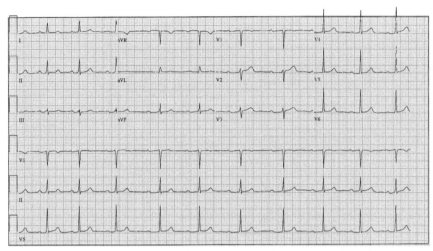

Fig. 2.11 Sinus arrhythmia with P-R prolongation during sinus slowing. P-R prolongation during sinus slowing is most likely caused by vagal effect on the atrioventricular node.

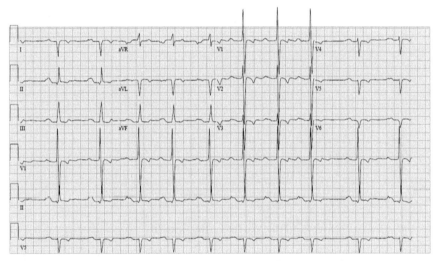

Fig. 2.12 Electrocardiogram depicts sinus arrhythmia with slight change in sinus P wave morphology during sinus slowing in a patient with dextrocardia. This is a normal respiratory variation of P wave in inferior leads.

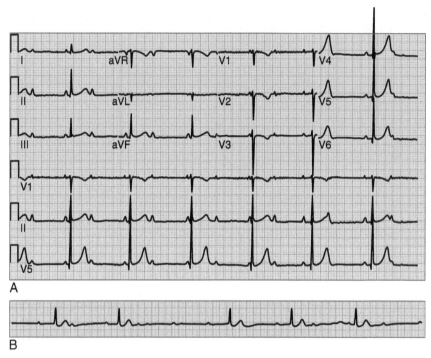

Fig. 2.13 Ventriculophasic sinus arrhythmia in the presence of advanced atrioventricular (AV) block. P-P intervals are shorter when they enclose QRS complexes, and P-P intervals are longer when no QRS complexes are enclosed in the presence of complete heart block (A). The rhythm strip shows advanced AV block with intermittent AV conduction (B).

TABLE 2.2   Sinus Node Dysfunction

Sinus Node Dysfunction	Electrocardiogram Findings	Comments
Sinus bradycardia	Sinus rate <60 bpm.	Sinus rate <40 bpm not during sleep is considered SND (Figs. 2.1 through 2.8). However, well-conditioned athletes can normally exhibit resting sinus rates in the 30s.
Sinus pauses or sinus arrest	Complete cessation of sinus activity.	It results from sinus arrest or SAN exit block. A reading >3 sec is considered abnormal, although it may not always be abnormal (Figs. 2.14 through 2.16). Prolonged asystole can cause syncope or sudden cardiac death.
Sinoatrial exit block		
First-degree	Abnormal prolongation of the sinoatrial conduction time, usually with a delay at a fixed interval.	Cannot be detected on surface ECG.
Second-degree type 1	Intermittent failure of the sinus impulse to exit the sinus node with Wenckebach periodicity of the P wave.	Progressively decreasing P-P intervals before a pause caused by an absent "dropped" P wave. The pauses associated with this type of sinoatrial exit block are less than twice the shortest sinus cycle (Figs. 2.17 and 2.18).
Second-degree type 2	Abrupt absence of one or more P waves because of failure of the impulse to exit the sinus node, without previous progressive prolongation of sinoatrial conduction time (without progressive shortening of the P-P intervals).	The sinus pause should be an exact multiple (2:1, 3:1, 4:1) of the immediately preceding P-P interval (Figs. 2.19 and 2.20).
Third-degree or sinus arrest	Absence of P waves owing to failure of the sinus impulse to conduct to the atrium.	Long pauses resulting in lower pacemaker escape rhythm. It cannot be differentiated from sinus arrest on a 12-lead ECG.
Tachycardia-bradycardia syndrome	Tachycardia alternating with sinus bradycardia or junctional rhythm.	Often tachycardia (paroxysmal AF, AFL, AT) terminates with a long sinus pause with lower pacemaker escape rhythm (Fig. 2.21).
Chronotropic incompetence	Inability to accelerate to 70% to 75% of the age-predicted maximum heart rate (220 − age) appropriately during exercise.	The response during stress test may also include early peaking of heart rate, fluctuation in heart rate and peak heart rate during recovery, or inability to achieve a sinus rate of 100 to 120 bpm at maximum effort during exercise (Fig. 2.22).
Carotid sinus hypersensitivity	An abnormal slowing in response to CSM (pause longer than 3 seconds) can indicate SND.	Abnormal response to CSM can also occur in asymptomatic elderly; therefore it should be correlated with symptoms. Other responses to CSM include atrioventricular block and hypotension (Fig. 2.23).

AF, Atrial fibrillation; AFL, atrial flutter; AT, atrial tachycardia; CSM, carotid sinus massage; ECG, electrocardiogram; SAN, sinoatrial node; SND, sinus node dysfunction.

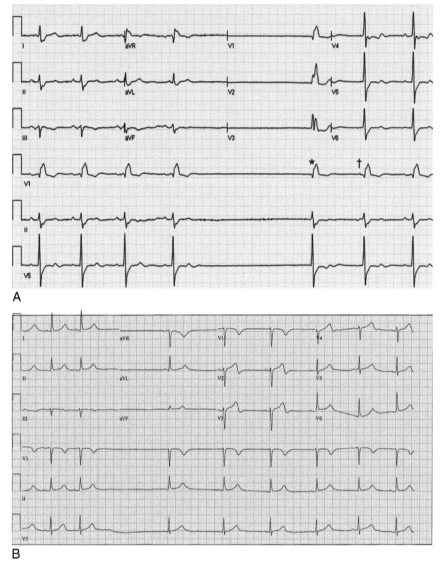

A

B

Fig. 2.14 (A) Electrocardiogram (ECG) shows sinus rhythm for four beats followed by a sinus pause and the junctional escape beat (*). The next beat is nonsinus atrial beat (†), which is followed by a sinus beat. (B) Sinus rhythm is present for two beats followed by a sinus pause. The sinus rate is slower after the sinus pause. It is a manifestation of sinus node dysfunction. (C) Telemetry rhythm strip shows progressive sinus slowing followed by spontaneous sinus pauses with a maximum pause being 4.2 seconds and then progressive increase in heart rate in a patient with sinus node dysfunction. It can also occur during intense vagal stimulation. (D) A 34-year-old man received an insertable loop recorder for infrequent syncope was found to have a 12-second sinus pause during syncope followed by brief convulsion (shown by movement artifact in the loop recorder interrogation strip).

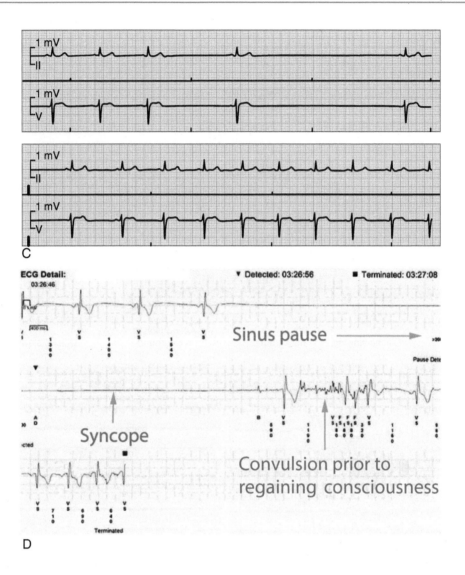

Fig. 2.14 (Continued)

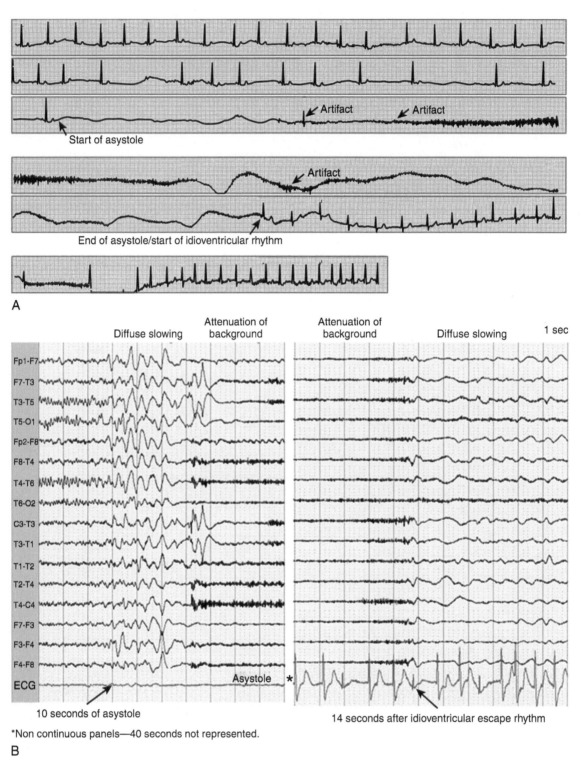

A

B

*Non continuous panels—40 seconds not represented.

Fig. 2.15 Sinus node dysfunction presenting as seizure disorder. Electrocardiogram (*upper panel*) shows sinus rhythm with slowing and junctional escape followed by a prolonged sinus pause followed by an idioventricular beat, then junctional escape rhythm and sinus rhythm. Prolonged asystole was associated with cerebral hypoxia and convulsions. The simultaneous electroencephalography during the first 10 seconds of asystole revealed diffuse slowing followed by background attenuation of brain waves (A). Recording of first 14 seconds after asystole demonstrated attenuation of brain waves followed by diffuse slowing of brain waves, which normalized after a few seconds (B). Patient received a pacemaker, which resolved the symptoms.

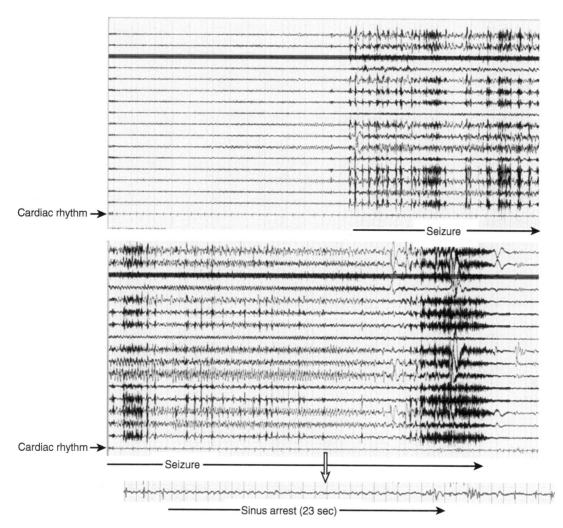

Cardiac rhythm →

← Seizure →

Cardiac rhythm →

← Seizure →

← Sinus arrest (23 sec) →

Fig. 2.16 Seizure disorder inducing sinus pause. Simultaneous electroencephalography (EEG) and electrocardiogram (ECG) recording in a patient with multiple seizure episodes shows the initiation of seizure waves associated with convulsions and sinus rhythm. The convulsion subsided for a few seconds and restarted during the prolonged asystole for 23 seconds (*lower panel*). This may be the vagal effect of the seizure causing prolonged cerebral hypoxia resulting in the recurrence of convulsions.

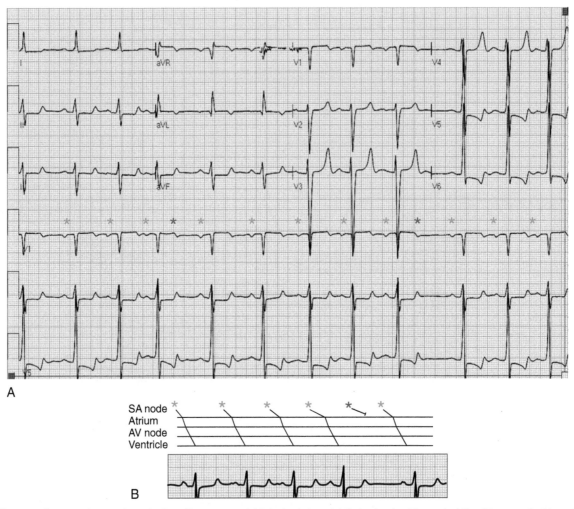

Fig. 2.17 Electrocardiogram shows sinus rhythm (P waves upright in lead 1 and inferior leads, *blue asterisk*) with normal atrioventricular (AV) conduction (A). There is progressive shortening of the P-P interval followed by an absent ("dropped") P wave (*red asterisk*) suggestive of second-degree type 1 (Wenckebach) sinoatrial (SA) block. The ladder diagram shows the typical pattern of SA conduction in type 1 second-degree SA block (B).

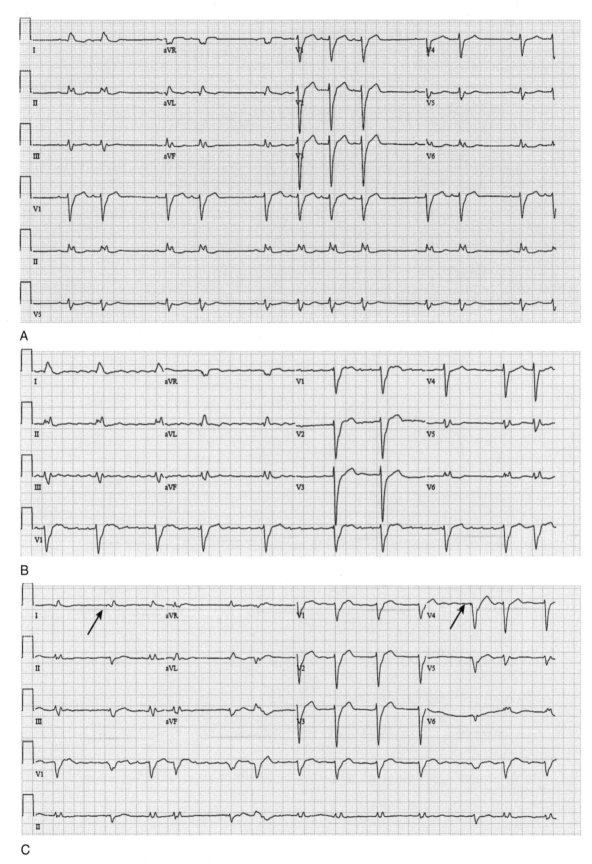

Fig. 2.18 Sinus node dysfunction manifesting as tachy-brady syndrome. (A) Electrocardiogram reveals type 2 second-degree sinoatrial block with a fixed P-P interval and absent or "dropped" P waves. Note the associated left bundle branch block. Patient with sinus node disease *can* have associated conduction disease of atrioventricular node or His-Purkinje system. Patient later developed atrial flutter (B) and atrial fibrillation with tachy-brady syndrome (C) requiring ventricular pacing (*arrows* show paced ventricular complexes).

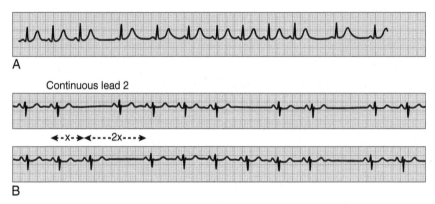

Fig. 2.19 (A) Type 1 second-degree sinoatrial block. Rhythm strip shows sinus rhythm with progressive shortening of P-P interval followed by absent or "dropped" P wave. (B) Type 2 second-degree sinoatrial block. Rhythm strip shows sinus rhythm with fixed P-P intervals with intermittent absent P waves. The longer P-P intervals (2 ×) are double the P-P interval (X). This is an example of a type 2 exit block.

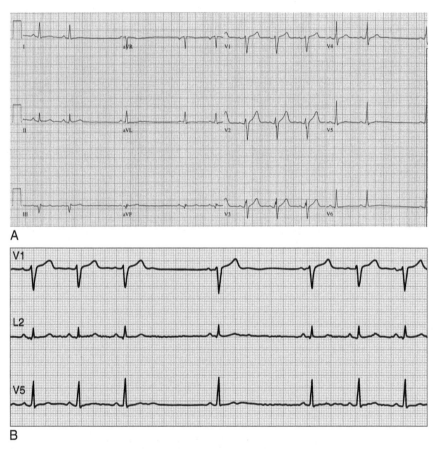

Fig. 2.20 Type 2 second-degree sinoatrial block. Electrocardiogram (A) and rhythm strip (B) show fixed P-P interval with "dropped" P waves. The longer P-P intervals are double the P-P interval.

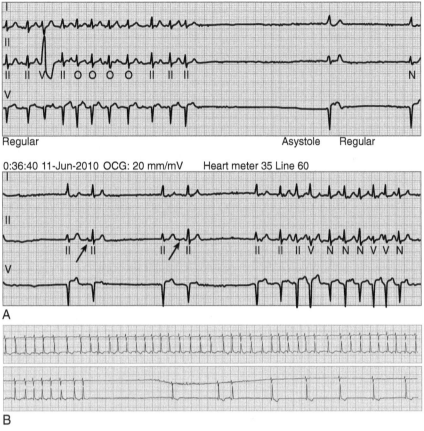

Fig. 2.21 Tachycardia-bradycardia syndrome. (A) Rhythm strip shows atrial fibrillation followed by multiple pauses and junctional escape rhythm along with intermittent single sinus complexes (*arrow*). Fibrillation is reinitiated. (B) Rhythm strip shows atrial fibrillation that terminates in a prolonged pause followed by a slow junctional rhythm.

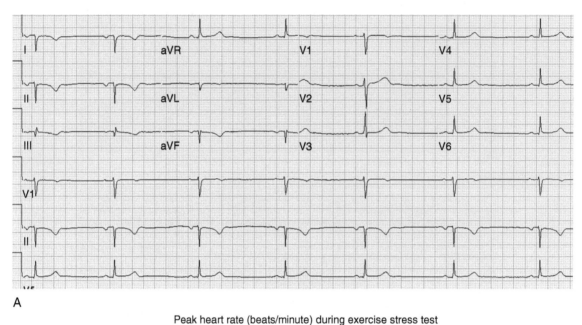

A

Peak heart rate (beats/minute) during exercise stress test

Peak heart rate 86   Peak heart rate 158 with AAIR pacing

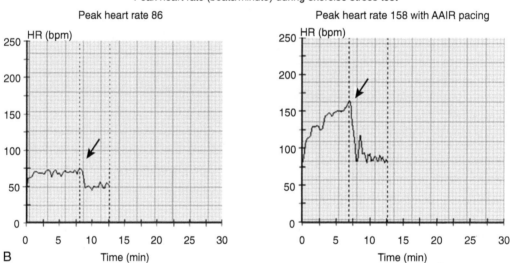

B   Time (min)

Fig. 2.22 Electrocardiogram of a 28-year-old female patient with mitochondrial myopathy. (A) Patient presented with symptomatic bradycardia, exercise intolerance, and syncope. Telemetry revealed sinus bradycardia as low as 34 bpm. (B) Exercise stress test revealed severe chronotropic incompetence with a maximum heart rate (HR) of 86 bpm (*arrow*). Patient received a permanent pacemaker programmed to AAIR during the follow-up stress test. She achieved a maximum HR of 158 bpm (*arrow*) during peak exercise.

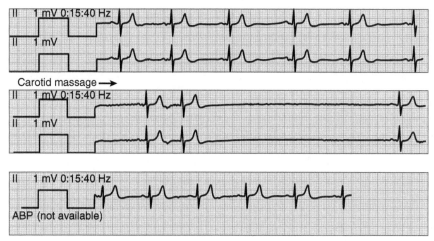

Fig. 2.23 Carotid sinus hypersensitivity. Right carotid sinus massage in a patient with syncope shows a 4.5-second symptomatic sinus pause. *ABP*, arterial blood pressure.

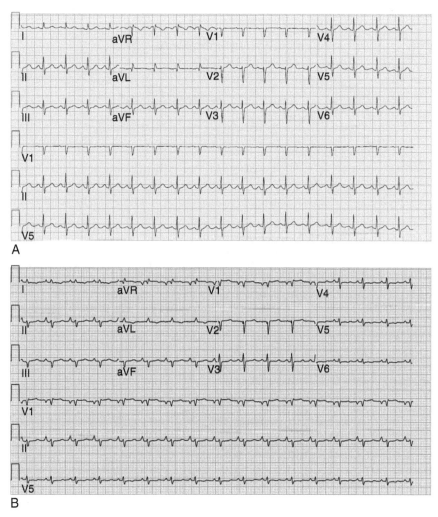

Fig. 2.24 Sinus tachycardia in a patient with normal heart (A) and in another patient with nonischemic cardiomyopathy (B) who presented with heart failure.

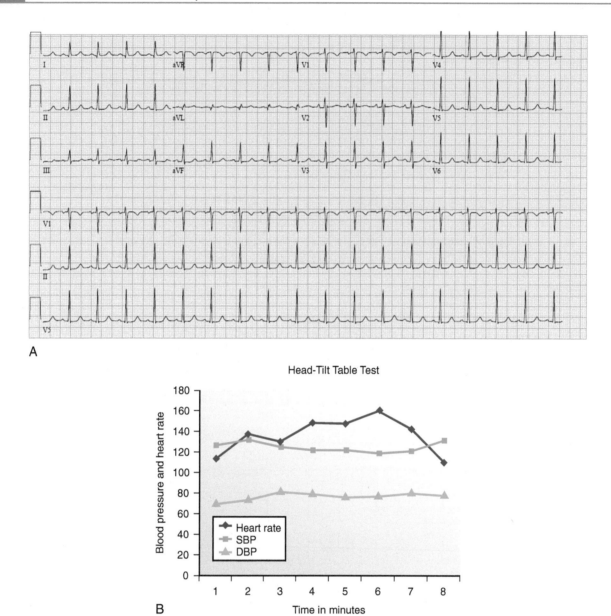

Fig. 2.25 Postural orthostatic tachycardia syndrome. (A) Electrocardiogram depicting baseline sinus tachycardia in a 38-year-old patient with orthostatic intolerance. During the head-tilt table test (B), the heart rate increased to 160 bpm without any significant change in blood pressure. Patient became very symptomatic and complained of dizziness, palpitations, and presyncope. *DBP*, diastolic blood pressure; *SBP*, systolic blood pressure.

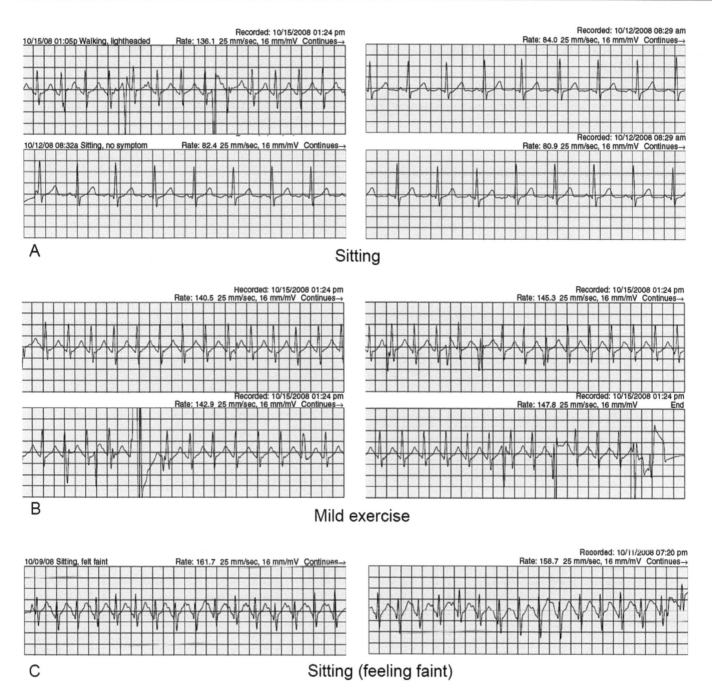

Fig. 2.26 Baseline electrocardiogram in another patient with postural orthostatic tachycardia syndrome. Baseline heart rate is 84 bpm during sitting (A). During mild exercise (walking inside her home), the heart rate increased to 145 bpm, and the patient became light-headed (B). Sometimes she was symptomatic, even during sitting, with a maximum heart rate of 162 bpm (C).

POSTURAL ORTHOSTATIC TACHYCARDIA SYNDROME AND INAPPROPRIATE SINUS TACHYCARDIA

Patients with inappropriate sinus tachycardia have persistent elevated average resting heart rate (>90−95 bpm) and an exaggerated heart rate (usually increase >25 bpm) in response to low levels of physical activity, such as walking. Some affected patients have increased responsiveness to infusions of isoproterenol (Fig. 2.27). In some patients, heart rate can increase just on upright posture in the absence of orthostatic arterial hypotension. It is called *orthostatic intolerance* or *POTS*. By definition, POTS occurs when the heart rate increases by more than 30 bpm or more than 120 bpm within 10 minutes of upright posture during a tilt table test. P wave morphology is identical during tachycardia and sinus rhythm.

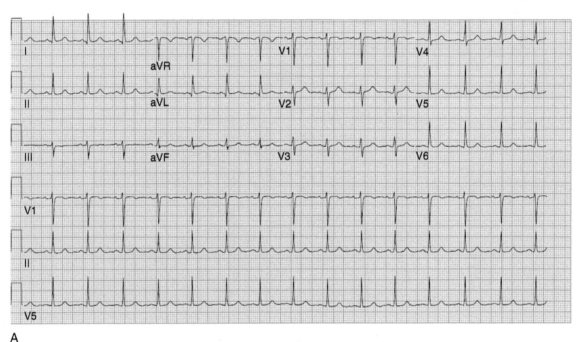

A

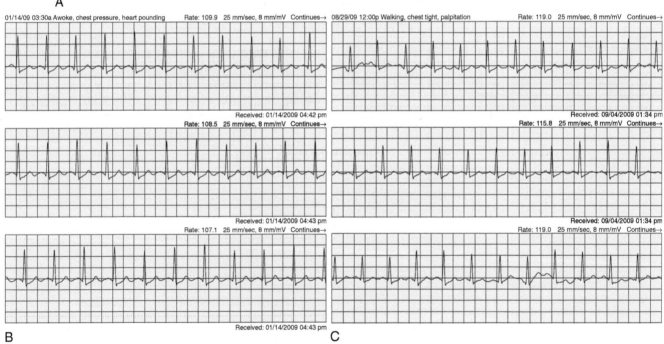

B   C

Fig. 2.27 Syndrome of inappropriate sinus tachycardia. Electrocardiogram of a 32-year-old patient with structurally normal heart depicts a baseline sinus rate of 91 bpm (A). During event monitoring the patient complained of chest tightness and palpitations with a baseline heart rate of 102 bpm (B). During walking her heart rate increased to 119 bpm, and she became more symptomatic (C).

BIBLIOGRAPHY

Goldberger AL. *Clinical Electrocardiography: A Simplified Approach.* 9th ed. St. Louis, MO: Mosby; 2017.

Issa ZF, Miller JM, Zipes DP, eds. *Clinical Arrhythmology and Electrophysiology: A Companion to Braunwald's Heart Disease.* 3rd ed. Philadelphia, PA: WB Saunders; 2019.

Kasumoto FM, et al. ACC/AHA/HRS Guideline on the Evaluation and Management of Patients With Bradycardia and Cardiac Conduction Delay: Executive Summary. *Heart Rhythm.* 2018;. 2018, S1547-5271(18) 31127-5.

Zipes DP, Jalife J, eds. *Cardiac Electrophysiology: From Cell to Bedside.* 7th ed. St. Louis, MO: WB Saunders; 2018.

3

Atrioventricular Conduction Abnormalities

Atrioventricular (AV) block can be defined as a delay or interruption in the transmission of an impulse from the atria to the ventricles caused by an anatomic or functional impairment in the conduction system. AV nodal conduction abnormalities can be classified in three types: first, second, and third degree. First-degree AV block is simply prolongation of the P-R interval longer than 200 ms. In second-degree AV block, some atrial impulses fail to reach the ventricles. Wenckebach initially, and later Mobitz, divided second-degree AV block into types 1 and 2. In third-degree (complete) heart block, all atrial impulses fail to conduct to the ventricles that have a rate less than 40 bpm (acquired) (Table 3.1). Sometimes the term *advanced AV block* is used when two or more consecutive P waves block and do not fit the usual type 1 or type 2 AV block classification noted previously. In addition, 2:1 AV block cannot be classified as type 1 or type 2 and is simply called *2:1 AV block*.

PATHOPHYSIOLOGY OF ATRIOVENTRICULAR BLOCK

AV block can be transient or permanent. Cardiac conduction disease (CCD) causes a potentially life-threatening alteration in normal impulse propagation through the cardiac conduction system. CCD can result from a number of physiologic mechanisms ranging from acquired to congenital and occur with or without structural heart disease. Progressive CCD, also known as *Lev-Lenègre disease*, is one of the most common cardiac conduction disturbances in the absence of overt structural heart disease. It is characterized by progressive (age-related) alteration of impulse propagation through the His-Purkinje system, with bundle branch block (right or left) and widening of the QRS complex leading to complete AV block, syncope, and occasionally sudden death. Acute myocardial infarction (MI) is associated with AV block in 12% to 25% of patients (first-degree AV block occurs in 2% to 12%, second-degree AV block in 3% to 10%, and third-degree AV block in 3% to 7%). Chronic ischemic heart disease can result in persistent AV block. Transient AV block can occur during angina pectoris and Prinzmetal angina. Inferior wall MI is associated with vagally mediated AV block and type 1 second-degree AV block that usually resolves within 2 or 3 days. Rarely, type 2 AV block occurs in inferior MI as a result of AV node involvement and can be persistent. Type 2 second-degree AV block occurring during an acute anterior MI is typically associated with bundle branch ischemia or infarction and frequently progresses to complete heart block. Complete AV block occurs in 8% to 13% of patients with acute MI. AV nodal blocking drugs and class III antiarrhythmic drugs can cause AV block or exacerbate AV block in patients with pre-existing conduction disease. Class I and class III antiarrhythmic drugs can also affect conduction in the His-Purkinje system, resulting in infranodal block. Infiltrative cardiomyopathies, such as amyloidosis, sarcoidosis, and hemochromatosis, can cause heart block. Autoimmune diseases, such as rheumatic fever, scleroderma, rheumatoid arthritis, and systemic lupus erythematosus, can cause AV block. Neuromuscular degenerative diseases, such as Becker muscular dystrophy, peroneal muscular dystrophy, Kearns-Sayre syndrome, and myotonic muscular dystrophy, are also associated with conduction system disease. Infections, such as aortic root abscess in infective endocarditis, Chagas disease, and Lyme disease, can cause AV block. AV block can be congenital and can also occur after aortic valve surgery, transcatheter aortic valve replacement, or surgery for the repair of congenital heart disease.

FIRST-DEGREE ATRIOVENTRICULAR BLOCK

First-degree AV block is manifested electrocardiographically as prolongation of the P-R interval. Electrophysiologically, the P-R interval is the sum of sinus node to AV nodal conduction (intraatrial conduction) time, nodal (AV node and AV node to His bundle) conduction time, and His bundle to ventricular conduction time. Therefore delay in any of the components alone or in combination can prolong the P-R interval. Most commonly, first degree AV block results from AV nodal disease and less commonly from His-Purkinje disease (Figs. 3.1 and 3.2).

SECOND-DEGREE ATRIOVENTRICULAR BLOCK TYPE 1

Type 1 block (Wenckebach) is progressive P-R interval prolongation preceding a nonconducted P wave. The electrocardiogram (ECG) typically shows group beating (3:2, 4:3, 5:4) with a pause shorter than two R-R intervals. It occurs because the cycle of the nonconducted ("dropped") beat is less than the summed cycles of any two previous cycles. This results because the absolute amount of conduction delay *decreases* in each subsequent cycle (Fig. 3.3).

ATYPICAL TYPE I SECOND-DEGREE ATRIOVENTRICULAR BLOCK

The classic AV Wenckebach structure depends on a stable atrial rate and a maximal increment in AV conduction time for the second P-R interval of the Wenckebach cycle, with a progressive decrease of AV conduction time in subsequent beats. Unstable or unusual alterations in the increment of AV conduction time or in the atrial rate, often seen with long Wenckebach cycles (e.g., 8:7), results in atypical forms of type 1 AV block in which the last R-R interval can lengthen because the PR increment increases or R-R intervals can fluctuate as a result of fluctuating P-R intervals (Fig. 3.4). Sometimes it occurs when a junctional escape ends the pause following a nonconducted P wave, resulting in an apparent shortening of the P-R interval. Concealed discharge from the His bundle can mimic first-degree (A), type 1 (B), and type 2 (C) second-degree AV block (Fig. 3.5). Examples of typical and atypical type 1 second-degree AV block are shown in Figs. 3.5 through 3.11.

TABLE 3.1   Electrocardiographic manifestations of AV block

| TYPE | ELECTROCARDIOGRAPHIC MANIFESTATION | SITE OF BLOCK | | COMMENTS |
		AV NODE	HIS-PURKINJE SYSTEM	
First degree	PR >200 ms, each P is followed by a QRS with a fixed P-R interval.	Most common site of block, especially when the QRS complex is narrow and PR is >300 ms.	Prolonged PR with BBB; occurs in 45% of cases.	Caused by intraatrial or interatrial conduction delay (broad P wave); block can occur at multiple levels.
Second degree type 1	Progressive PR prolongation preceding a nonconducted P wave; P-R interval prolongs at a decreasing interval.	Most common site of block.	Rare.	Atypical Wenckebach occurs in >50% type 1 block.
Second degree type 2	P-R interval remains unchanged prior to the nonconducted P wave.	Less common.	Almost always infranodal; occurs in His bundle in 30% of cases.	
Third degree	Failure of conduction of all P waves.	Narrow QRS usually congenital; rate 40–60 bpm; block lessens with atropine or exercise.	Wide QRS usually acquired; rate 20–40 bpm; block does not improve with atropine.	Site can be either AV node or His-Purkinje system.

AV, Atrioventricular; *BBB*, bundle branch block.

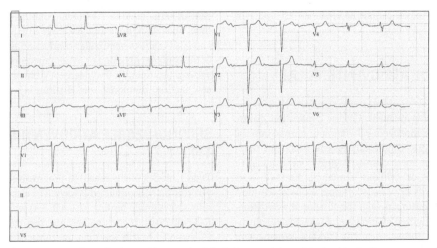

Fig. 3.1 Electrocardiogram demonstrates sinus rhythm with a marked first-degree atrioventricular block. P waves are closer to the previous QRS (i.e., the R-P interval is shorter than the P-R interval); however, it cannot be a junctional rhythm with retrogradely conducted P waves because P waves are upright in the inferior leads. Retrogradely conducted P waves are negative in inferior leads.

SECOND-DEGREE ATRIOVENTRICULAR BLOCK TYPE 2

In type 2 AV block, the P-R interval remains unchanged before the P wave suddenly fails to conduct to the ventricles (Fig. 3.3B). A true Mobitz type 2 AV block occurs mostly as a result of infranodal disease and is usually associated with a wide QRS complex caused by associated conduction system disease (Figs. 3.12 and 3.13). Therefore type 2 second-degree block in conjunction with a narrow QRS complex is relatively rare and occurs without sinus slowing and without Wenckebach phenomenon. Coexistence of intermittent type 1 and type 2 block with a narrow QRS practically excludes His-Purkinje disease as the cause of block. Exercise-induced second-degree AV block is most commonly infranodal and rarely is secondary to AV nodal disease or cardiac ischemia. Apparent Mobitz type 2 AV block can also be caused by concealed junctional extrasystoles (confined to the specialized conduction system and not propagated to the myocardium) (Fig. 3.5).

ATRIOVENTRICULAR BLOCK

The distinction between type 1 and type 2 AV block cannot be made easily from the ECG when 2:1 AV block is present (Box 3.1). In this situation every other beat is nonconducted, and there is no opportunity to observe the PR prolongation that is characteristic of type 1 block (Fig. 3.14). To aid in the diagnosis, a long rhythm strip should be

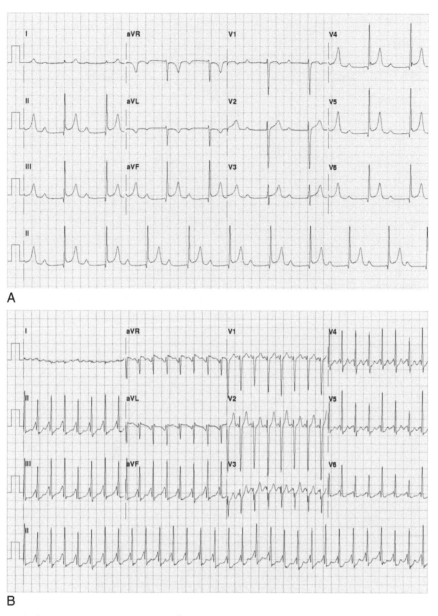

Fig. 3.2 First-degree atrioventricular (AV) block. (A) Electrocardiogram (ECG) of a patient with a markedly prolonged P-R interval with 1:1 AV conduction. (B) ECG of the same patient showing a long RP tachycardia with a very short P-R interval. The P-R interval is too short for an atrial impulse to conduct by way of the AV node unless it is a rare condition of enhanced AV nodal conduction. This ECG was recorded during a treadmill exercise test. The markedly prolonged baseline P-R interval becomes further prolonged during an exercise stress test. Note that there is progressive prolongation of the P-R interval during exercise (owing to the decremental property of the AV node in C). *Black arrows* show P waves that conduct to the next QRS complex (*red arrows*). During the peak exercise there is "crossover" of P and R waves so that the P wave conducting via the AV node gives rise to the QRS not immediately following the P wave, but the QRS complex (*red arrow*, fourth strip in C and D) following the next QRS; that is, the P-R interval exceeds the P-P interval, a phenomenon called "skipped P waves." During recovery, the PR shortens, and crossover ends (C *bottom strip*).

obtained or a previous ECG showing any Wenckebach pattern may be helpful. Atropine may be tried in an attempt to induce 3:2 AV conduction. Carotid sinus massage may improve type 2 AV block and worsen type 1 AV block.

ADVANCED ATRIOVENTRICULAR BLOCK

AV block is considered high-grade or advanced second-degree AV block if two or more consecutive P waves fail to conduct when AV synchrony is otherwise maintained. This block occurs because of AV nodal

or His-Purkinje disease and not because of retrograde concealment in the AV node or His-Purkinje system caused by junctional or ventricular escape complexes (Figs. 3.15 through 3.18).

THIRD-DEGREE (COMPLETE) ATRIOVENTRICULAR BLOCK

The majority of examples of third-degree heart block result from conduction system disease in the His-Purkinje system. When third-degree

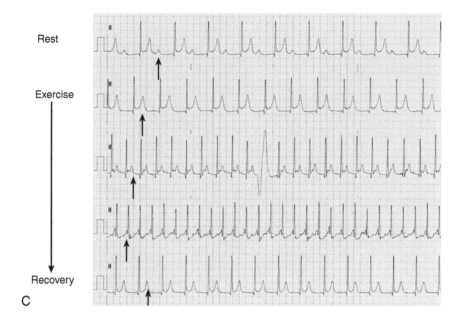

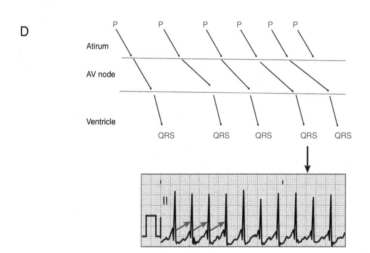

Fig. 3.2 (Continued).

AV block occurs in the AV node, approximately two-thirds of the escape rhythms have a narrow QRS complex (i.e., a junctional or AV nodal rhythm). The site of block is usually AV node in congenital third-degree AV block or during transient AV block associated with acute inferior wall MI or induced by beta blockers, calcium channel blockers, and digitalis toxicity. As a general rule, the more distal the block, the slower the escape rhythm. The rate of junctional escapes increases with exercise and atropine and catecholamine infusion and slows with vagal maneuvers. Lower escape sites are less responsive to autonomic manipulation (Figs. 3.19 through 3.29).

Congenital Heart Block

Congenital complete AV block is thought to result from embryonic maldevelopment of the AV node. The defect usually occurs proximal to the His bundle. These patients usually have an escape rhythm from the His bundle. Therefore the QRS duration is narrow (<120 ms). Less

frequently, the defect occurs in the His-Purkinje system and the escape rhythm is slow with wide QRS. Neonatal lupus, caused by maternal antibodies that cross the placenta to affect the fetal heart, accounts for 60% to 90% of cases of congenital complete AV block. Approximately half of the patients with congenital AV block have concurrent congenital heart disease (Fig. 3.30).

ALTERNATE LEFT BUNDLE BRANCH BLOCK AND RIGHT BUNDLE BRANCH BLOCK, OR RIGHT BUNDLE BLOCK WITH ALTERNATE FASCICULAR BLOCK

Alternating right bundle branch block and left bundle branch block, or right bundle branch block with alternating fascicular block at rest or during exercise, signifies severe His-Purkinje disease (Fig. 3.31).

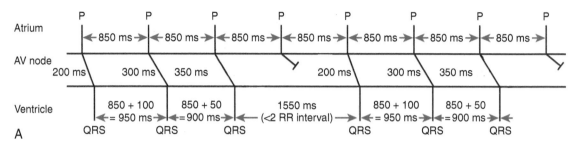

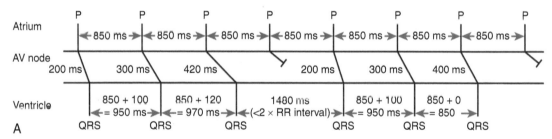

Fig. 3.3 (A) Type 1 second-degree atrioventricular (AV) block: typical 4:3 Wenckebach cycle. P waves (A tier) occur at a cycle length of 850 ms. The P-R interval (AV tier) is 200 ms for the first beat and generates a ventricular response (V tier). The P-R interval increases by 100 ms in the next complex, which results in an R-R interval of 950 ms (850 + 100). The increment in the P-R interval is only 50 ms for the third cycle, and the P-R interval becomes 350 ms. The R-R interval shortens to 900 ms (850 + 50). The next P wave is blocked, and an R-R interval is created that is less than twice the P-P interval by an amount equal to the increments in the P-R interval. (B) Type 2 AV block. The ladder diagram shows 4:3 type II second-degree AV block, the P-R interval remains constant before the blocked P wave, and the R-R interval between the blocked P wave is twice the P-P cycle length.

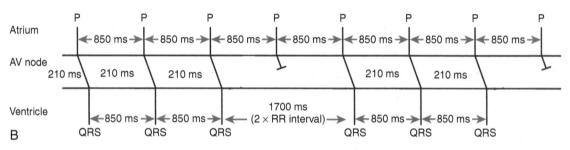

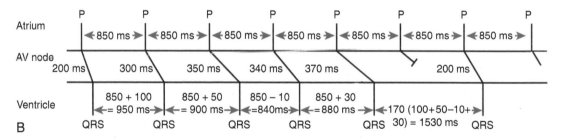

Fig. 3.4 Atypical type 1 second-degree atrioventricular (AV) block. This is unlike the classic AV Wenckebach with a maximal increment in AV conduction time for the second P-R interval of the Wenckebach cycle, with a progressive decrease in subsequent beats. The typical Wenckebach pattern changes when an unstable or unusual alteration in the increment of AV conduction time or in the atrial rate occurs. For example, in (A) the increment in the P-R interval of the last conducted complex increased rather than decreased (e.g., 120 ms rather than 100 ms), the last R-R interval before the block therefore increases (970 ms) rather than decreases. In (B) another example of atypical Wenckebach pattern is shown, with a fluctuating P-R interval, and therefore fluctuating R-R interval before the nonconducted P wave. This is most likely due to variation in vagal tone.

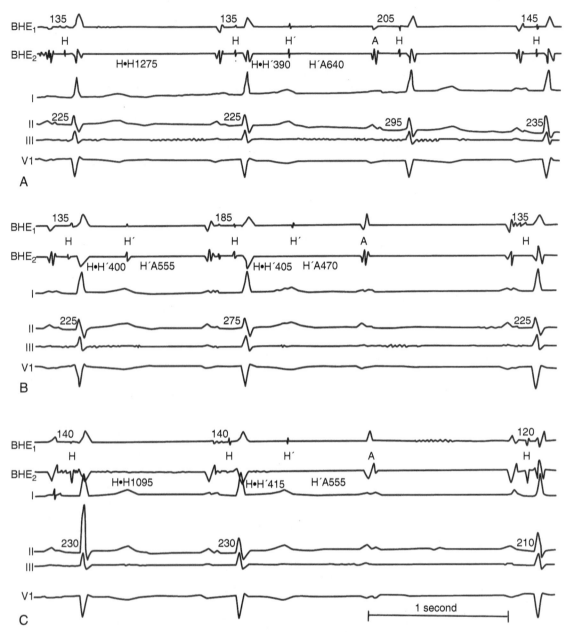

Fig. 3.5 Concealed discharge from the His bundle mimicking first-degree (A), type 1 (B), and type 2 (C) second-degree atrioventricular (AV) block. Numbers are in ms, and timelines are 1 second (magnification differs in the three panels; numbers in the bipolar His electrogram [*BHE₁*] indicate A-H intervals; the H-V interval is constant). Numbers in lead 2 indicate P-R interval. *H-H*, Interval between His responses in normal conducted cycles; *H-H'*, interval between the last normal His discharge and the premature His discharge; *H'-A*, interval between the premature His depolarization and the next normal sinus-initiated atrial discharge. *H'* invaded the AV node and lengthened the A-H interval or produced AV nodal block of the next atrial depolarization. (From Bonner AJ, Zipes DP. Lidocaine and His bundle extrasystoles. His bundle discharge conducted normally, conducted with functional right or left branch block, or blocked entirely [concealed]. *Arch Intern Med.* 1976;136:700-704.)

EXERCISE-INDUCED HEART BLOCK AND PAROXYSMAL ATRIOVENTRICULAR BLOCK

Paroxysmal heart block can result from AV nodal disease or His-Purkinje disease. Patients with AV nodal disease usually have narrow QRS complexes, and patients with His-Purkinje disease often have baseline bundle branch block. However, the block can be at multiple levels in patients with conduction system disease (Fig. 3.32).

ATRIOVENTRICULAR DISSOCIATION

AV dissociation results from dissociated or independent depolarization of the atria and ventricles. It is not a primary disturbance of rhythm but is an underlying rhythm disturbance produced by one of three causes or combination of causes that prevent the normal transmission of impulses from atrium to the ventricles. These include (1) sinus bradycardia with junctional/ventricular escapes, (2) junctional/ventricular tachycardia, (3) AV block allowing junctional/ventricular escapes, and (4) various combinations of the preceding (Figs. 3.33 through 3.40).

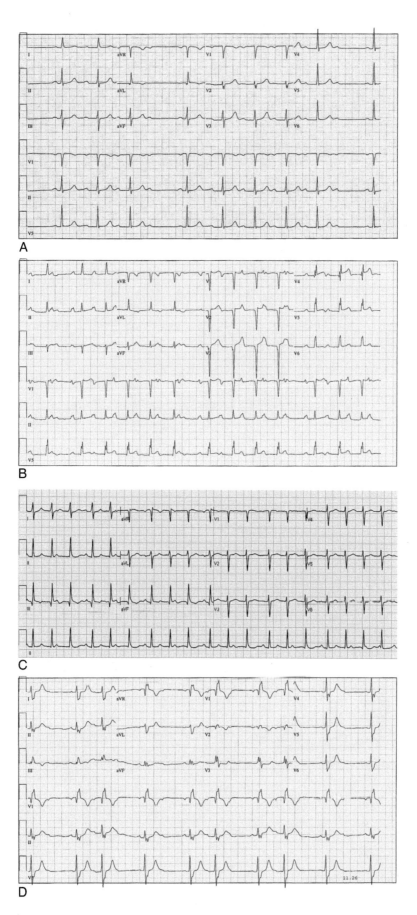

Fig. 3.6 Sinus rhythm with type 1 second-degree atrioventricular (AV) block. Electrocardiograms (ECGs) showing typical Wenckebach pattern during sinus rhythm with progressive prolongation of the P-R interval followed by a nonconducted P wave. The P-R interval after the blocked beat is shortest, and the P-R interval before the nonconducted sinus beat (by way of the AV node) is longest because of the increment (albeit at a decreasing value) in the P-R interval. ECGs (A through C) depict sinus rhythm with typical Wenckebach pattern of AV block with variable AV block (4:3 to 6:5 AV conduction). (D) ECG shows sinus rhythm with type 1 second-degree AV block and right bundle branch block with right axis deviation indicating associated His-Purkinje disease.

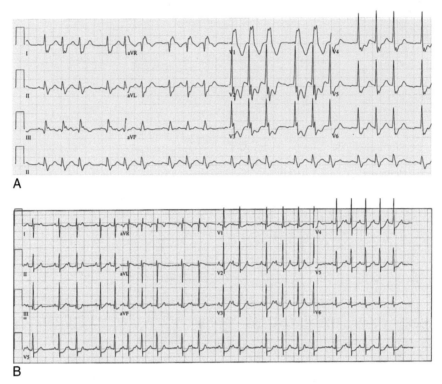

A

B

Fig. 3.7 Sinus rhythm with type 1 second-degree atrioventricular (AV) block. (A) Atrial tachycardia with 4:3 AV block and right bundle branch block. (B) Atrial tachycardia with 3:2 to 6:5 second-degree type 1 AV nodal block.

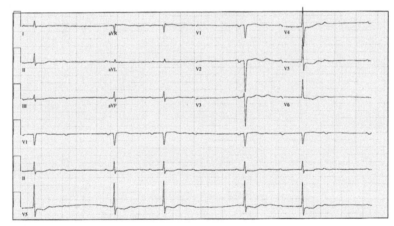

Fig. 3.8 Sinus bradycardia with type 1 second-degree atrioventricular block. Electrocardiogram was recorded during vagal stimulation.

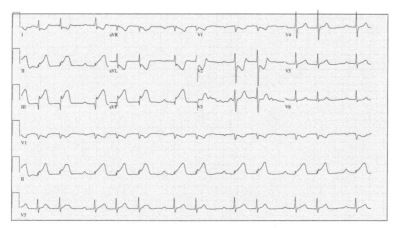

Fig. 3.9 Type 1 second-degree heart block associated with acute inferior myocardial infarction. This usually results from a high vagal tone and resolves spontaneously.

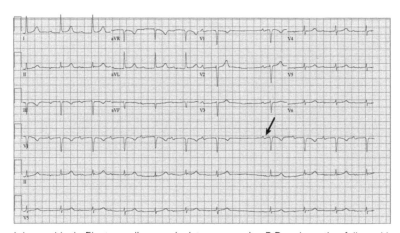

Fig. 3.10 Atypical type 1 second-degree block. Electrocardiogram depicts progressive P-R prolongation followed by the loss of a sinus beat owing to a sinus pause that is followed by a sinus beat conducted at a shorter P-R interval (*arrow*) compared with the immediately previous P-R interval. The sinus pause allows the atrioventricular node to recover, and therefore the P-R interval shortens.

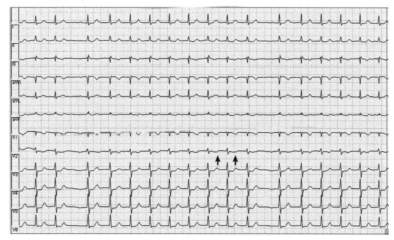

Fig. 3.11 Atypical type 1 second-degree atrioventricular (AV) block. The rhythm shows a long AV node Wenckebach (10:9) pattern with two conducted (*arrows*) beats in which P-R intervals are not prolonged. Sometimes P-R interval can fluctuate during type 1 AV block and is designated as atypical AV node Wenckebach pattern.

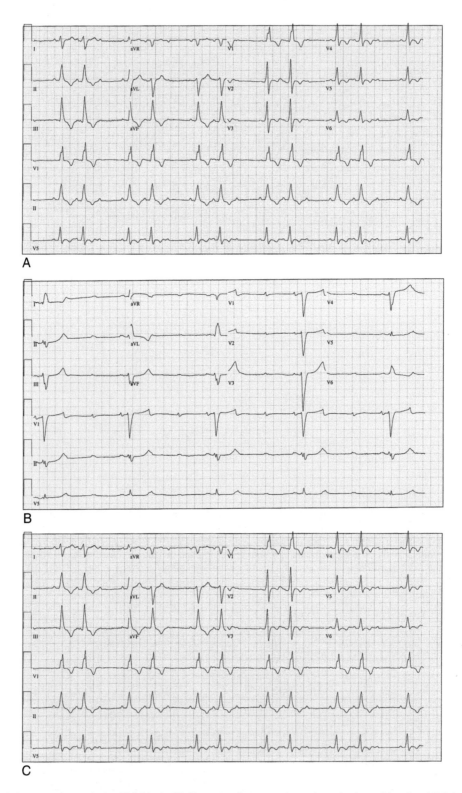

Fig. 3.12 Type 2 second-degree atrioventricular (AV) block. (A) Electrocardiograms show sinus rhythm with a fixed P-R interval and 3:2 AV block. (B) 3:1 AV block. (C) 3:2 AV block. (D) 10:9 AV block. (E) 2:1 AV block.

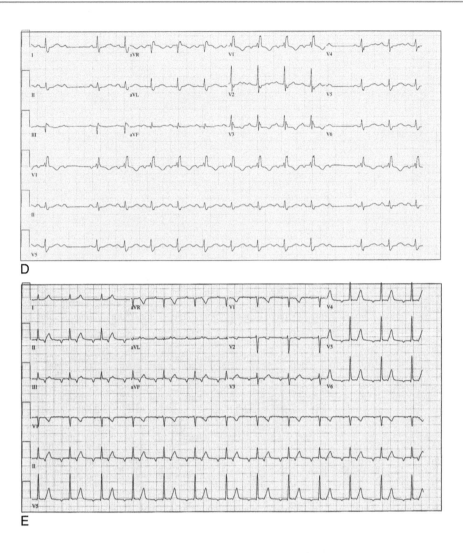

Fig. 3.12 (Continued).

1. AV dissociation by default: Slowing of the primary pacemaker allows a subsidiary to arise by default. It usually occurs during sinus bradycardia, which allows escape of a subsidiary or latent pacemaker and permits an independent AV junction rhythm to arise (Fig. 3.33).

2. AV dissociation by usurpation: Acceleration of a latent pacemaker, which usurps control of the ventricles, can cause AV dissociation even if the sinus node function is normal. An abnormally enhanced discharge rate of a usually slower subsidiary pacemaker is pathologic and commonly occurs during nonparoxysmal AV junctional tachycardia or ventricular tachycardia without retrograde atrial capture.

3. AV block: The heart block is defined as AV block, which generally occurs at the AV junction, prevents impulses formed at a normal rate in a dominant pacemaker (sinus) from reaching the ventricles, and allows the ventricles to beat under the control of a subsidiary pacemaker. Junctional or ventricular escape rhythms during AV block, without retrograde atrial capture, are a common example in which block gives rise to AV dissociation. Complete AV block is not synonymous with complete AV dissociation. Patients who have complete AV block have complete AV dissociation, but patients who have complete AV dissociation may or may not have complete AV block.

4. A combination of causes mentioned in the preceding paragraphs: A combination of the aforementioned causes can occur in pathologic condition. The common example is digitalis toxicity resulting in nonparoxysmal AV junctional tachycardia associated with sinoatrial or AV block.

VENTRICULOPHASIC SINUS ARRHYTHMIA

Ventriculophasic sinus arrhythmia can be observed during second- or third-degree AV block. The two P waves with a QRS complex in-between have a shortened interval compared with the two P waves that occur sequentially without an intervening QRS complex (Fig. 3.41). The mechanism of this phenomenon is not certain. It is suggested that ventricular contractions enhance sinus node automaticity by increasing the pulsatile blood flow through the sinus nodal artery or, alternatively, reflex slowing for P-P interval following the QRS complex that results in systolic ejection of the blood causing stretch of the carotid sinus with reflex slowing of sinus node.

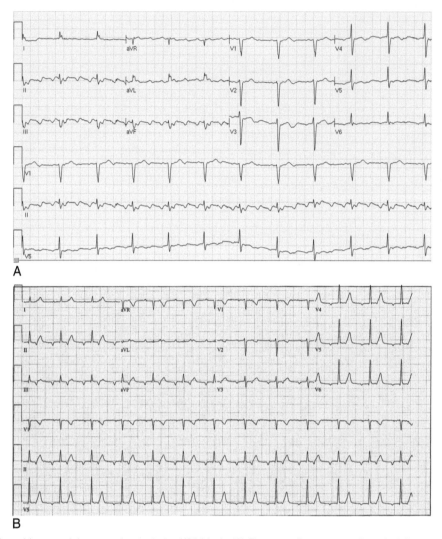

Fig. 3.13 Atrial arrhythmias with second-degree atrioventricular (AV) block. (A) Electrocardiogram reveals typical flutter with uncommon pattern of second-degree AV block (3:1). The usual pattern of AV block in typical flutter is 2:1, 4:1, or variable. (B) Atrial tachycardia with 2:1 AV block.

BOX 3.1 **Site of block (AV node vs. His-Purkinje system) in 21 AV block**	
LIKELY AV NODE	**LIKELY HIS-PURKINJE SYSTEM**
Type 1 Wenckebach pattern preceding the 2:1 block	PR fixed despite varying RP interval
PR >300 ms	PR <160 ms
Narrow QRS	Wide QRS[a]
Improvement of block with atropine or exercise	No improvement of block with atropine[b]

AV, Atrioventricular.
[a]Site of block could still be AV node.
[b]Absence of such response does not exclude intranodal block.

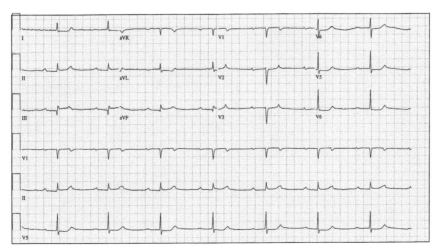

Fig. 3.14 Electrocardiogram of a patient who suffered from inferior wall myocardial infarction (ST segment elevation in inferior leads) shows sinus rhythm with 2:1 atrioventricular (AV) block and narrow QRS complexes. Intermittent type 1 second-degree AV block was also noted during telemetry, suggesting that the site of block is at the AV node level, as does the lack of a bundle branch block.

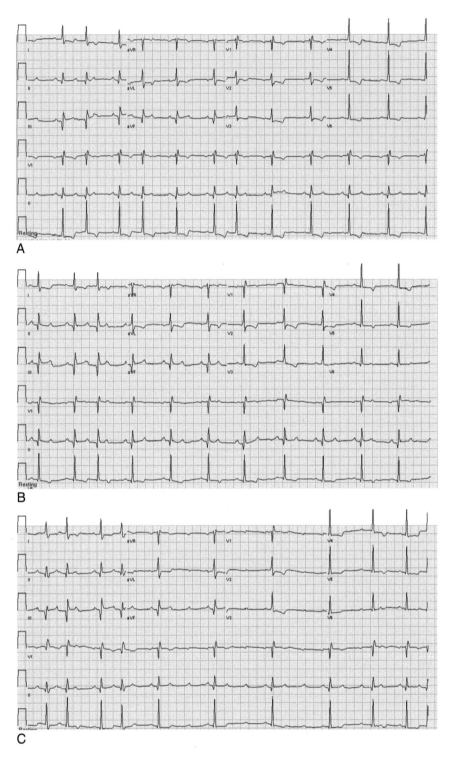

Fig. 3.15 (A) Electrocardiogram depicts sinus tachycardia with type 1 second-degree atrioventricular (AV) block that progresses to 2:1 AV block with narrow QRS complexes (B). However, within a few minutes the rhythm shows AV nodal Wenckebach followed by 3:1 AV block, which is followed by 2:1 AV block (C). Narrow QRS complexes suggest that the block is most likely at the level of AV node.

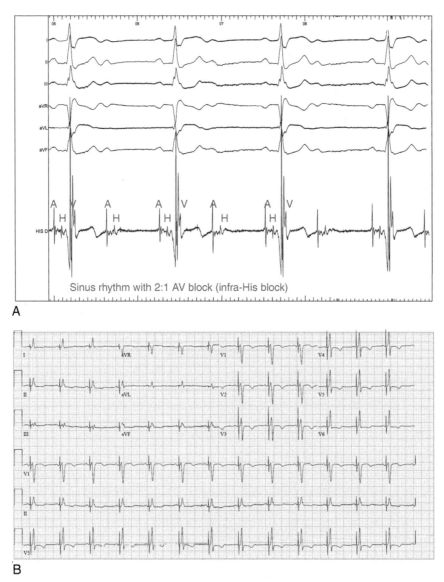

A

B

Fig. 3.16 (A) The electrocardiogram shows sinus rhythm with 2:1 atrioventricular block and left bundle branch block. The intracardiac recording shows that the block is infra-His level (A = atrial potential, H = His bundle recording, V = ventricular potential) (B). The patient received an His bundle pacing with resulting narrow QRS paced complexes.

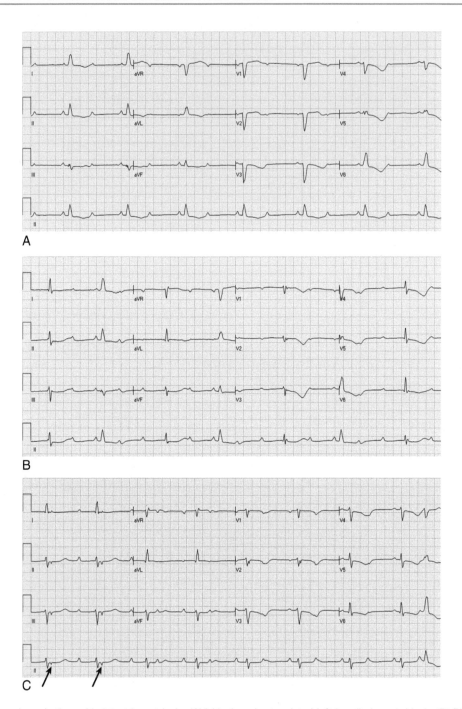

Fig. 3.17 (A) Patient has sinus rhythm with 2:1 atrioventricular (AV) block and rate-related left bundle branch block. (B) Rhythm later changed to advanced AV block with intermittent ventricular escape rhythm with narrow QRS complexes. (C) Electrocardiogram depicts complete heart block. There are two consecutive P waves followed by retrograde atrial conduction (negative P waves in inferior leads) demonstrating intact ventriculoatrial conduction (*arrows*), despite anterograde AV block.

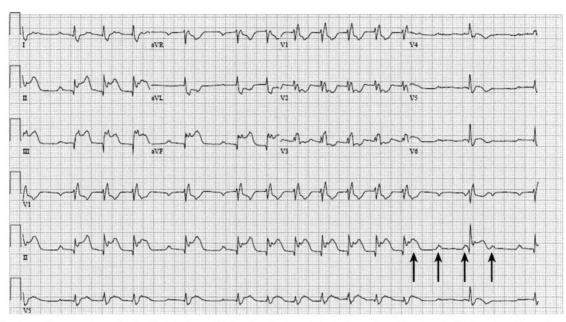

Fig. 3.18 Electrocardiogram of a patient with inferior wall infarction depicts sinus tachycardia with a long P-R interval and type 1 atrioventricular block with group beating. The rhythm later shows three consecutive nonconducted P waves followed by junctional escape. The P wave immediately following the junctional rhythm also does not conduct. The *arrows* point to P waves.

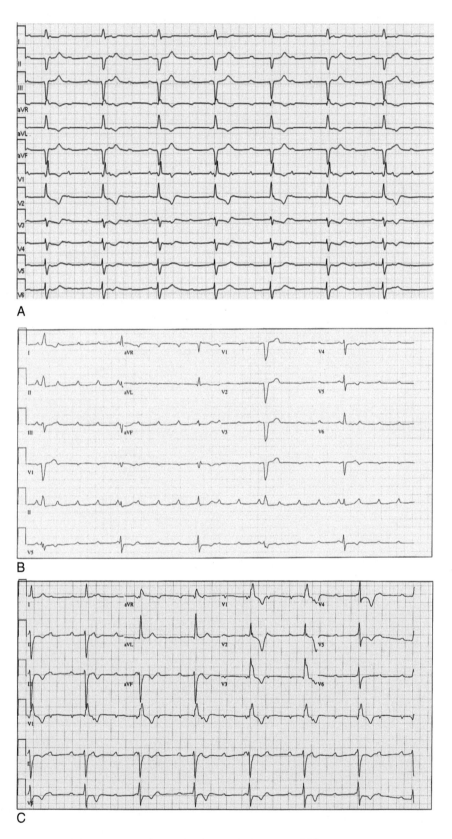

Fig. 3.19 Sinus rhythm and complete atrioventricular (AV) block with relatively narrow QRS complexes (A), intermittent narrow and wide QRS complexes (B), and wide (C) ventricular escape beats. Complete AV block with narrow QRS complexes suggests that the site of the AV block is at the AV node. Complete AV block with wide QRS complexes suggests that the site of the AV block is at the His-Purkinje level.

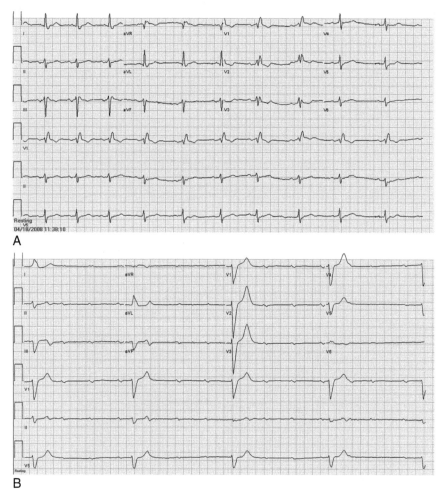

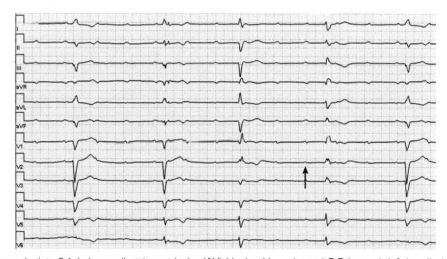

Fig. 3.20 (A) Electrocardiogram of a 74-year-old male patient shows sinus rhythm with prolonged P-R interval, right bundle branch block, and left axis deviation suggestive of bifascicular block. (B) Atrioventricular block later progressed to third-degree (complete), and all the P waves failed to conduct. Note the slow ventricular escape rhythm with a wide QRS complex (ventricular escape) and a rate of 25 bpm, consistent with block in the His-Purkinje system.

Fig. 3.21 Electrocardiogram depicts 3:1 (advanced) atrioventricular (AV) block with prolonged P-R interval, left bundle branch block, and left axis deviation. The first two QRS complexes are conducted. These are followed by two nonconducted ventricular complexes. The first is slightly premature, but the second ventricular complex occurred as an escape rhythm because the native P wave (*arrow*), which should have conducted as a part of baseline 3:1 AV conduction, did not conduct.

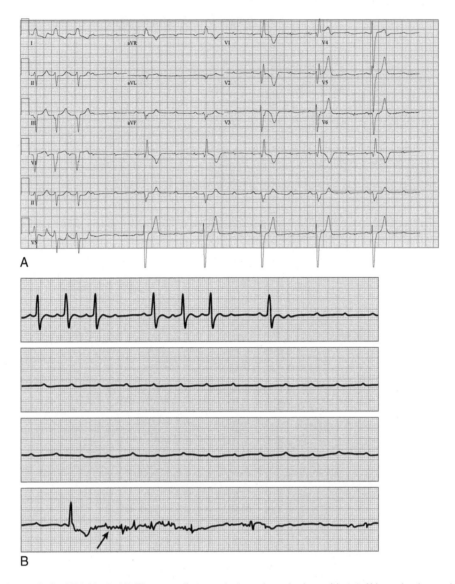

A

B

Fig. 3.22 Paroxysmal atrioventricular (AV) block. (A) Electrocardiogram depicts sinus rhythm with 1:1 AV conduction and left bundle branch block (first three beats) followed by 3:1 AV block with right bundle branch block pattern. Long P-R interval with alternate left bundle branch block and right bundle branch block signifies severe His-Purkinje disease. (B) The rhythm strip shows sinus rhythm with 2:1 AV block followed by complete AV block and a spontaneous junctional escape after 17 seconds followed by five more slow, irregular junctional escapes. During this period, the patient developed cerebral hypoxia with convulsions manifested as an artifact in the lower strip (*arrow*).

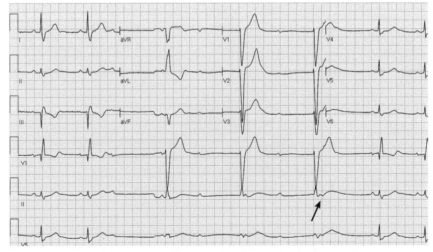

Fig. 3.23 Electrocardiogram shows sinus rhythm with two initial beats conducted by way of the atrioventricular (AV) node. It is followed by sinus slowing and transient AV block with three consecutive ventricular escape beats. The third ventricular escape beat is followed by retrograde conduction with atrial depolarization (retrograde P wave [*arrow*]), and then resumption of AV nodal conduction occurs. Such changes can occur spontaneously or during a vagal maneuver. Episode of syncope recorded by an implantable loop recorder.

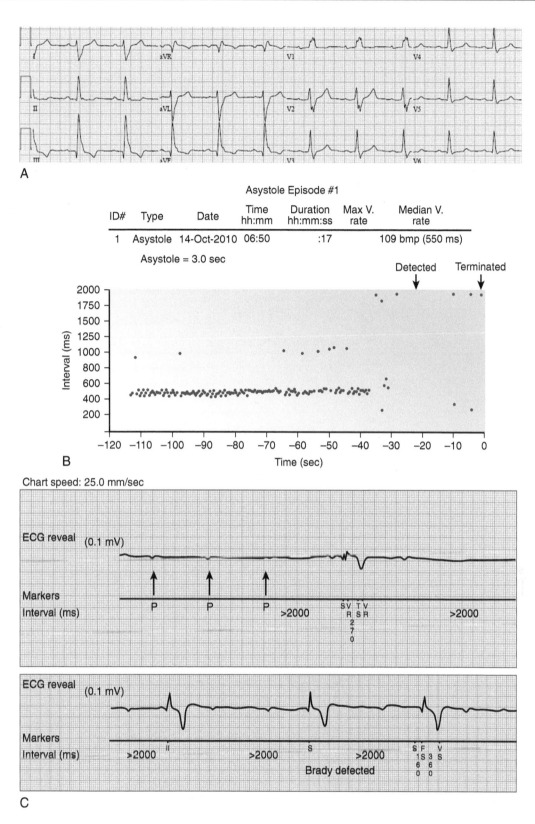

Fig. 3.24 (A) Electrocardiogram (ECG) of a 70-year-old male patient presenting with syncope shows sinus rhythm with prolonged P-R interval, right bundle branch block, and right posterior axis suggestive of trifascicular block. Patient underwent electrophysiology study that showed a moderately prolonged H-V interval of 75 ms (normal, 35–55 ms) that prolonged to 85 ms after procainamide infusion. He did not qualify for pacemaker implant because the H-V prolongation of greater than 100 ms is considered the marker of severe His-Purkinje disease. Patient presented with syncope 3 months later. A loop recorder was implanted. Patient had recurrence of syncope 1 week later. (B) Interrogation of loop recorder revealed two episodes of sinus rhythm with complete atrioventricular block, which correlated with patient's syncopal episodes. The longer episode is shown here. The rhythm is sinus with complete atrioventricular block and ventricular pauses up to 17 seconds. (C) *Arrows* indicate nonconducted P waves. Patient received a pacemaker. *V,* Ventricular.

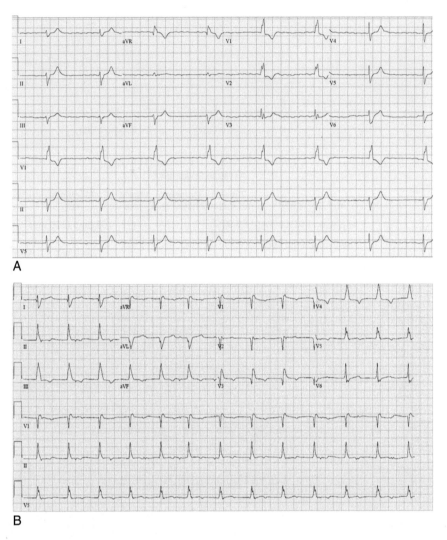

Fig. 3.25 (A) Electrocardiogram shows atrial fibrillation with a fixed ventricular rate and ventricular escape of 43 bpm indicating complete heart block, typically seen in severe conduction system disease or drug effect, such as digoxin toxicity. (B) Electrocardiogram depicts an atrial rhythm with atrioventricular dissociation and nonparoxysmal junctional tachycardia resulting from digitalis toxicity.

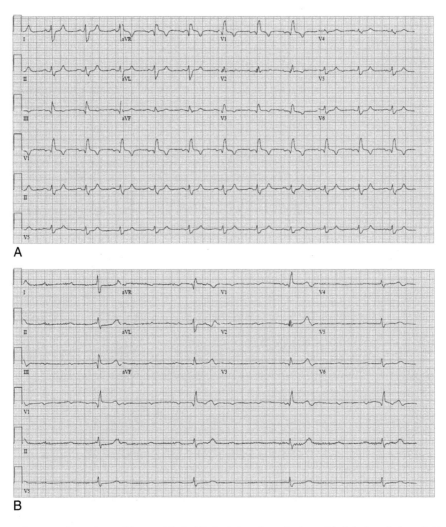

Fig. 3.26 Baseline electrocardiogram of a patient with sarcoidosis (A) depicting sinus rhythm with right bundle branch block and probable posterior fascicular block, later progressing to complete heart block (B).

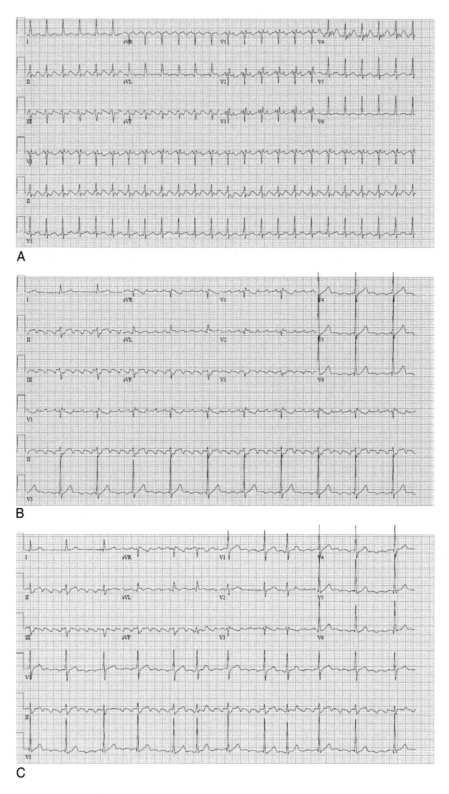

Fig. 3.27 Electrocardiogram of a patient who presented with the typical counterclockwise right atrial flutter with 2:1 atrioventricular (AV) block (A). AV block progressed with calcium blocker therapy to 4:1 AV conduction (B), and later, variable AV conduction (C).

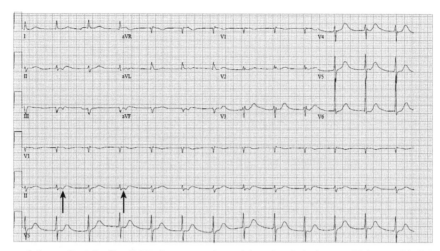

Fig. 3.28 Electrocardiogram of the patient in Fig. 3.18 shows accelerated junctional rhythm at 76 bpm with 2:1 ventriculoatrial block after atrioventricular nodal—blocking therapy. The *arrows* point to retrogradely conducted P waves.

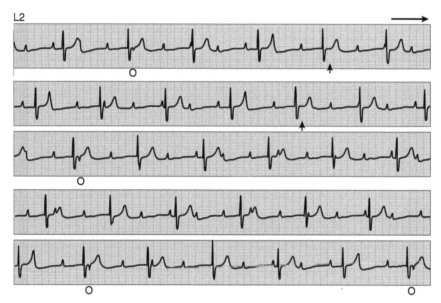

Fig. 3.29 Lead 2 rhythm strip shows complete heart block with intermittent ventriculoatrial conduction when atrium is not refractory. Antegrade P waves (embedded in QRS wave) blocks the retrograde conduction via the atrioventricular node, after the same QRS (expected timing of the retrograde P wave is marked by *arrows*), therefore there is no compensatory pause in the next P-P cycle. Retrograde P waves marked by *small circles* depolarize the atrium earlier than the expected sinus wave, and therefore result in a compensatory pause due to resetting of the sinus node (from Dr. Charles Fisch collection).

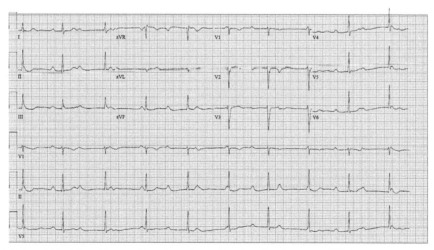

Fig. 3.30 Congenital complete heart block in a 17-year-old male patient with a junctional escape of 58 bpm.

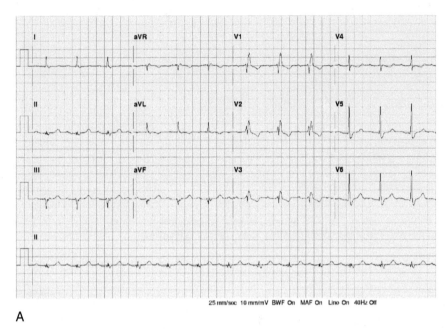

25 mm/sec 10 mm/mV BWF On   MAF On   Line On   40Hz Off

A

Fig. 3.31 Baseline electrocardiogram (A) demonstrated first-degree atrioventricular block, right bundle branch block, and left anterior fascicular block (left axis deviation). During the stress test (B and C), frequent changes in QRS axis suggested alternating right and left fascicular blocks. QRS axis returned to baseline during recovery phase (D). Electrophysiology study (E) revealed an A-H interval of 70 ms (normal, 60–120 ms) and a markedly prolonged H-V interval of 140 ms (normal, 35–55 ms), confirming severe His-Purkinje disease.

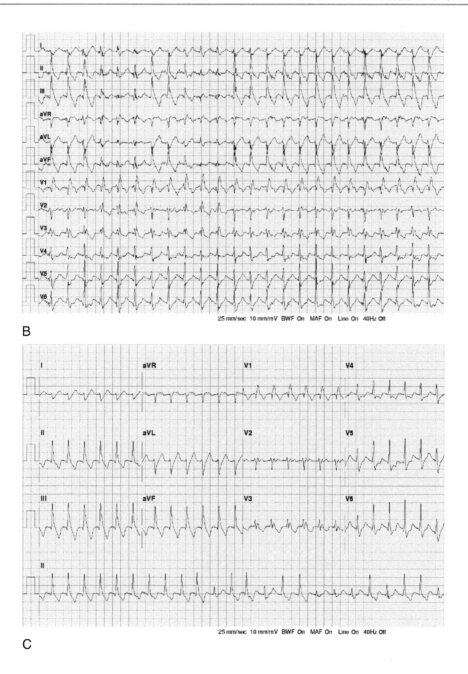

Fig. 3.31 (Continued).

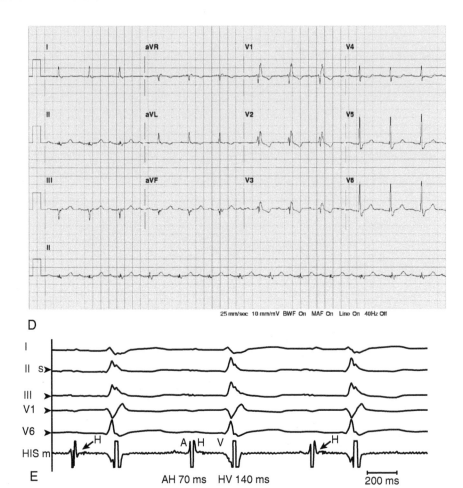

Fig. 3.31 (Continued).

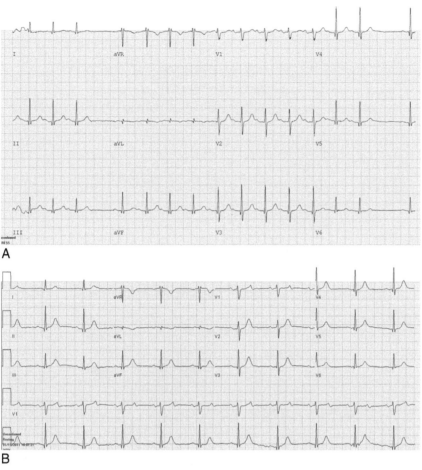

Fig. 3.32 (A) Baseline electrocardiogram (ECG) during treadmill exercise of a 70-year-old man who developed syncope during physical activity is essentially unremarkable. During continued exercise, the patient developed advanced (2:1 followed by 3:1) atrioventricular (AV) block (B and C). This is followed by complete AV block (D) and presyncope recorded as motion artifacts during heart block. Electrophysiology study (E and F) showed 3:1 AV nodal block during atrial pacing (A) at 590 ms (102 bpm) with block at two levels but predominantly at His-Purkinje (His) level (F) First complex of A is followed by His-bundle deflection (H) and ventricular electrogram (V). The second A is not followed by H, indicating block at the AV nodal level. The third A complex is followed by H, which is not followed by V, confirming His bundle disease. (F) Infra-His block (H without a following A) during every second and third atrial paced beats at a pacing rate of 109 bpm (550 ms). Surface ECG demonstrates 3:1 AV block. There are pacing artifacts on the surface ECG and intracardiac recording. *HRA*, High right atrium.

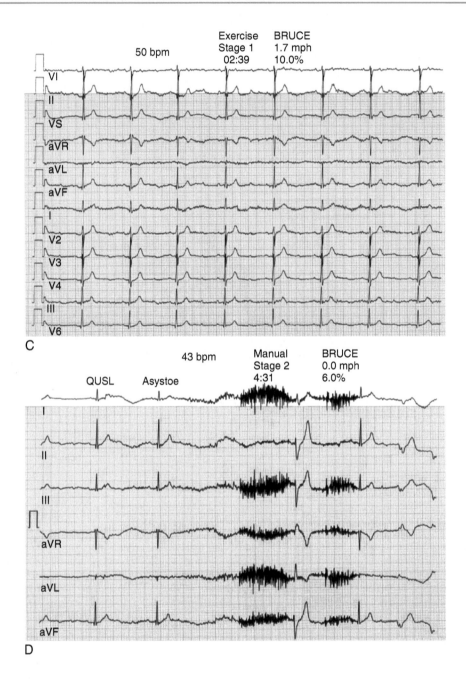

Fig. 3.32 (Continued).

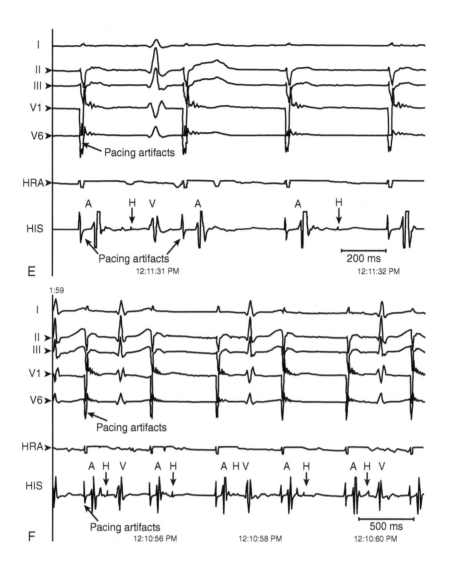

Fig. 3.32 (Continued).

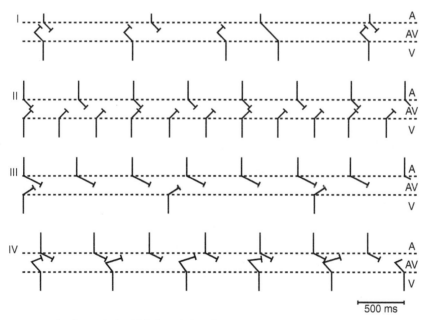

Fig. 3.33 Diagram of the four causes of atrioventricular (AV) dissociation. Sinus bradycardia allowing escape of an AV junctional rhythm that does not capture the atria retrogradely illustrates type 1 intermittent sinus captures (third P wave) to produce incomplete AV dissociation (*I*). Ventricular tachycardia without retrograde atrial capture produces complete AV dissociation (*II*). Complete AV block with a ventricular escape rhythm (*III*). The combination of type 2 and 3 represents a nonparoxysmal AV junctional tachycardia and some degree of AV block (*IV*). (Modified from Zipes DP, Libby P, Bonow RO, Mann DL, Tomaselli G. *Braunwald's Heart Disease: A Textbook of Cardiovascular Medicine.* 11th ed. Philadelphia, PA: WB Saunders; 2019.)

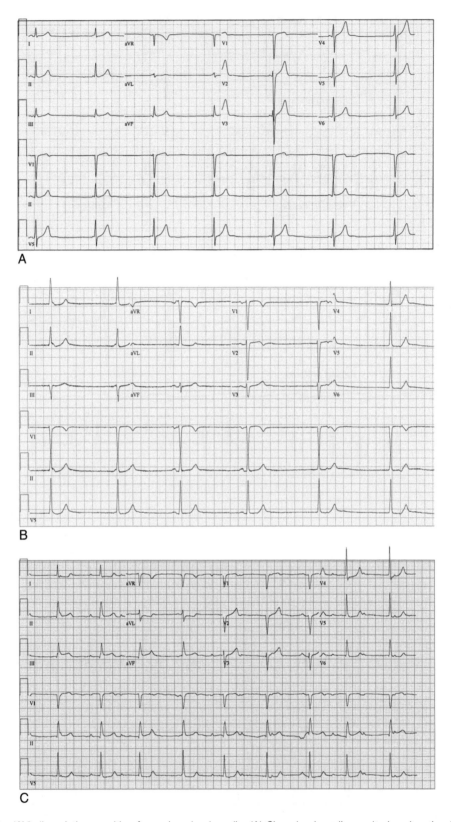

Fig. 3.34 Atrioventricular (AV) dissociation resulting from sinus bradycardia. (A) Sinus bradycardia results in a junctional escape rhythm slightly faster than the sinus rate. (B) AV dissociation and sinus bradycardia and junctional escape rhythm with two sinus capture beats. This occurs in the setting of sinus arrhythmia. (C) Acute inferior myocardial infarction associated with AV dissociation with junctional escape rhythm and intermittent AV conduction.

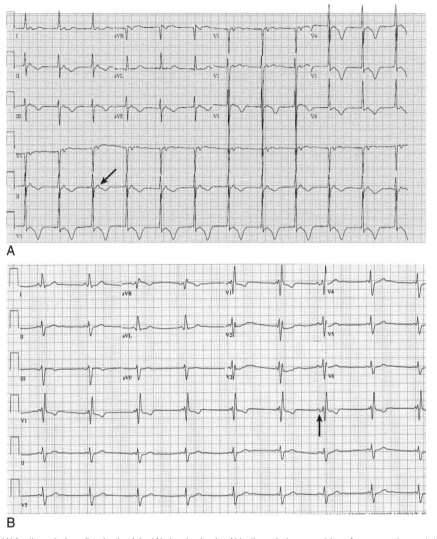

Fig. 3.35 Atrioventricular (AV) dissociation (isorhythmic). (A) Isorhythmic AV dissociation resulting from accelerated junctional rhythm without retrograde AV conduction. The P wave (*arrow*) is upright in leads 1 and 2, indicating sinus rhythm. P wave should be inverted in lead 2 if retrogradely captured during a junctional rhythm. (B) Isorhythmic AV dissociation resulting from sinus bradycardia accelerated junctional rhythm. The P wave is upright in leads 1 and 2, indicating sinus rhythm. Single sinus beat is conducted to the ventricle (*arrow*), resulting in a short RR interval.

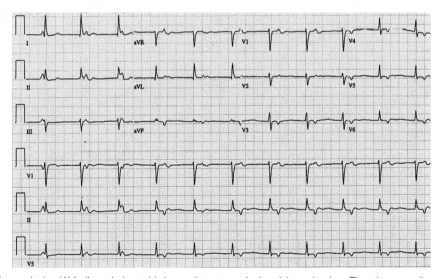

Fig. 3.36 Incomplete atrioventricular (AV) dissociation with intermittent ventriculoatrial conduction. The electrocardiogram demonstrates sinus P waves (first three beats) and AV dissociation resulting from a junctional tachycardia. Subsequently, the junctional tachycardia captures the atria retrogradely, with retrograde P waves, thereby ending the AV dissociation. Note that the sinus rhythm P waves are upright in lead 2. P waves become negative during retrograde ventriculoatrial conduction (fourth complex onward). The fifth P wave is an atrial fusion complex of the retrograde conduction from the junctional rhythm and an atrial premature complex.

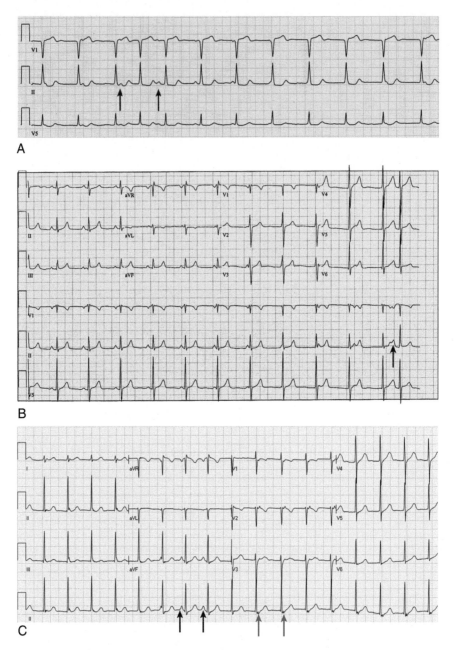

Fig. 3.37 Atrioventricular (AV) dissociation resulting from accelerated junctional rhythm. (A) Rhythm strip shows sinus rhythm with accelerated junctional rhythm resulting in AV dissociation. AV dissociation is intermittent because the third and fourth P waves (*black arrows*) conduct to the ventricle. (B) Electrocardiogram (ECG) shows sinus rhythm with accelerated junctional rhythm. One sinus beat in this ECG depicts ventricular capture (*black arrow*). (C) ECG reveals sinus rhythm with AV dissociation resulting from accelerated junctional rhythm. Two sinus beats show ventricular capture (*black arrows*). It is followed by AV dissociation with junctional rhythm and ventriculoatrial conduction (*red arrows*).

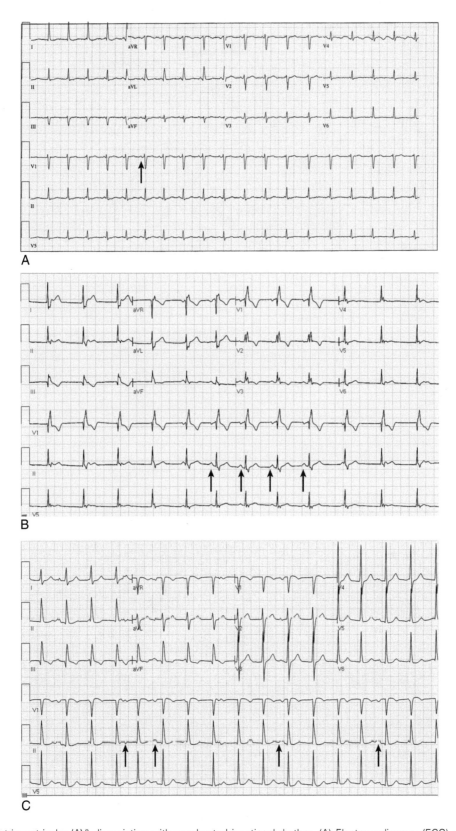

Fig. 3.38 Intermittent atrioventricular (AV) dissociation with accelerated junctional rhythm. (A) Electrocardiogram (ECG) shows sinus tachycardia along with junctional tachycardia with AV dissociation in the first four beats. After that (*arrow*), eight consecutive P waves are conducted. It is followed by sinus slowing and accelerated junctional rhythm with AV dissociation. (B) ECG demonstrated sinus rhythm with right bundle branch block and AV dissociation. Normal AV conduction resumed for four beats with P waves (*arrows*) conducted to the ventricle (sixth to ninth complexes) when the sinus rate is relatively faster than the junctional rhythm. (C) ECG demonstrates AV dissociation caused by accelerated junctional rhythm and intermittent sinus capture beats (*arrows*) during junctional tachycardia.

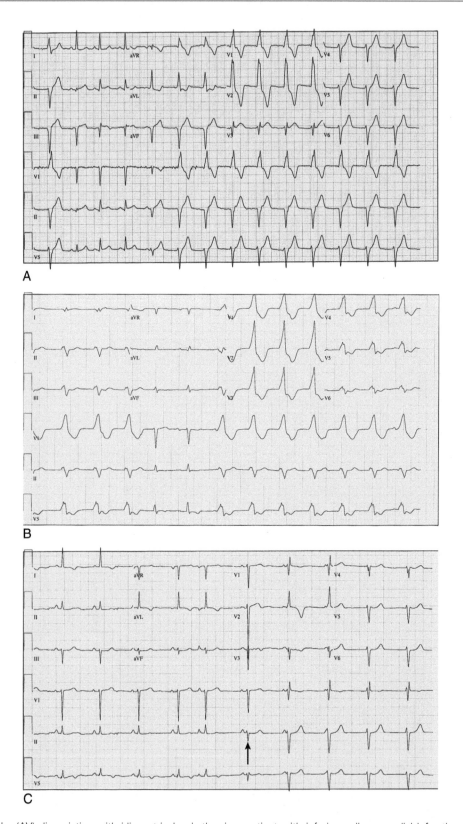

Fig. 3.39 Atrioventricular (AV) dissociation with idioventricular rhythm in a patient with inferior wall myocardial infarction. (A) Electrocardiogram (ECG) depicts single ventricular complex followed by sinus rhythm (first three beats) with 1:1 AV conduction and then sinus slowing, allowing the escape of an idioventricular rhythm and resulting in AV dissociation. (B) ECG demonstrates idioventricular rhythm with AV dissociation and two captured beats during sinus rhythm. (C) ECG shows sinus rhythm with normally conducted QRS complexes. The fifth P wave is an atrial premature complex. The QRS complex following the sixth P wave (sinus) is a fusion beat (*arrow*), which is followed by AV dissociation resulting from an idioventricular rhythm.

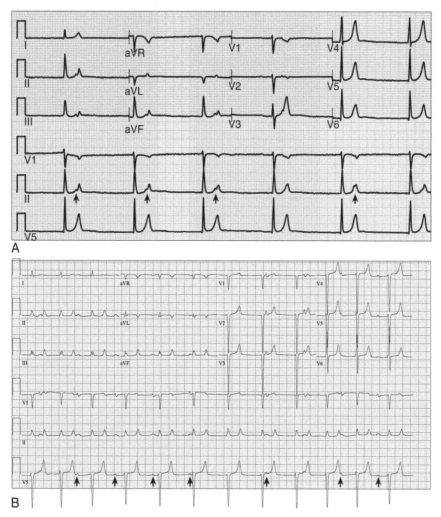

Fig. 3.40 (A) Atrioventricular dissociation resulting from a sinus bradycardia with junctional escape and peaked T waves in midprecordial leads in a patient with renal failure and hyperkalemia. P waves are shown by *arrows*. (B) Sinus rhythm with atrioventricular dissociation caused by a junctional tachycardia. Note the prominent and peaked T waves in leads V3-V5 and inferior leads associated with hyperkalemia.

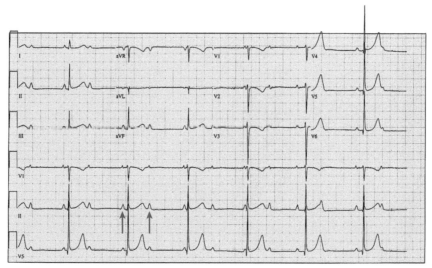

Fig. 3.41 Electrocardiogram shows sinus rhythm with complete atrioventricular block. The P-P interval containing QRS is shorter than the P-P interval without QRS in-between, which is consistent with ventriculophasic sinus arrhythmia. P waves are shown by *arrows*.

BIBLIOGRAPHY

Bonner AJ, Zipes DP. Lidocaine and His bundle extrasystoles. His bundle discharge conducted normally, conducted with functional right or left branch block, or blocked entirely [concealed]. *Arch Intern Med.* 1976;136:700–704.

Zipes DP, Libby P, Bonow RO, Mann DL, Tomaselli G. *Braunwald's Heart Disease: A Textbook of Cardiovascular Medicine.* 11th ed. Philadelphia, PA: WB Saunders; 2019.

4

Junctional Rhythm

JUNCTIONAL ESCAPE RHYTHM

The atrioventricular (AV) node is located at the right lower septum near the AV ring. The areas surrounding the AV node are called the *AV junction*. The inherent AV junctional rate in adults is between 40 and 60 bpm. Junctional rate greater than 60 is called *junctional tachycardia* (JT). The impulse from the AV junction travels anterogradely by way of the His bundle to the bundle branches and then to the Purkinje fibers to activate the ventricles. Therefore in the absence of bundle branch block (BBB), the QRS complex is narrow in a junctional rhythm (<120 ms) because the ventricle is excited normally by the His-Purkinje system. However, in the presence of BBB or intraventricular conduction delays, the QRS can be wide (>120 ms) (Figs. 4.1 through 4.3). Junctional rhythm with a wide QRS complex can mimic an idioventricular rhythm. A prior electrocardiogram may help establish the baseline QRS morphology and duration during sinus rhythm to show that it is similar to that of the junctional rhythm. An idioventricular rhythm generally can be differentiated from a junctional beat with BBB by QRS morphology. Usually, BBB QRS complexes have a typical RSR pattern with a rapid initial upstroke and are less than 140 ms in the presence of right BBB and less than 160 ms in the presence of left BBB.

The junctional impulse can also travel to the atrium if there is no ventriculoatrial conduction block. Retrogradely conducted P waves are negative in the inferior leads and are relatively narrower than the sinus P wave because of septal exit of the impulse from the AV node with rapid spread to both atria. (Depending on the rapidity of conduction from the junction to the atria, P waves during junctional rhythm can precede, be buried [hidden], or follow the QRS complexes [Fig. 4.4].) Junctional rhythm can occur in the setting of sinus or AV nodal dysfunction. In children it occurs more commonly in the presence of sinus node dysfunction after repair of transposition of the great vessels and in patients with congenital AV block.

Junctional rhythm can also cause AV dissociation (see Chapter 3) when the sinus rate is slower than the junctional rhythm. When the sinus rate and junction rates are the same or nearly the same, isorrhythmic AV dissociation may result (Figs. 4.5 through 4.10). Junctional beats can conduct retrogradely to the atria as 1:1, 2:1, or in Wenckebach pattern (Figs. 4.11 through 4.15). His bundle ectopy that fails to conduct to both the atria and ventricles, with retrograde concealment in the AV node, can manifest as first-degree or type 2 second-degree AV block (see Chapter 3, Fig. 3.12). Such a phenomenon may be difficult to differentiate from actual AV block without electrophysiology testing. Electrocardiogram clues to concealed junctional extrasystoles include (1) abrupt, unexplained prolongation of the P-R interval; (2) the presence of apparent Mobitz type 2 AV block in the presence of a normal QRS; (3) the presence of both type 1 and type 2 AV block in the same tracing; and (4) the presence of manifest junctional extrasystoles elsewhere in the tracing.

Myocardial ischemia, digitalis toxicity, and adrenergic drug infusion (e.g., isoproterenol) are also associated with fast junctional rhythms (Figs. 4.16 through 4.18). Septal ventricular tachycardia may have a QRS duration of less than 120 ms and mimic junctional rhythm. (Fig. 4.19).

JUNCTIONAL TACHYCARDIA

JT is also called junctional ectopic tachycardia, rapid automatic tachycardia, rapid JT, accelerated junctional rhythm, accelerated junctional ectopic tachycardia, and His bundle tachycardia (Figs. 4.20 and 4.21). JT is a narrow QRS complex tachycardia, usually with AV dissociation and slower atrial than ventricular rate. This tachycardia originates in or near the His bundle with normal QRS complexes at a rate exceeding 170 bpm (170–260 bpm).[1] JT usually occurs after surgery for congenital heart disease (incidence, 5.6%) in infants and children. Postoperative dopamine use and younger age are associated with JT.[2] Rarely, JT occurs in adults after cardiac surgery or in patients with normal hearts. It can also present with 1:1 retrograde ventriculoatrial conduction.

Junctional rhythm can cause an AV nodal echo beat in patients with dual AV nodal pathway (Fig. 4.22). Junctional rhythm or fast junctional rhythm is noted during slow pathway modification for AV nodal reentrant tachycardia using radiofrequency energy (Figs. 4.23 through 4.26). Application of radiofrequency energy in the fast AV nodal pathway region results in fast JT, usually greater than 120 bpm, which may result in fast pathway ablation or AV node block. Cryoablation of slow AV nodal pathway for AV nodal reentrant tachycardia does not result in junctional rhythm. JT should be considered when there is a long R-P with a very short P-R interval or short R-P tachycardia.

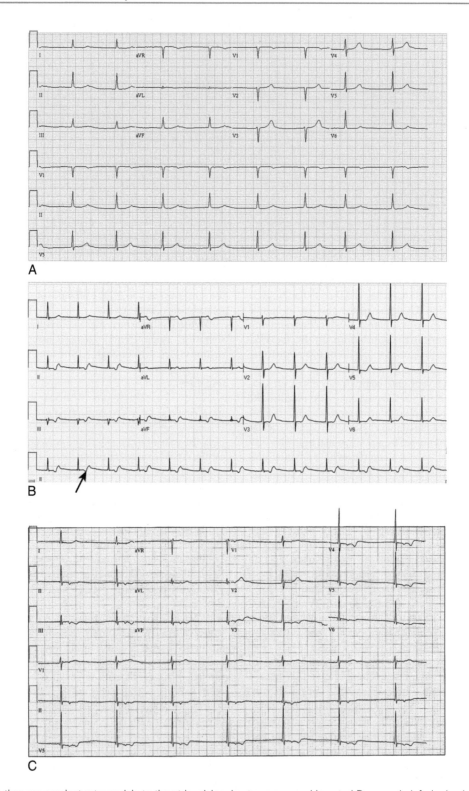

A

B

C

Fig. 4.1 Junctional rhythm can conduct retrogradely to the atria, giving rise to narrow and inverted P waves in inferior leads. (A) Junctional rhythm at 51 bpm without ventriculoatrial (VA) conduction. Note that narrow retrograde P waves may not be visible on a 12-lead electrocardiogram when it is superimposed on the QRS complex. (B) Junctional rhythm with a VA interval of 120 ms. *Arrow* points to retrograde P wave. (C) Junctional rhythm with a prolonged VA time of 200 ms. (D) Junctional rhythm with intraventricular conduction delay. *Arrow* points to retrograde P wave. (E) Junctional rhythm with right bundle branch block pattern of QRS. The patient has right bundle branch block during sinus rhythm. *Arrow* points to retrograde P wave. (F) Junctional rhythm with left bundle branch block pattern mimicking an idioventricular rhythm. The patient has left bundle branch block during sinus rhythm.

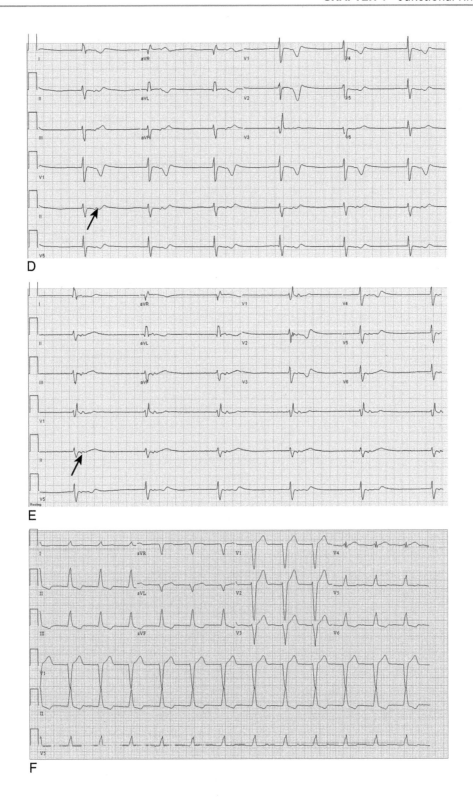

Fig. 4.1 (Continued).

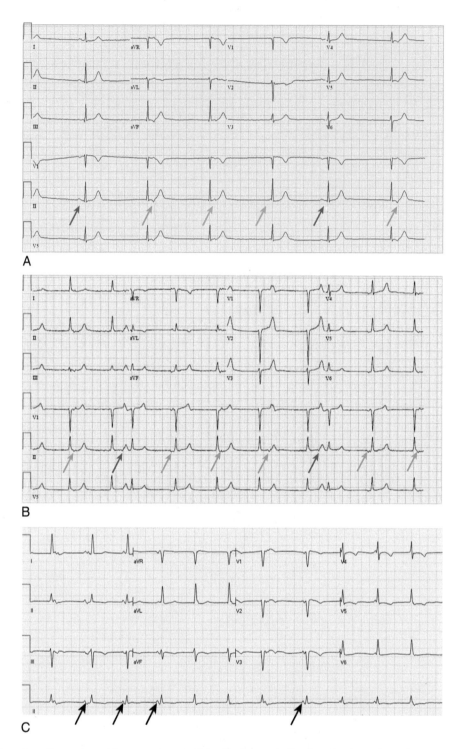

Fig. 4.2 (A) Sinus bradycardia with conducted beats to the ventricles (*red arrows*). The junctional rate is similar to the sinus rate and conducts retrogradely (*blue arrows*) to the atria. In two beats, the junctional impulse could not conduct retrogradely due to simultaneous sinus-initiated atrial complexes (*green arrows*). (B) Sinus bradycardia and junctional rhythm without ventriculoatrial conduction. Two sinus-initiated impulses capture the ventricles (*red arrows*) and a few junctional beats with retrograde conduction with inverted P waves in inferior leads (*blue arrows*). (C) Sinus arrhythmia associated with accelerated junctional rhythm sinus-initiated impulses capture the ventricles during faster rates (during inspiration). *Arrows* point to sinus P wave.

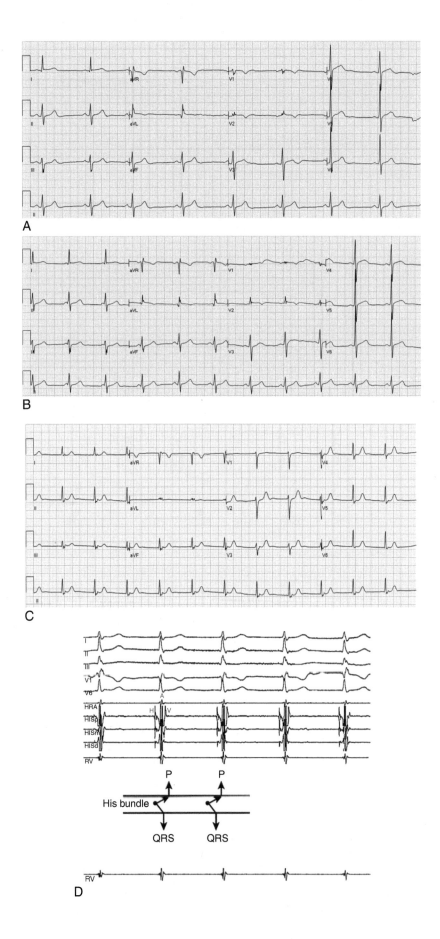

Fig. 4.3 (A) Sinus rhythm with a normal P-R interval. (B) Isorhythmic atrioventricular dissociation occurs during junctional tachycardia at 70 bpm in the first four beats in the patient in panel (A). (C) Electrocardiogram shows junctional rhythm of a patient who underwent electrophysiology study. (D) The intracardiac recording shows His bundle recording (*H*), which results in ventricular (*V*) activation, and retrograde atrial activation (*A*). HRA, high right atrium; RV, right ventricle.

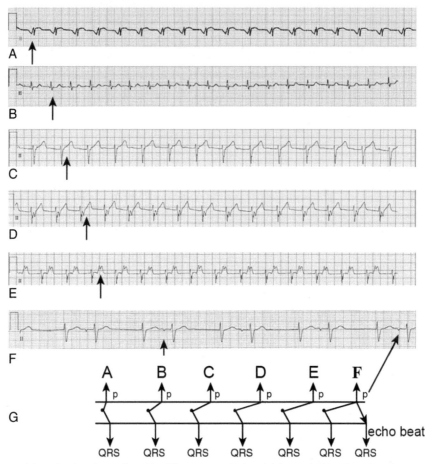

Fig. 4.4 Junctional rhythm and junctional tachycardia with different ventriculoatrial intervals (A–E) and during an echo beat (F). (A) P wave precedes the QRS because of relatively rapid conduction of the junctional impulse retrogradely to the atria compared with the anterograde conduction to the ventricle. (B) Because P wave and QRS complexes occur simultaneously, the P wave is not visible on the surface electrocardiogram. (C–E) During junctional rhythm, QRS complexes precede the P waves because of a relatively longer conduction time from the junction to the atria compared with the time taken for the impulse that travels from the junction to the ventricle. The QRS-P interval is longer in (D) than in (C), and longer in (E) than in (D). P waves occur on T waves. (F) The junctional beat is associated with a long R-P interval because the impulse travels to the atria by way of the slow atrioventricular (AV) nodal pathway. The same impulse then travels down to the ventricle by way of the fast AV nodal pathway (retrograde echo beat). This suggests dual AV nodal pathways. The ladder diagram (G) represents relative position of retrograde P waves during a junctional rhythm from strips A to F.

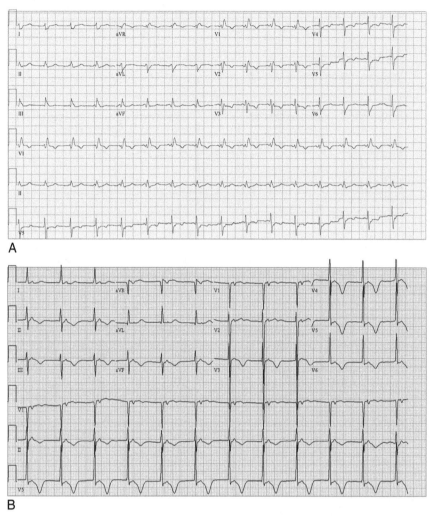

Fig. 4.5 (A) Sinus rate is similar to the junctional rate with P waves preceding QRS complexes in the latter half of the rhythm strip (lead II). It is isorhythmic atrioventricular dissociation because the P-R interval is shorter than the baseline P-R interval, and therefore cannot be conducting to the ventricles. (B) Junctional tachycardia with QRS preceding the P waves. P waves originate from the sinus node because they are upright in the inferior leads and lead I, and therefore these cannot be retrogradely conducted from the junctional focus.

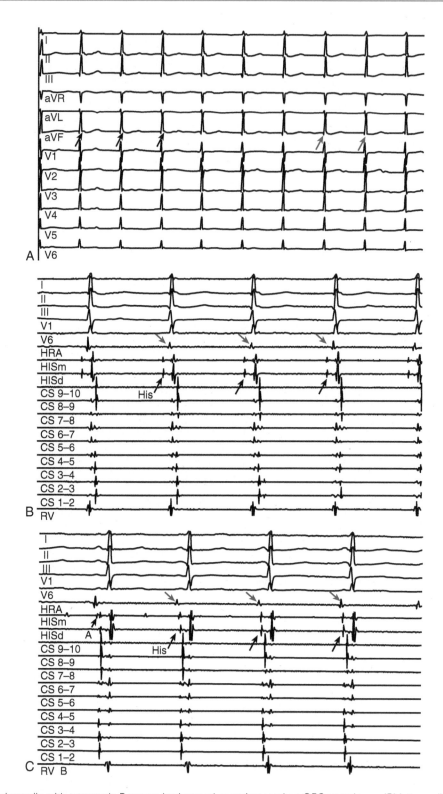

Fig. 4.6 (A) Junctional tachycardia with retrograde P waves (*red arrows*) superimposed on QRS complexes. (B) Intracardiac recordings confirm that the rhythm is a junctional tachycardia with isorhythmic atrioventricular dissociation. Retrograde P waves (*red arrows*) are not visualized distinctly because they occur during the QRS complex. *Black arrows* show intracardiac His bundle recording. (C) Intracardiac recordings show P waves (*red arrows*) preceding the QRS. However, a short and varying A-H interval (normal A-H interval, 60–120 ms) confirms that it is an accelerated junctional rhythm with isorhythmic atrioventricular dissociation. *Black arrows* show intracardiac His bundle recording.

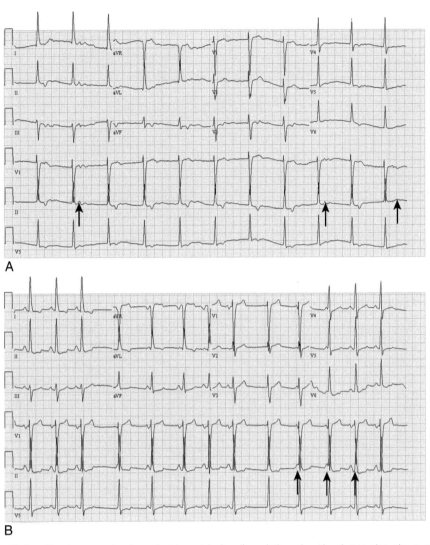

Fig. 4.7 Sinus arrhythmia with junctional escape beats and atrioventricular dissociation. Junctional rate also slows and then increases (*arrows* show sinus P waves) along with the sinus rate (A). Sinus bradycardia in the same patient is associated with junctional rhythm with retrograde atrial capture. *Arrows* show sinus P waves (B).

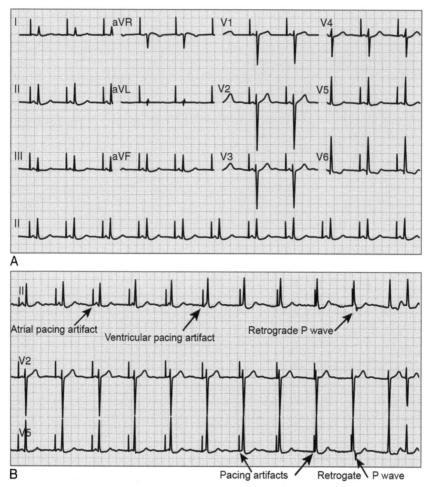

Fig. 4.8 Junctional tachycardia in a patient with atrial pacing. (A) Atrial paced rhythm with intact atrioventricular conduction. (B) Atrial paced rhythm (*arrow*) with progressive shortening of P to QRS interval followed by an atrial paced event on the QRS (*arrow*) with retrograde P wave (*arrow*), another junctional beat, and an atrial premature complex or an echo beat.

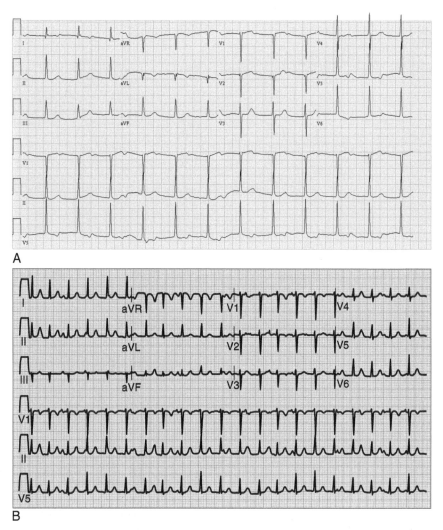

Fig. 4.9 (A) Sinus rhythm with atrioventricular dissociation and junctional escape rate of 72 bpm. (B) Sinus tachycardia at 105 bpm and junctional tachycardia at 120 bpm with atrioventricular dissociation.

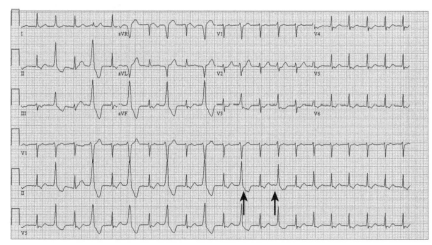

Fig. 4.10 Junctional tachycardia with premature ventricular complexes with varying QRS interval (narrow to wide) depending on the degree of fusion.

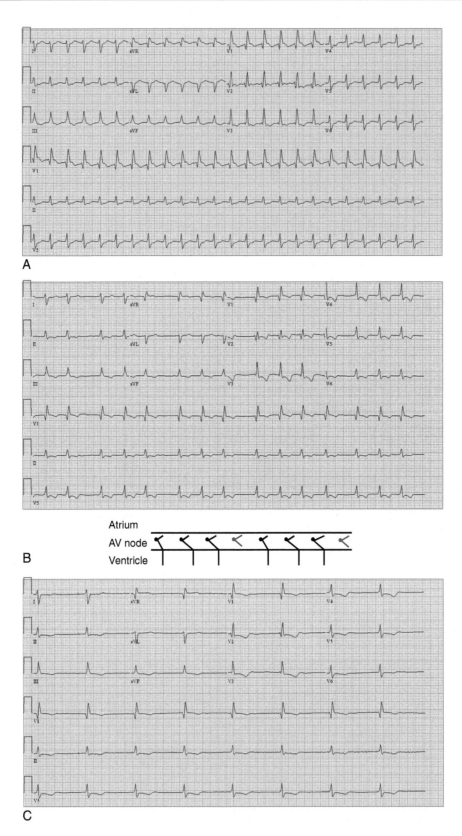

Fig. 4.11 (A) Electrocardiogram of a female patient with atrial fibrillation with junctional tachycardia at 148 bpm causing atrioventricular dissociation. (B) The rhythm later changed to junctional tachycardia with 4:3 to 5:4 Wenckebach pattern of ventricular-to-atrial conduction. (C) The junctional rate was later controlled with amiodarone therapy.

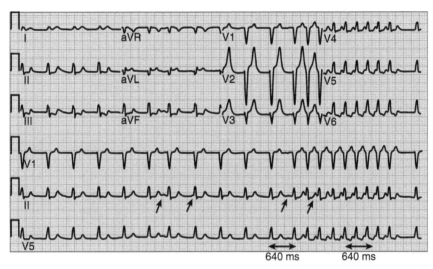

Fig. 4.12 Junctional tachycardia (JT) with 2:1 ventricular conduction in a patient who underwent Ross procedure for severe aortic stenosis. Rhythm strip shows JT with cycle length (CL) of 640 ms followed by a 9-beat run of JT at the CL of 320 ms. This suggests 2:1 conduction (CL, 640 ms) followed by 1:1 conduction to the ventricle. The last conducted ventricular beats are the result of 2:1 conduction from the junction to the ventricle. There are a few premature atrial complexes (*arrows*), which conducted to the ventricle, causing the R-R interval to shorten. Horizontal arrows show cycle length of junctional rhythm.

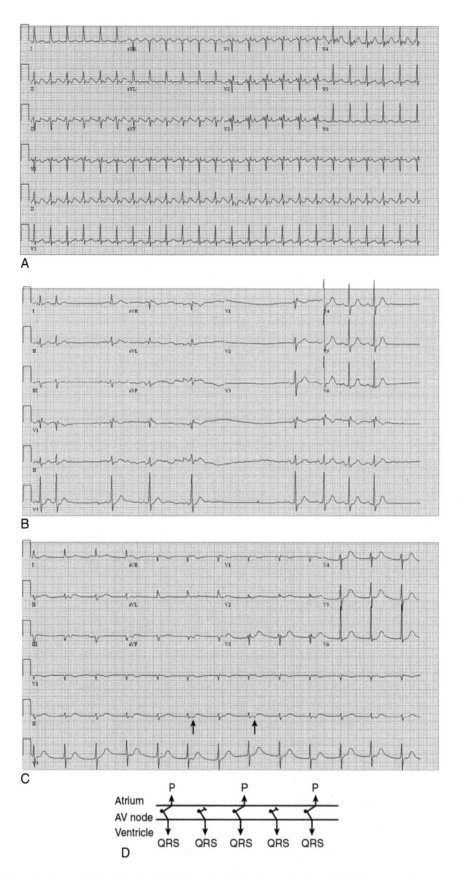

Fig. 4.13 (A) Electrocardiogram shows atrial flutter with 2:1 atrioventricular block. (B) The arrhythmia converted spontaneously to sinus rhythm, with multiple sinus pauses, during diltiazem infusion. (C) The rhythm later changed to junctional rhythm with 2:1 junctional conduction to the atria (*arrows* show retrograde P waves), shown in the ladder diagram (D).

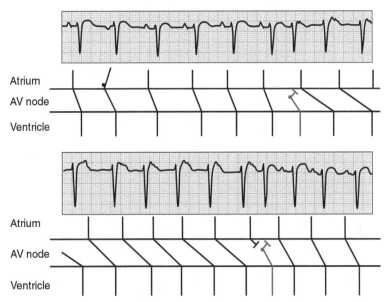

Fig. 4.14 Rhythm strip shows sinus rhythm, a single late atrial premature complex (second atrial complex), and a junctional beat that conducts retrogradely by way of the fast atrioventricular (AV) nodal pathway but fails to reach the atria (*red lines*). The sinus conduction then continues down the slow AV nodal pathway because the fast pathway is now refractory (long P-R compared with the baseline P-R interval) for a few beats. A second junctional beat (*red lines*) concealed in the slow AV nodal pathway allowed time for the fast pathway to recover, and the sinus rhythm following the junctional beat conducts with a normal P-R interval by way of the fast AV nodal pathway. The rhythm strip provides explanation of the dual AV nodal pathways.

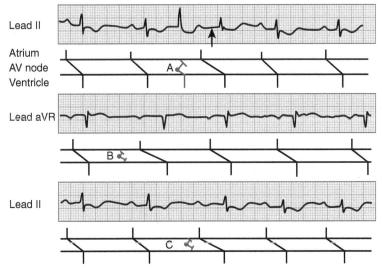

Fig. 4.15 The rhythm strip shows sinus rhythm with three junctional impulses marked in *red* in the ladder diagram. The first junctional impulse conducts to the ventricles with slight aberrancy and conceals retrogradely into the atrioventricular node, causing a delay in conduction of the next sinus impulse, as shown by a long P-R interval (*arrow* shows lack of sinus P wave generation). The next two junctional impulses (*red*) do not conduct to the ventricles or back to the atria but cause concealment in the atrioventricular node, resulting in P-R prolongation in the following beats (see also Fig. 1.43).

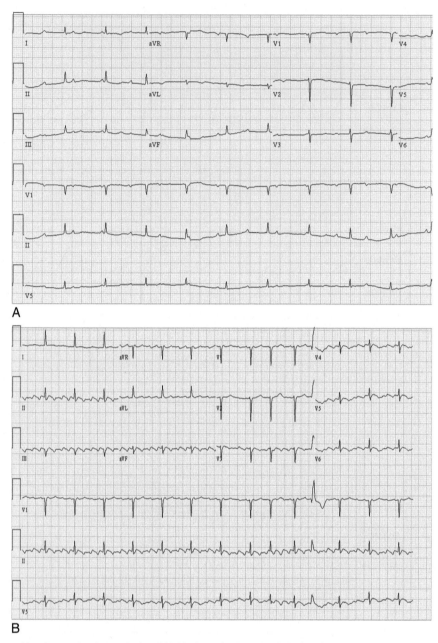

Fig. 4.16 (A) Sinus rhythm with advanced atrioventricular (AV) block and a junctional rhythm at 72 bpm after aortic valve surgery. In general, to make a diagnosis of acquired complete AV block, the ventricular escape rate should be slower than 72 bpm, or approximately 40 bpm, to ensure that the AV node—His bundle has sufficient time to conduct an impulse if it is going to conduct. There could have been some conduction if the ventricular rate in this electrocardiogram had been slower. (B) Consistent with this reasoning, the AV conduction later improved, and the patient developed typical atrial flutter with variable AV block.

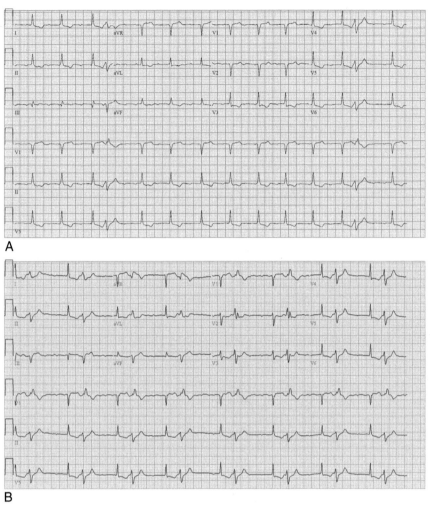

Fig. 4.17 (A) Atrial tachycardia (cycle length, 260 ms) with atrioventricular block (cycle length, 720 ms) and two premature ventricular complexes. (B) Electrocardiogram of the same patient showing atrial tachycardia, atrioventricular block, and ventricular bigeminy caused by digoxin toxicity.

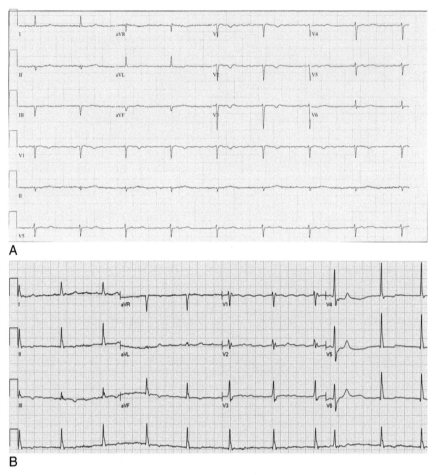

Fig. 4.18 Atrial fibrillation (A) and flutter (B) with complete atrioventricular block and a junctional escape rhythm.

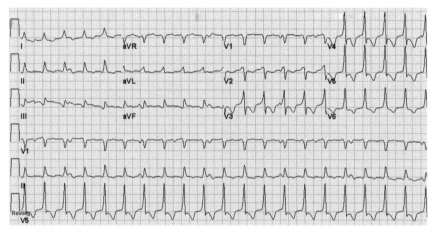

Fig. 4.19 Electrocardiogram depicting a relatively narrow QRS complex and atrioventricular dissociation due to a ventricular tachycardia that was mapped to originate from the midseptum of the left ventricle during an electrophysiologic study. The QRS is relatively narrow because of its septal origin with almost simultaneous activation of both ventricles.

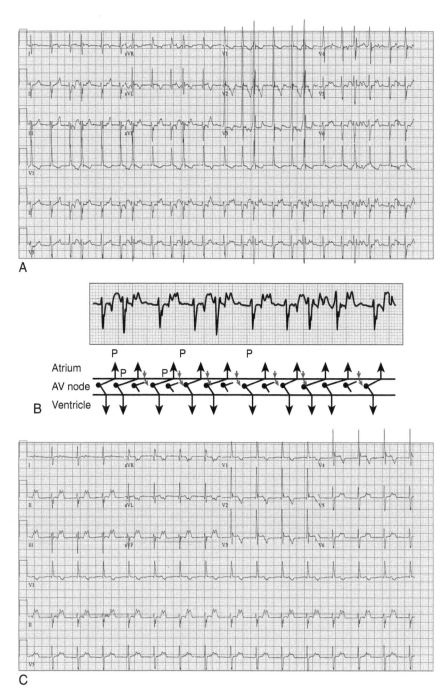

Fig. 4.20 Junctional tachycardia (JT) with serial electrocardiograms of a child with a complex congenital heart disease, including isolated levocardia situs ambiguous, left-sided inferior vena cava, bilateral superior vena cava into a common atrium, asymmetric atrioventricular (AV) canal, double-outlet right ventricle and pulmonary stenosis, and status post bidirectional Glenn procedure. (A) Atrial tachycardia (AT) at 150 bpm and JT at 205 bpm. Rhythm strip in lead II shows the AT with varying ventriculoatrial conduction times resulting from retrograde block or delay of junctional impulse because atrial impulses from the AT conceal in the AV node (but do not conduct to the ventricles). There is a variable block of the conduction from the JT to the ventricles. The QRS before pauses shows right bundle branch block aberrancy. (B) Ladder diagram of the most likely conduction pattern during simultaneous JT and AT. The *red arrows* depict sinus impulse that is blocked in AV node by junctional impulse. (C–E) The AT slowed spontaneously with the gradual improvement in retrograde conduction time to the atria, as shown by progressive decrease in QRS-P interval with slowing of the junctional rate. The AT subsided with diltiazem therapy.

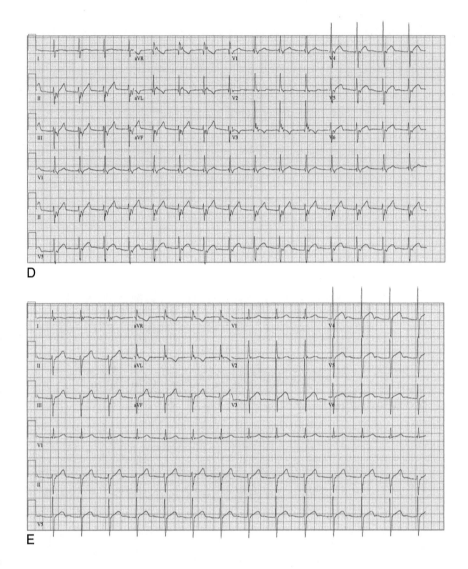

D

E

Fig. 4.20 (Continued).

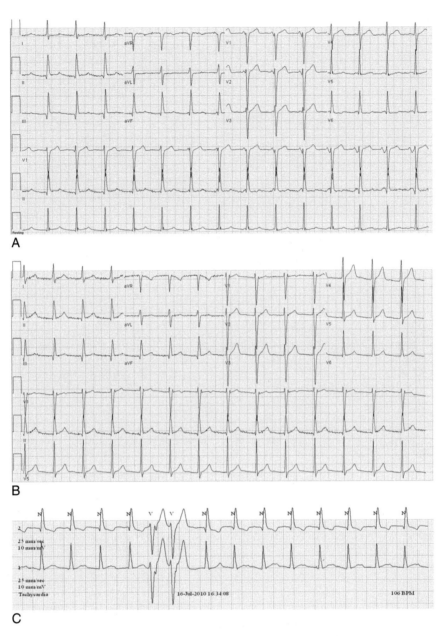

Fig. 4.21 Paroxysmal junctional tachycardia (JT) observed in a patient after aortic valve surgery. The junctional rate increases to 120 bpm. (A) JT with atrioventricular dissociation because the sinus rate is slightly lower than the junctional rate. (B) JT at 82 bpm. (C) JT at 106 bpm and two premature ventricular contractions during a Holter recording. The second premature ventricular complex resets the JT by retrograde conduction to the His bundle.

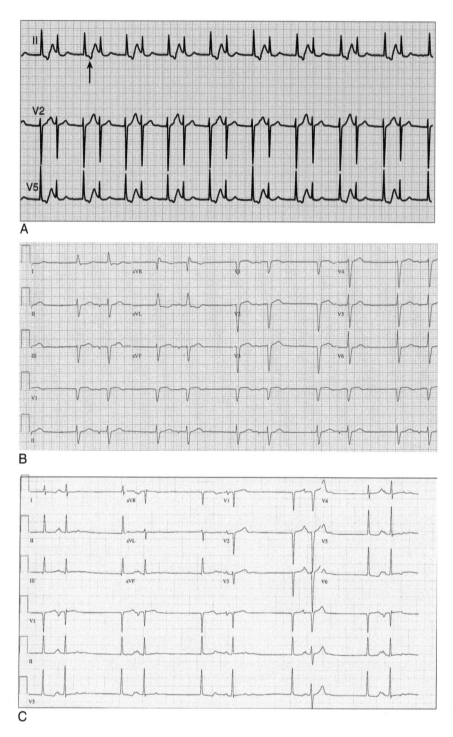

Fig. 4.22 (A) Retrograde echo beats versus atrial bigeminy. Electrocardiogram (ECG) shows a junctional rhythm with retrograde atrial echo (*arrow*) via the fast atrioventricular (AV) nodal pathway (short R-P interval with inverted P waves in the inferior leads), which conducts to the ventricle via a slow AV nodal pathway (long R-P interval). This is evidence for a dual AV nodal pathway. Because the retrograde fast pathway is refractory and cannot conduct to the atrium again, an AV nodal reentrant tachycardia does not begin. (B) ECG depicts a junctional rhythm with retrograde atrial echoes via the slow AV nodal pathway (long R-P interval with inverted P waves in inferior leads), which conduct to the ventricle via the fast AV nodal pathway (long R-P interval). This is evidence for a dual AV nodal pathway. Because the retrograde slow pathway is refractory and cannot conduct to the atria, an AV nodal reentrant tachycardia does not begin. (C) ECG shows junctional rhythm with atrial bigeminy with upright P waves in lead II, unlike an echo beat, which should generate negative P waves in the inferior leads.

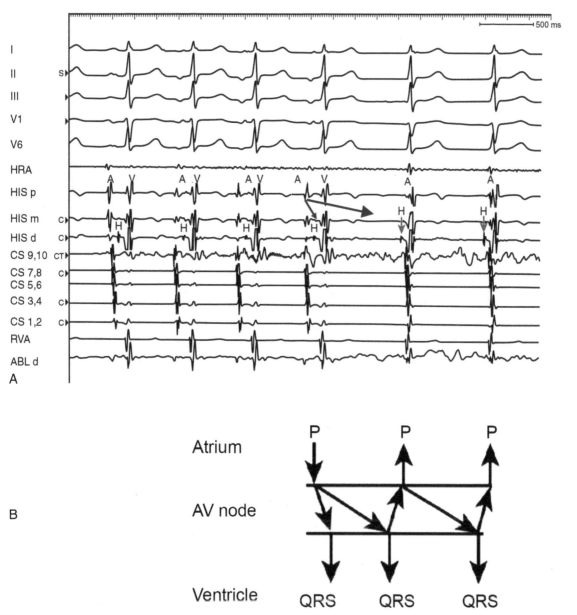

Fig. 4.23 (A) The first atrial beat conducts down the fast pathway and also down the slow pathway, resulting in 1:2 atrioventricular (AV) conduction (1:2 AV response) and initiation of atypical AV nodal reentrant tachycardia. The AV nodal reentrant tachycardia terminates after three beats. It is followed by two junctional beats, shown by *red arrows*. (B) Atrial beat conducts down the fast pathway, followed by slow pathway conduction resulting in 1:2 AV conduction (1:2 response) confirmed with other electrophysiologic maneuvers during the electrophysiology study. (C) During modification of slow pathway by radiofrequency catheter ablation, a junctional rhythm is seen, which occurs in most cases at the site of successful catheter ablation. Atrial pacing is usually initiated to confirm the intactness of AV conduction during ablation because slow pathway modification can rarely result in complete AV block. *A*, atrial; *H*, His bundle; *V*, ventricle.

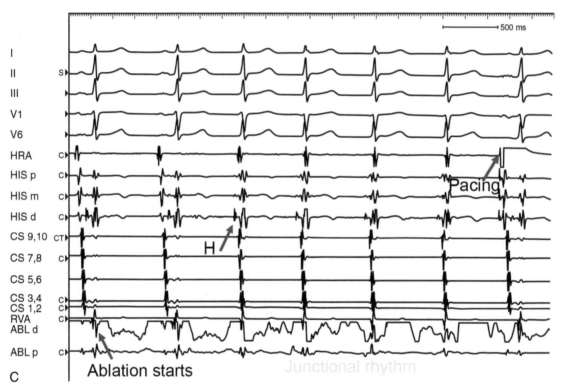

Fig. 4.23 (Continued).

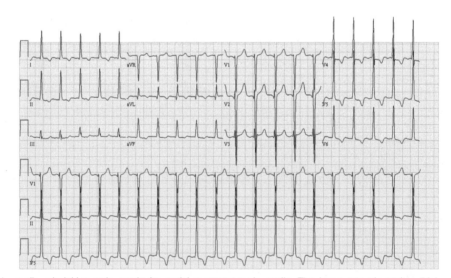

Fig. 4.24 Junctional tachycardia mimicking atrioventricular nodal reentrant tachycardia. The heart rate slowed to 80 bpm with a calcium channel blocker, which proved that this was a junctional tachycardia because atrioventricular nodal reentrant tachycardia slows down after a few beats and usually terminates with the use of a calcium channel blocker.

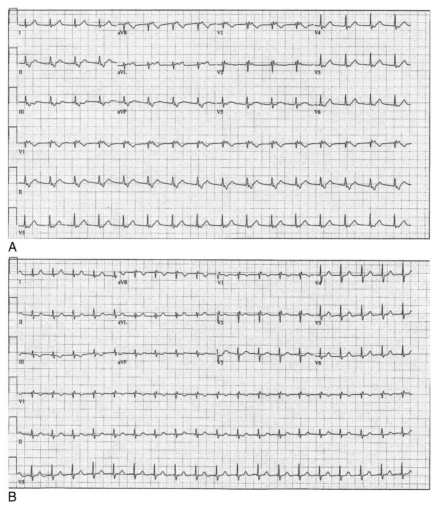

Fig. 4.25 (A) Electrocardiogram shows a short R-P′ tachycardia and suggests an atrioventricular nodal reentrant tachycardia (AVNRT), atrioventricular reentrant tachycardia (AVRT), or junctional tachycardia with retrograde atrial conduction. The rate is 102 bpm, which is unusual for an AVRT and rare for an AVNRT. (B) The rate of the tachycardia later increased to 115 bpm with no discernible P waves on the electrocardiogram. This change is not consistent with an AVNRT because the R-P′ interval (conduction via the fast atrioventricular nodal pathway) usually does not change in an AVNRT. This is most likely a junctional tachycardia with retrograde block to the atrium at the faster rate.

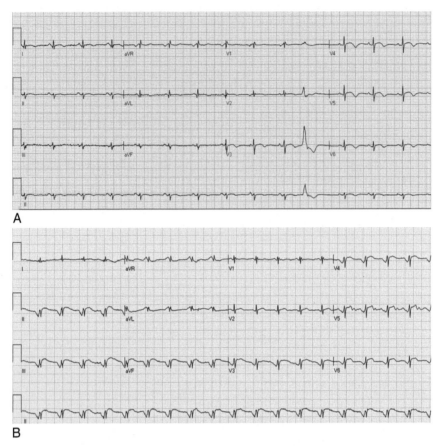

A

B

Fig. 4.26 Long R-P tachycardia. (A) Baseline electrocardiogram showing sinus rhythm with a normal P-R interval. (B) A long R-P′ tachycardia with inverted P waves in inferior leads. The differential diagnosis of the rhythm is atrial tachycardia (see Chapter 7), atypical atrioventricular nodal reentrant tachycardia (AVNRT) (see Chapter 5), persistent form of junctional reciprocating tachycardia (PJRT) (see Chapter 6), and junctional tachycardia with retrograde atrial conduction over a slow pathway. The short P-R interval (100 ms) rules out an atrial tachycardia. The tachycardia did not terminate with intravenous adenosine, making an AVNRT or a PJRT unlikely. The rhythm is most likely a junctional tachycardia.

REFERENCES

1. Haas NA, Plumpton K, Justo R, Jalali H, Pohlner P. Postoperative junctional ectopic tachycardia (JET). *Zeitschrift fur Kardiologie.* 2004;93:371–380.

2. Hoffman TM, Bush DM, Wernovsky G, et al. Postoperative junctional ectopic tachycardia in children: incidence, risk factors, and treatment. *Ann Thorac Surg.* 2002;74(5):1607–1611.

Atrioventricular Nodal Reentrant Tachycardia

SUPRAVENTRICULAR TACHYCARDIA

Supraventricular tachycardia (SVT) is broadly defined as a narrow QRS complex (generally, unless aberrant conduction of the QRS complex occurs) tachycardia that requires atrial tissue or the atrioventricular (AV) node as an integral part of the arrhythmia substrate. SVT is classified as short RP' or long RP' tachycardia according to the timing of the P wave in relation to the R-R cycle (note that the letter R is used to indicate the QRS complex). During tachycardia, if the interval from the R wave to the next P wave exceeds the interval from that same P wave to the next R wave, the SVT is termed *long R-P' tachycardia* (Box 5.1). If the interval from the R wave to the next P wave is shorter than the interval from that same P wave to the next R wave, the SVT is called *short R-P' tachycardia*. The classification is just a broad guideline. Approximately 90% of AV nodal reentrant tachycardia (AVNRT) cases and 87% of AV reentrant tachycardia (AVRT) cases are short R-P' tachycardias.[1] Only 11% of atrial tachycardias present as a short R-P' tachycardia.

ATRIOVENTRICULAR NODAL REENTRANT TACHYCARDIA

AVNRT is the most common form of paroxysmal SVT. AVNRT is two to three times more common in women than in men. It occurs more commonly in young adults (25–35 years of age) but can occur at any age. The exact anatomy and physiology of the AV node and its extension are incompletely defined. The circuit of the tachycardia mainly involves the AV node, all or a component of adjacent atrial myocardium, and at least two atrionodal connections or inputs (dual AV nodal physiology). The superior (anterior) input has a longer refractory period and faster conduction (fast pathway) than the inferior (posterior) input, which has a shorter refractory period but slower conduction (slow pathway). During sinus rhythm in people with dual AV nodal physiology, conduction to the ventricle occurs by way of the fast pathway, AV node, and His-Purkinje system. The conduction down the slow pathway fails to reach the His bundle because it finds the AV node refractory insofar as the impulse via the fast pathway has just conducted down to the His bundle (Fig. 5.1). The common type of AVNRT (slow-fast) involves anterograde conduction down the slow AV nodal pathway and retrogradely by way of the fast AV nodal pathway. Typically, a premature atrial complex (PAC) initiates AVNRT by blocking anterogradely in the fast pathway, conducting down the slow pathway to the His bundle, and retrogradely to the atria (retrograde P wave) by way of the fast pathway that has now recovered excitability. This retrograde P wave is called the *echo beat*. If the impulse that reaches the atrium by way of the fast pathway can conduct down the slow pathway again, the AVNRT circuit is complete and the tachycardia continues until a PAC or premature ventricular complex (PVC)

enters the circuit to block conduction (Figs. 5.2 through 5.4). Alternatively, a change in autonomic tone can alter conduction or refractoriness of one of the pathways (usually the slow pathway) to terminate the tachycardia. The less common fast-slow type of AVNRT involves conduction anterogradely down the fast pathway and retrogradely up the slow pathway. A slow-slow or slow-intermediate form of AVNRT with the retrograde P wave occurring midcycle probably involves reentry by way of the slow and an intermediate pathway. In none of the forms of AVNRT does the circuit involve the ventricular myocardium. Single echo anterograde or retrograde beats without initiation of AVNRT is typically seen after a PAC or PVC (Fig. 5.5).

ELECTROPHYSIOLOGIC CHARACTERISTICS OF ATRIOVENTRICULAR NODAL REENTRANT TACHYCARDIA

1. Rate: The tachycardia rate can vary between 100 and 280 bpm but is generally 200 to 250 bpm, commonly at the faster rates in young and at the slower rates in older persons. The tachycardia rate is not diagnostic of AVNRT because an AVRT or atrial tachycardia also can have similar heart rates.
2. Relative position of the P wave within the R-R interval (Fig. 5.6):
   a. Typical AVNRT: During typical AVNRT, because the impulse conducts in parallel via the fast pathway retrogradely to the atrium and via the His bundle anterogradely to the ventricles, there is almost simultaneous activation of the atrium (retrograde P wave) and the ventricles (QRS). The timing of the initiation of the P wave in relation to the QRS wave depends on the rapidity of conduction to the atrium via the fast pathway and also the conduction down the His-Purkinje system (which is usually unchanged at rapid rates if there is no conduction system disease). Therefore the P wave (1) can be negative (mimicking a Q wave), (2) can be buried in the QRS wave (inapparent), or, more commonly, (3) can manifest at the end or just after the S wave (mimicking an additional R' in lead V1 and additional S wave in inferior leads). The R-P interval usually varies between −40 and 70 ms. In elderly subjects the R-P interval can be greater than 70 ms owing to the age-related slowed conduction in the fast pathway (Figs. 5.7 through 5.9).
   b. Atypical AVNRT: During an atypical AVNRT, anterograde conduction via the fast pathway rapidly reaches the ventricle, but the conduction takes longer retrogradely to reach the atrium by way of the slow pathway, so it becomes a long R-P' tachycardia (Fig. 5.9).

BOX 5.1 Short R-P versus long R-P tachycardia

SHORT R-P TACHYCARDIA	LONG R-P TACHYCARDIA
Atrioventricular nodal reentrant tachycardia	Sinus tachycardia
Atrioventricular reentrant tachycardia	Atrial tachycardia
Junctional tachycardia with retrograde atrial capture	Atypical (fast-slow) atrioventricular nodal reentrant tachycardia
Atrial tachycardia with a long P-R interval	Permanent junctional reciprocating tachycardia

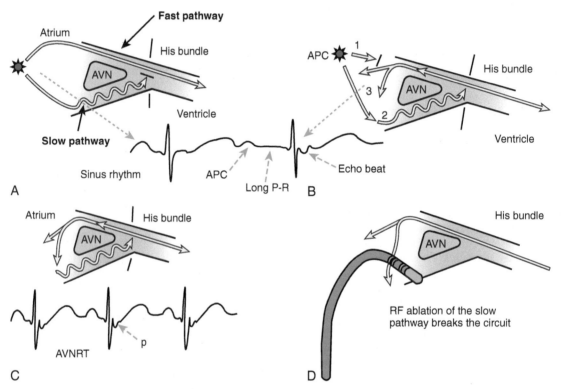

Fig. 5.1 Dual atrioventricular (AV) nodal physiology and mechanism of AV nodal reentrant tachycardia (AVNRT). (A) Conduction from the sinus node reaches both fast and slow AV nodal pathway inputs. However, as a result of the faster conduction property of the fast pathway, the conduction reaches the His bundle and then the ventricle via the fast pathway. Conduction down the slow pathway is blocked in the AV node (AVN) as a result of the refractoriness of the tissue because the fast pathway conduction has just occurred. (B) Premature atrial premature complex (APC) following the sinus beat finds the fast pathway refractory (*1*), but the slow pathway is able to conduct the impulse (*2*) via the His bundle to the ventricles and almost simultaneously (retrogradely) to the atrium via the fast pathway. The subsequent atrial depolarization (*3*) manifests as negative P wave (the echo beat) in inferior leads. (C) Retrograde conduction via the fast pathway may conduct down the slow pathway again if the slow pathway is not refractory and the AVNRT ensues. (D) Catheter modification of slow pathway region, which is typically at the lower tricuspid annular region anterior to the coronary sinus, usually abolishes the tachycardia circuit. In 7% of cases, the slow pathway has left posterior extension in the coronary sinus and may require ablation at the mitral annulus. *RF*, radiofrequency.

c. Slow-slow or slow-intermediate AVNRT: Rarely, dual AV nodal physiology can result from conduction over two slow pathways or a slow pathway with an intermediate pathway and one fast pathway (Fig. 5.10). P wave timing in relation to the R wave can vary accordingly. In slow-slow AVNRT, the R-P interval is usually shorter than, and sometimes equal to, the P-R interval. Occasionally, the P wave is inscribed in the middle of the R-R cycle, mimicking atrial flutter if the tachycardia rate is 150 bpm, or a slowly conducting posteroseptal accessory pathway (AP), such as in a permanent junctional reciprocating tachycardia (PJRT) (Fig. 5.11). Because both PJRT and AVNRT have the earliest atrial activation in the posteroseptal region, conduction time from that site to the upper septum (near the His bundle) is significantly longer in AVNRT than PJRT, resulting in a significantly longer R-P interval in V1 and a significantly greater difference in the R-P interval between V1 and inferior leads during AVNRT. Therefore finding a ΔR-P interval (lead V1 to lead III) greater than 20 ms suggests slow-slow AVNRT (sensitivity: 71%, specificity: 87%).

3. Mode of onset, variation in the heart rate, and mode of termination of the SVT: AVNRT commonly starts after a PAC that conducts to the ventricle with a very long P-R interval (via the slow pathway because the fast pathway is refractory) (Fig. 5.12). Similarly, a single PVC can also initiate the AVNRT by retrogradely conducting into the fast pathway but blocking before it reaches the atrium (concealed conduction; Chapter 1)

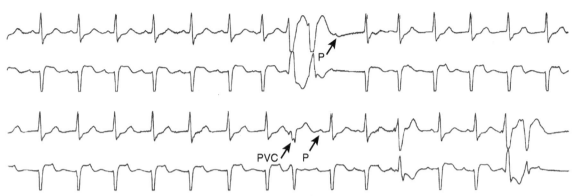

Fig. 5.2 Dual atrioventricular nodal physiology. Rhythm strips (top two leads recorded simultaneously, continuous tracing with bottom two leads) shows sinus rhythm with normal P-R interval. After a ventricular couplet, P-R interval prolongs as a result of retrograde concealment in the fast pathway with block of anterograde conduction and partial concealment in the slow pathway, which conducts with a prolonged P-R interval (*first arrow*). The slow pathway conduction continues until a premature ventricular complex (PVC) (*second arrow*) conducts retrogradely, resulting in concealment and block in the slow pathway, and allows the fast pathway to resume anterograde conduction with normal P-R interval.

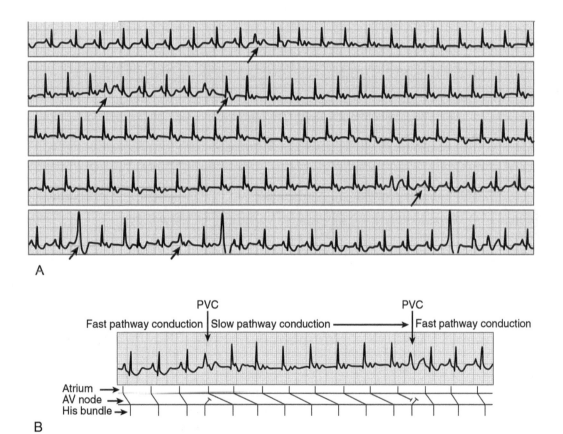

Fig. 5.3 Dual atrioventricular (AV) nodal physiology. (A) Sinus rhythm with normal P-R interval. After a premature ventricular complex (PVC) (*arrow*), P-R interval prolongs as a result of retrograde concealment in the fast pathway with block of anterograde conduction and partial concealment in the slow pathway, which conducts with a prolonged P-R interval. The slow pathway conduction continues until a PVC (*second arrow*) conducts retrogradely, resulting in concealment and block in the slow pathway, which allows the fast pathway to resume anterograde conduction with a normal P-R interval. This phenomenon occurs several times after a PVC. (B) The impulse from the first PVC conceals into the fast atrioventricular nodal pathway retrogradely; therefore the next sinus impulse conducts via the slow pathway with a prolonged P-R interval. The slow pathway conduction continues in subsequent beats until the second PVC conceals conduction in the slow pathway retrogradely. It results in the resumption of anterograde fast pathway conduction with normal P-R interval.

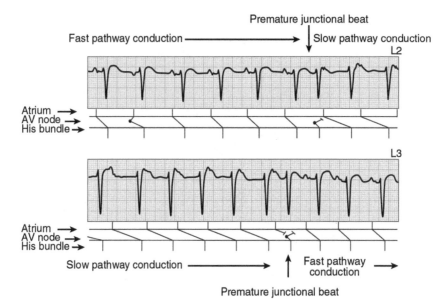

Fast pathway conduction ⟶ Premature junctional beat ↓ Slow pathway conduction

Fig. 5.4 Dual atrioventricular (AV) nodal physiology unmasked by a premature junctional beat. Diagram depicts sinus rhythm with normal P-R interval because of anterograde conduction via the fast AV nodal pathway. The impulse from the first premature junctional beat conceals into the fast AV nodal pathway retrogradely, and the next sinus impulse conducts anterogradely via the slow pathway with a prolonged P-R interval. The slow pathway conduction continues until the second junctional beat conceals conduction in the slow pathway retrogradely. This results in resumption of anterograde fast pathway conduction with normal P-R interval. *L2*, Lead 2; *L3*, lead 3.

(Fig. 5.13). This then prevents the next sinus impulse from conducting via the fast pathway. However, the same sinus impulse can conduct anterogradely down the slow pathway, return retrogradely in the fast pathway (which is no longer refractory), and initiate the tachycardia. AVNRTs often show cycle length variation during the initiation and termination phase of the tachycardia because of changes in conduction in the slow AV nodal pathway. However, such a phenomenon is not diagnostic of AVNRT because it can also occur during an AVRT. The AVNRT usually terminates after a PVC or PAC. It sometimes terminates as a result of alteration in the conduction property of the slow pathway that blocks the conduction via the slow pathway (Fig. 5.14). In that case the P-R interval usually prolongs before the termination of SVT at the slow pathway.

4. P wave morphology and axis: During an AVNRT, the atrium is activated retrogradely via one of the pathways; therefore the P wave is negative in the inferior leads (sometimes manifesting as pseudo Q waves when it occurs earlier than the initiation of the QRS complex) and positive in lead V1 (pseudo R wave) (Fig. 5.15). A positive P wave in the inferior leads is inconsistent with a diagnosis of AVNRT. It is important to remember that a negative P wave can also occur during an AVRT with a posteroseptal or posterior AP or during an atrial tachycardia originating low in the atrium. In AVNRT, the atrial activation occurs from the septum to the right and left atria, and therefore the P wave is narrower than during the sinus rhythm.

5. Effect of spontaneous PVC or a PVC introduced during electrophysiology study, during a short R-P' tachycardia when the His bundle is refractory: During sinus rhythm, retrograde atrial conduction after a PVC can occur via the AV node, when the His bundle is not refractory. Retrograde conduction can also occur simultaneously (with anterograde conduction via the His bundle) via the AP when present. During AVNRT, retrograde conduction after a spontaneous or stimulated PVC, when the His bundle is refractory, cannot reach the atrium because there is

no alternate pathway. Therefore the AVNRT cycle is not changed, and the P-P interval is unchanged after the PVC, although the ventricle is excited earlier. This proves that the ventricles are not part of the circuit. During AVRT, retrograde conduction after a PVC, at a time when the His bundle is refractory, cannot reach the atrium by way of the AV node but can reach the atrium by way of the AP, and the subsequent atrial depolarization (P wave on surface electrocardiogram [ECG]) will occur earlier. This indicates that an AP is present. This is one of the major features that differentiates an AVNRT from a septal AVRT (Figs. 5.16 and 5.17).

6. Cycle length variations:
   a. Oscillations in tachycardia cycle length: Subtle oscillations in the cycle length can occur during an SVT. If cycle length variation occurs during an SVT and the QRS-P time (ventriculoatrial conduction time) does not change (i.e., if the R-R interval change precedes the P-P interval change), then it suggests that the SVT is AV node–dependent (AVNRT, AVRT, or junctional tachycardia) (Fig. 5.18). More important, it rules out an atrial tachycardia. However, if P-P interval changes precede R-R interval changes, it is less diagnostic for a particular SVT, although more commonly it suggests an atrial tachycardia.
   b. Cycle length prolongation with aberrancy: If tachycardia cycle length suddenly prolongs with the onset of rate-related aberrancy (bundle branch block [BBB]), it suggests an AVRT involving the AP ipsilateral to the site of the BBB. If the cycle length remains unchanged during a short R-P tachycardia, it may be an AVRT with BBB contralateral to the site of the AP, AVNRT, or atrial tachycardia.
   c. Cycle length alternans: Cycle length alternans can occur during AVNRT as a result of alternate slowing of the conduction by way of the slow pathway. It may also result from participation of more than two AV nodal pathways during AVNRT with alternate conduction by way of the slow-slow or slow-intermediate pathways anterogradely or retrogradely (Fig. 5.19).

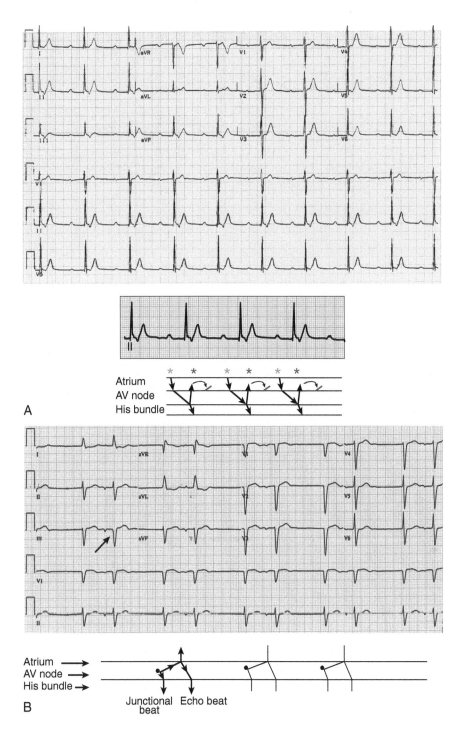

Fig. 5.5 Anterograde and retrograde echo beats. (A) Electrocardiogram shows sinus rhythm with single echo beat. Alternatively, it may be an atrial bigeminy. The baseline P-R interval was shorter (fast pathway conduction), which increased during the present rhythm, suggesting dual atrioventricular (AV) nodal physiology. The ladder diagram depicts anterograde conduction down the slow pathway (*blue asterisk*) and retrograde conduction to the atria (*red asterisk*) up the fast pathway, producing a single echo beat that is unable to reexcite the slow pathway because it is refractory (*red line*). Therefore the AV nodal reentrant tachycardia circuit cannot be completed, and AV nodal reentrant tachycardia is not initiated. (B) Electrocardiogram and V1, lead II rhythm strips show junctional escape beats that retrogradely activate the atria via the slow pathway with a long R-P interval. The impulse then conducts to the ventricle via the fast AV nodal pathway to produce a single AV nodal echo beat (*arrow*). This pattern continues in a bigeminal fashion.

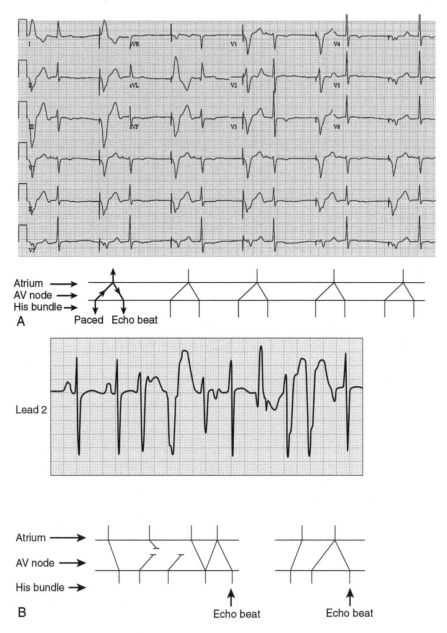

Fig. 5.6 (A) Ventricular paced beats result in retrograde slow pathway conduction to the atrium (inverted P waves in inferior leads) with a long R-P interval. The impulse also conducts to the ventricle via the fast atrioventricular (AV) nodal pathway (single AV nodal echo beat). This pattern continues in a bigeminal fashion. (B) Rhythm strip reveals that the first premature ventricular complex results in anterograde block of the sinus impulse. The second premature ventricular complex results in concealment in the fast pathway retrogradely followed by conduction of the next sinus impulse via the slow pathway, followed by a retrograde AV nodal echo. A similar phenomenon occurred after ventricular couplets at the end of the rhythm strip.

7. QRS morphology:
   a. Wide QRS during SVT: Preexisting BBB or rate-related BBB (aberrancy) results in a wide complex tachycardia. The P wave may not be manifest on the routine 12-lead ECG (Figs. 5.20 and 5.21).
   b. QRS alternans: QRS alternans is a phasic alteration in the amplitude of the QRS complex, which usually occurs at faster rates. It is a nonspecific finding of unknown mechanism (Fig. 5.22). Thus it most commonly occurs in conjunction with orthodromic AVRT (25%–38%) and less commonly with AVNRT (13%–23%).[2] QRS alternans usually does not occur with atrial tachycardia.

8. Left-sided AV nodal inputs: Right and left atria inputs of the AV node have been demonstrated to be involved in the anatomically complex AVNRT circuit. In approximately 5% of patients with slow-fast AVNRT, the anterograde limb of the circuit (slow pathway) appears to be formed by the leftward inferior extension of the AV node (Fig. 5.23). Postulated circuit of the left variant slow-fast AVNRT includes retrograde conduction over the fast pathway (right atrial or left atrial extension) that connects to the AV node. The slow pathway connection travels from the mitral annulus to the AV node via the coronary sinus and interatrial septum to the AV node. Ablation of slow

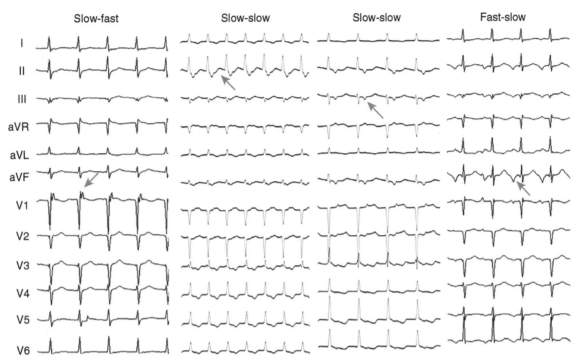

Fig. 5.7 Scalar electrocardiogram of the different types of atrioventricular nodal reentrant tachycardia (AVNRT). *Arrows* mark the P waves. In slow-fast (typical) AVNRT, the P wave may lie within the QRS (invisible) or distort the terminal portion of the QRS (mimicking an R wave in V1, first panel). In slow-slow AVNRT, the P wave lies outside the QRS in the ST-T wave, and the R-P interval is longer than that in slow-fast AVNRT (in middle panels the RP interval may vary depending on the conduction time in retrograde slow pathway). In fast-slow (atypical) AVNRT, the P wave lies before the QRS with a long R-P interval (last panel). In all varieties of AVNRT, the P wave is relatively narrow, negative in the inferior leads, and positive in V1.

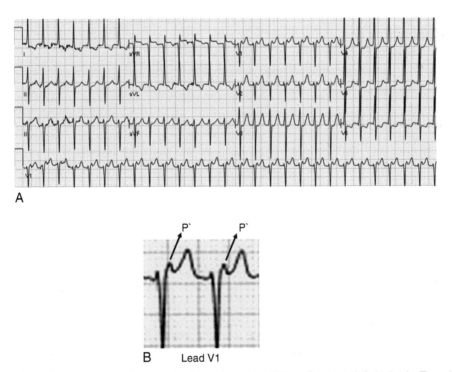

Fig. 5.8 Short R-P′ tachycardia. (A) Narrow complex tachycardia does not have an obvious P wave in inferior leads. There is a pseudo R′ in lead V1, which was not present during the sinus rhythm (*arrow*). It is a very short R-P′ interval suggestive of an atrioventricular nodal reentrant tachycardia. (B) Electrocardiogram of the same patient during sinus rhythm shows no evidence of incomplete right bundle branch block or a second R′ in lead V1 that was seen during supraventricular tachycardia (*arrow*).

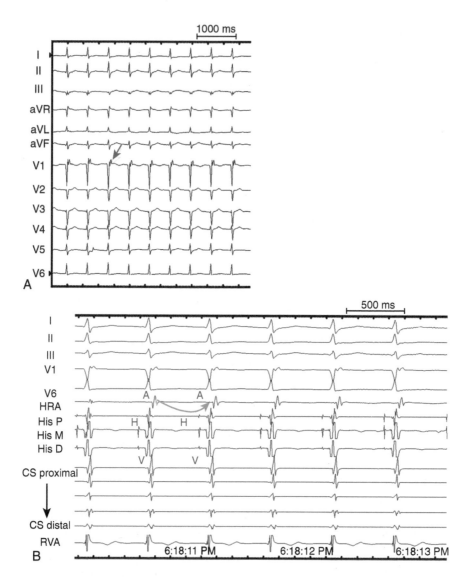

Fig. 5.9 Typical and atypical atrioventricular (AV) nodal reentrant tachycardia (AVNRT) in the same patient (A) AVNRT with pseudo R′ in lead V1. Electrocardiogram (ECG) shows a short R-P′ tachycardia at 110 bpm with an R-P interval of 40 ms. Retrograde P wave is not visible except in lead V1 (*red arrow*) and possibly in lead III. (B) Intracardiac electrograms reveal a short R-P′ tachycardia (cycle length: 500 ms) with a midline retrograde atrial conduction pattern. P waves in lead V1 on surface ECG and an R-P′ interval of 40 ms suggests an AVNRT. During a typical AVNRT, the conduction via the slow pathway is represented by the A-H interval, and conduction via the fast pathway is represented by the H-A interval (*arrow*). Other maneuvers during electrophysiology study, such as introduction of a premature ventricular complex during His bundle timing, entrainment from the right ventricle, measurement of A-H interval during supraventricular tachycardia versus A-H interval during atrial pacing at the tachycardia cycle length, initiation of the tachycardia with sudden prolongation of AH in response to progressively earlier premature atrial complexes, and parahisian pacing confirmed the mechanism of the tachycardia as a typical AVNRT. (C) Patient developed a long R-P′ tachycardia (atypical AVNRT; *red arrow* points to retrograde P wave). (D) Intracardiac electrograms during the long R-P′ tachycardia (C) show the midline retrograde atrial conduction pattern and inverted P waves in inferior lead on surface ECG suggestive of atypical AVNRT. (E) Schematic of atypical (fast-slow) AVNRT (D), which shows anterograde conduction via the fast AV nodal pathway and retrograde conduction via the slow AV nodal pathway during the tachycardia. *A,* Atrial electrogram; *AVN,* atrioventricular node; *CS,* coronary sinus; *H,* His bundle electrogram; *His D,* distal His; *His M,* middle His; *His P,* proximal His; *HRA,* high right atrium; *RVA,* right ventricular apex; *V,* ventricular electrogram.

pathway inside the coronary sinus is often successful, although slow pathway ablation is sometimes required at the mitral annulus to eliminate the AVNRT circuit.

9. AVNRT with lower and upper common pathway block: The distal junction of the fast and slow pathways in a typical (slow-fast) AVNRT has traditionally been considered to be located in the AV node, with a region of AV nodal tissue extending between the distal junction of the two pathways and the His

bundle (the lower common pathway). However, the anatomic correlate of the lower common pathway is not known. The presence of a lower common pathway consisting of AV nodal tissue would predict occasional block proximal to the His bundle during a typical (slow-fast) AVNRT, but this phenomenon is rare. This can present with 2:1 or a higher degree of AV block, mimicking an atrial tachycardia (Figs. 5.24 and 5.25). The proximal connection between the slow and fast pathway (the

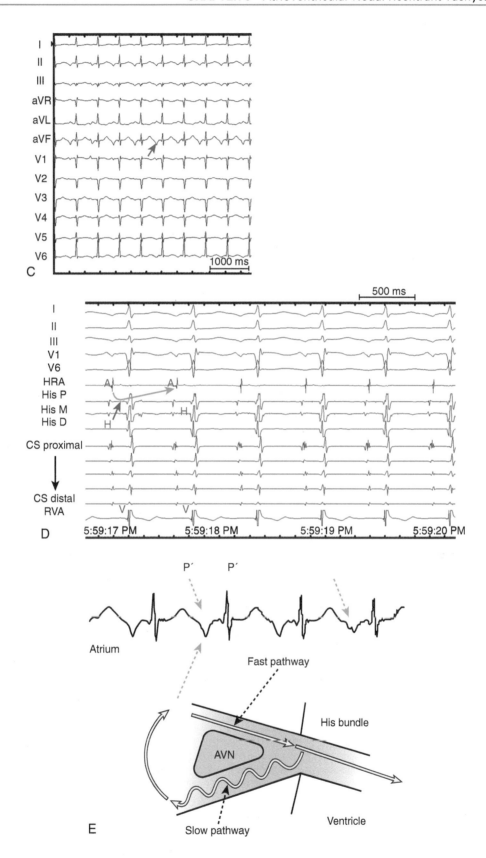

Fig. 5.9 (Continued).

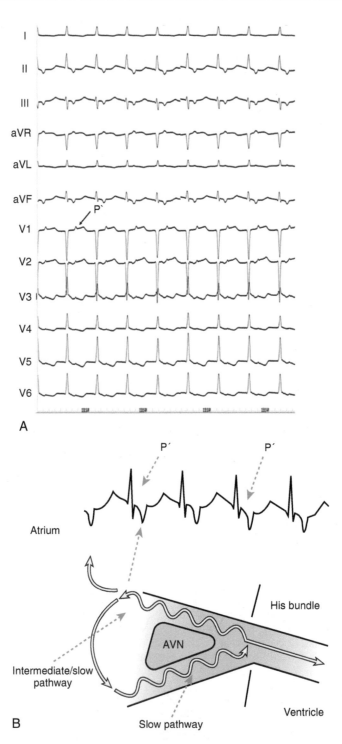

Fig. 5.10 Intermediate R-P′ atrioventricular (AV) nodal reentrant tachycardia (AVNRT). (A) Intermediate R-P′ tachycardia at 175 bpm. There are inverted P waves in inferior leads (*arrow*). This electrocardiogram is consistent with an atypical fast-slow AVNRT, an AV reentrant tachycardia with a slowly conducting posteroseptal accessory pathway, or an atrial tachycardia originating from a site in the lower right atrium. Electrophysiology study confirmed AVNRT. (B) The patient has two intermediate AV nodal pathways. Usually, a premature atrial complex blocks anterogradely at the anterior AV nodal pathway and engages the slow AV nodal pathway anterogradely, which initiates AVNRT. *AVN,* Atrioventricular node.

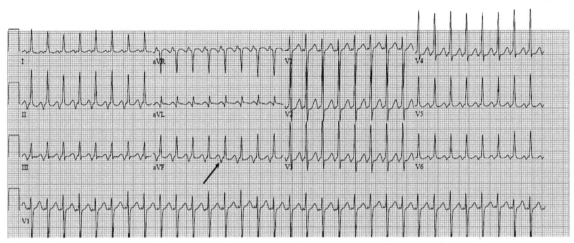

Fig. 5.11 Surface electrocardiogram depicts a long R-P′ tachycardia. In slow-slow or slow-intermediate atrioventricular nodal reentrant tachycardia, the P wave lies outside the QRS in the ST-T wave (*arrow*), and the R-P′ interval is longer than that of a typical slow-fast atrioventricular nodal reentrant tachycardia, a permanent form of reciprocating junctional tachycardia, or low right atrial tachycardia.

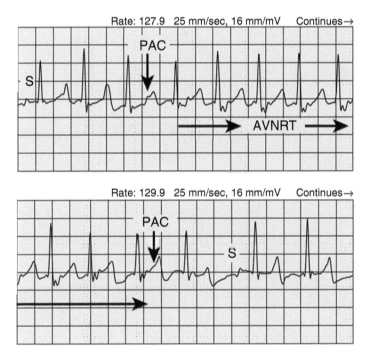

Fig. 5.12 Initiation and termination of atrioventricular nodal reentrant tachycardia (AVNRT). Electrocardiogram reveals sinus rhythm (S) with frequent premature atrial complexes (PACs) and slow-fast (typical) AVNRT. The AVNRT is initiated after a PAC with anterograde atrioventricular conduction via the slow pathway. Another PAC terminates the tachycardia by making the anterograde slow pathway refractory.

upper common pathway) can also present with 2:1 ventriculoatrial block during AVNRT. However, the existence of the upper common pathway is controversial.

10. Sinus rhythm with 1:2 ventricular response: Normally in patients with dual AV nodal physiology, conduction occurs over the fast pathway to the ventricles via the His bundle and, after activation of the fast pathway, conduction retrogradely conceals in the slow pathway, blocking before reaching the atrium. Such concealed conduction blocks anterograde conduction to the ventricle over the slow pathway. Anterograde conduction over the slow pathway can occur if retrograde concealment does not take place. If this occurs, 1:2 AV conduction to the ventricle results during sinus rhythm (Fig. 5.26). This patient had inducible AVNRT during electrophysiology study, and slow pathway ablation resulted in conduction to the ventricles via the fast pathway only.

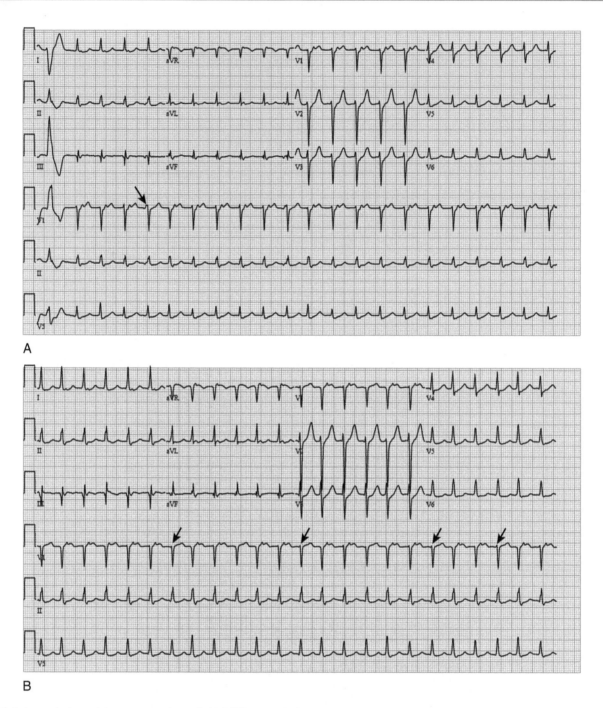

A

B

Fig. 5.13 Atrioventricular nodal reentrant tachycardia (AVNRT) initiated with a premature ventricular complex, which was preceded by sinus rhythm (not shown). The short R-P′ tachycardia (AVNRT) is induced by single premature ventricular complex. *Arrows* show frequent premature atrial complexes, which occur just before the QRS (A) or during QRS during supraventricular tachycardia (B).

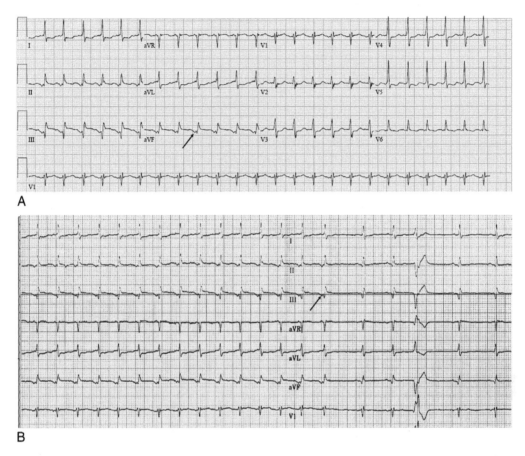

Fig. 5.14 Termination of atrioventricular (AV) nodal reentrant tachycardia. (A) Electrocardiogram during supraventricular tachycardia shows atypical (fast-slow) AV nodal reentrant tachycardia. The *arrow* shows retrograde P wave. (B) Tachycardia terminated spontaneously after prolongation of R-R interval with no preceding P wave as a result of slow pathway refractoriness (*arrow*). Similar termination can occur with carotid sinus massage and intravenous adenosine infusion. Usually, these are followed by sinus slowing, AV block, or both.

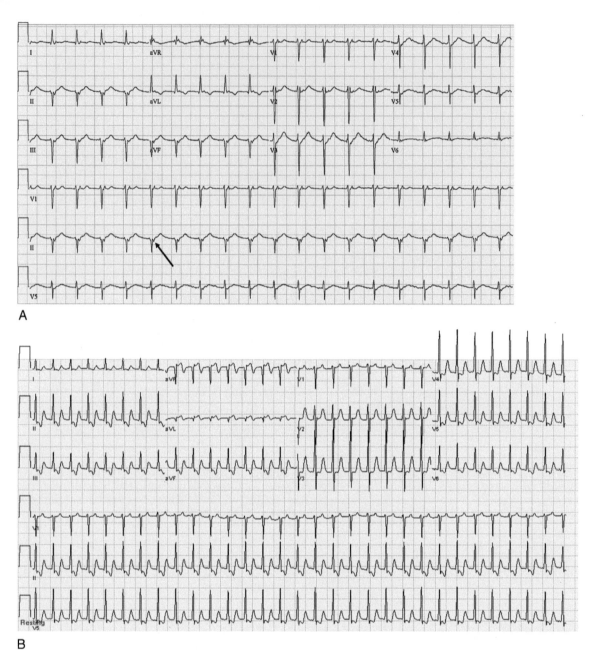

Fig. 5.15 P wave morphology and axis. During the typical (slow-fast) atrioventricular (AV) nodal reentrant tachycardia (AVNRT), the atrium is activated retrogradely via the fast pathway and during atypical (fast-slow) AVNRT via the slow pathway. Therefore the P wave is negative in the inferior leads and positive in lead V1 (pseudo R wave). Positive P wave in the inferior leads is inconsistent with a diagnosis of AVNRT (*arrow*). (A) Negative P waves in inferior leads with a short R-P (<70 ms) is consistent with typical AVNRT. The P wave duration in AVNRT is short because of simultaneous activation of both the atria from the septum. (B) Negative P waves in inferior leads after the QRS complexes end during the short R-P′ interval tachycardia is consistent with typical AVNRT or more commonly AV reentrant tachycardia. Tachycardia was confirmed to be AVNRT during the electrophysiology study. (C) Long R-P′ interval tachycardia with positive P waves (*arrow*) in inferior leads excluded AVNRT. This is an atrial tachycardia. (D) Long R-P′ tachycardia with a very short P-R′ interval and positive P waves in inferior leads exclude AVNRT and AV reentrant tachycardia involving a posterior accessory pathway. P waves (*arrow*) extend into next QRS waves and conduct to the subsequent QRS (skipped P waves; see Figure 3.2) as a result of first-degree AV block with markedly prolonged baseline P-R interval. This is sinus tachycardia with marked first-degree AV block recorded during exercise testing.

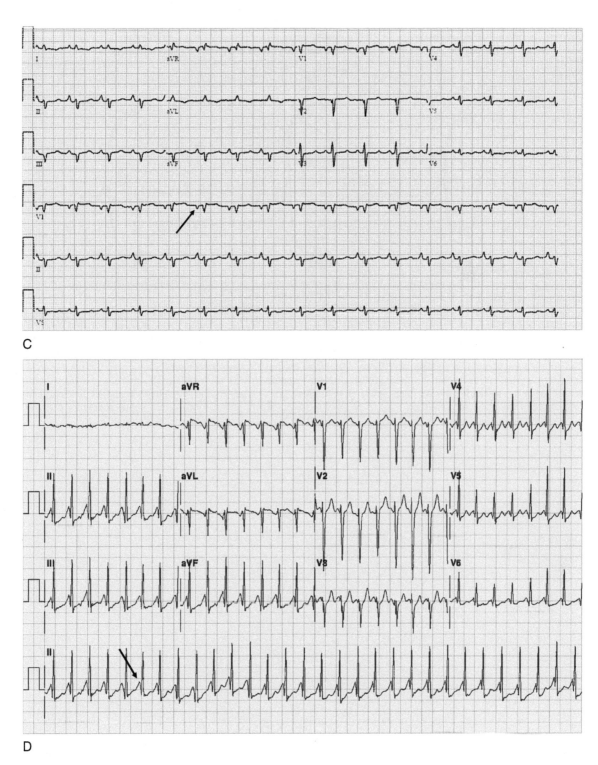

Fig. 5.15 (Continued).

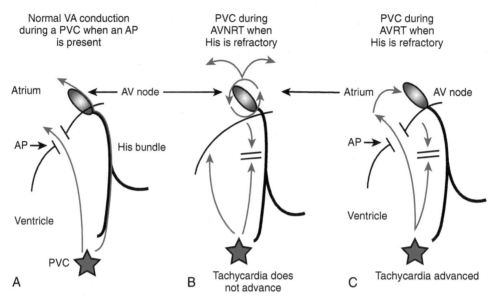

Fig. 5.16 The response to introduction of a ventricular extrastimulus at a time when His is refractory or spontaneous premature ventricular complex (PVC) during supraventricular tachycardia. (A) During sinus rhythm, retrograde atrial conduction after a PVC can occur via the atrioventricular (AV) node, when the His bundle is not refractory. Retrograde conduction can also occur simultaneously via the accessory pathway (AP) if one is present. (B) During AV nodal reentrant tachycardia (AVNRT), retrograde conduction after a PVC when the His bundle is refractory cannot reach the atrium because there is no alternate pathway. Therefore the next P wave does not occur early, and the tachycardia cycle length does not change (tachycardia is not advanced). (C) During AV reentrant tachycardia (AVRT), retrograde conduction after a PVC when the His bundle is refractory cannot reach the atrium via the AV node but can reach the atrium via the AP, and the subsequent atrial depolarization (P wave on surface electrocardiogram) will occur earlier. When this His-synchronous PVC occurs during AVRT with a septal accessory pathway, the next P wave should occur early, and the tachycardia cycle length will be changed (tachycardia is advanced). *VA*, ventriculoatrial.

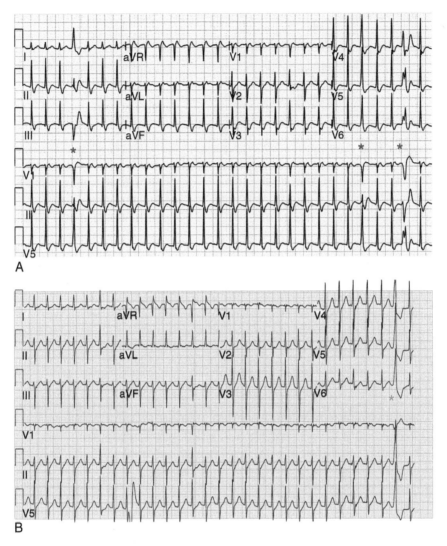

Fig. 5.17 Premature ventricular complex (PVC) when His is refractory during an atrioventricular nodal reentrant tachycardia (AVNRT). (A) Electrocardiogram shows a short R-P' tachycardia with inverted P waves in inferior leads and a pseudo R wave in lead V1. There are three PVCs (red asterisks). First and second PVCs are fusion complexes during the supraventricular tachycardia. The third complex (*red asterisk*) occurs 50 ms earlier than the anticipated QRS, but the timing of associated P' wave does not change. The third PVC occurs during the period when the His bundle is refractory (provided the His ventricular interval is normal, 35–55 ms). This argues against an atrioventricular reentrant tachycardia using a septal accessory pathway because when the His bundle is refractory, the retrograde atrial depolarization (after the PVC, as shown by a blue asterisk) would occur via the accessory pathway earlier than expected during the tachycardia. (B) Intracardiac electrograms reveal a short R-P' tachycardia with earliest activation in the proximal coronary sinus (CS). A PVC was introduced when His was refractory that did not advance next atrial activation (A). This is most consistent with an AVNRT, as shown in Fig. 5.16B. (C) Intracardiac electrograms show a long R-P' tachycardia with earliest activation in the CS proximal. A PVC was introduced when His was refractory that did not advance next atrial activation (A). This is most consistent with atypical AVNRT. (D) Intracardiac electrograms show a long R-P' tachycardia with earliest activation in the *CS proximal*. A PVC was introduced during His timing that did not advance next atrial activation (A). This proves that the His bundle is not a part of the tachycardia circuit, suggestive of atypical AVNRT. *A*, Atrial electrogram; *CS*, coronary sinus; *H*, His bundle electrogram; *His D*, distal His; *His M*, middle His; *His P*, proximal His; *HRA*, high right atrium; *RVA*, right ventricular apex; *V*, ventricular electrogram.

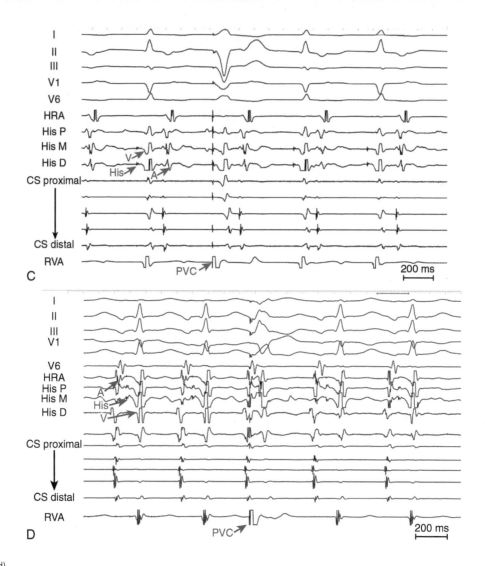

C

D

Fig. 5.17 (Conitinued).

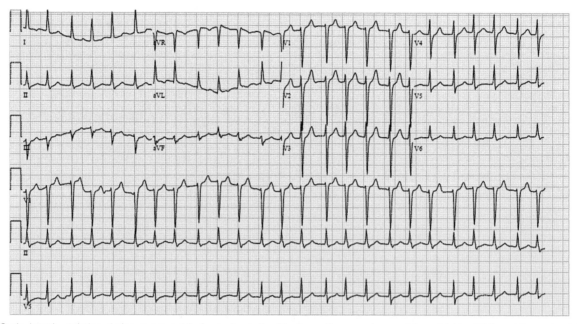

Fig. 5.18 Cycle length variation during supraventricular tachycardia. Electrocardiogram shows atrioventricular (AV) nodal reentrant tachycardia (AVNRT) with subtle oscillations in the cycle length. During a short R-P' tachycardia, if cycle length variation occurs with the QRS-P time (ventriculoatrial conduction time) unchanged, this suggests AV node–dependent supraventricular tachycardia (AVNRT, AV reentrant tachycardia, or junctional tachycardia). In AVNRT, this usually occurs during variation in slow pathway conduction time.

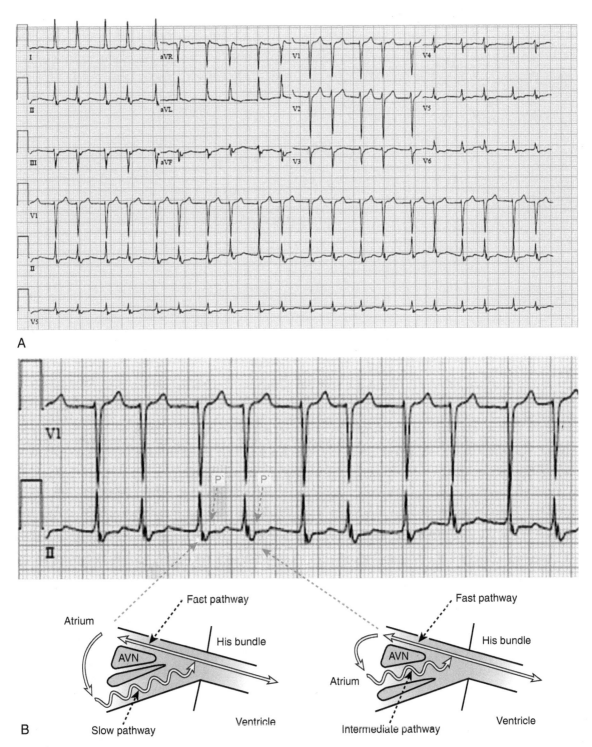

Fig. 5.19 Cycle length variation with alternate shortening and lengthening of R-R interval during supraventricular tachycardia. Electrocardiogram depicts a short R-P' tachycardia with alternate shortening and lengthening of R-R interval (A). This occurs in the presence of two slow pathways or a slow and an intermediate pathway. During tachycardia, alternate anterograde conduction via the two pathways with different conduction properties results in the variation of P-R interval, thus varying R-R interval (B). Note that the R-P' interval is fixed because the retrograde conduction always occurs via the fast pathway. *AVN,* Atrioventricular node.

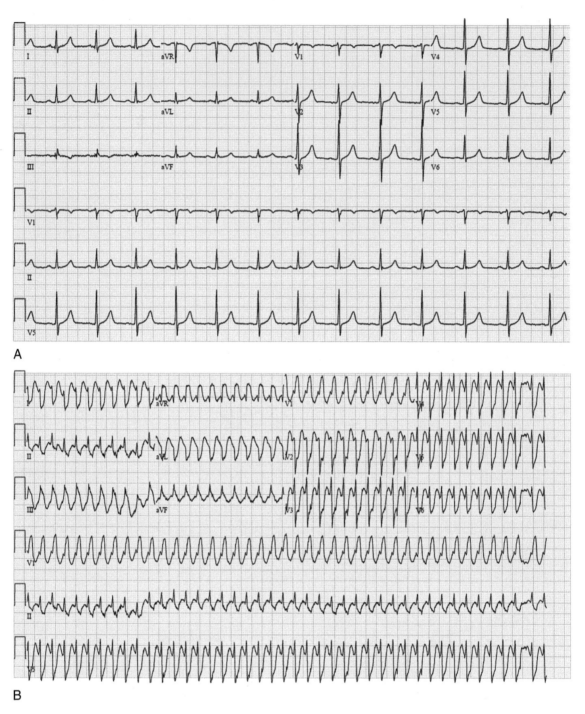

A

B

Fig. 5.20 Rate-related right bundle branch block aberrancy during atrioventricular nodal reentrant tachycardia. (A) Baseline electrocardiogram shows normal QRS duration during sinus rhythm. (B) At electrophysiology study, tachycardia was proved to be atrioventricular nodal reentrant tachycardia with right bundle branch block aberrancy.

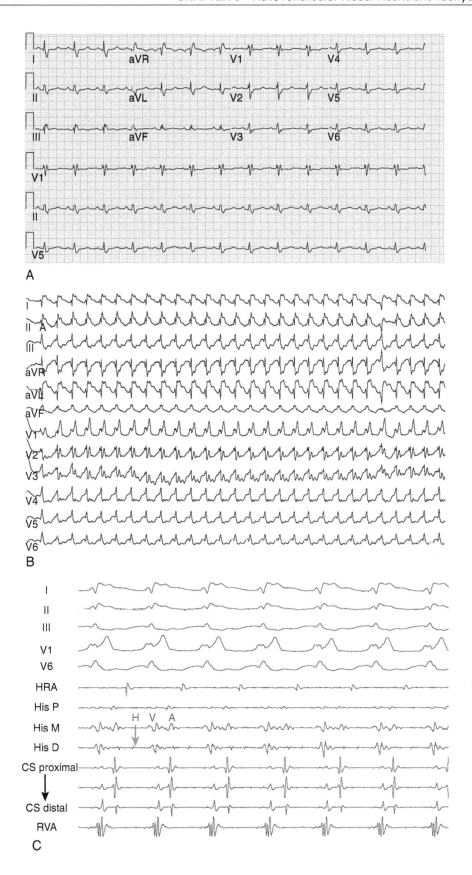

Fig. 5.21 Atrioventricular nodal reentrant tachycardia presenting with a wide complex tachycardia. (A) Baseline electrocardiogram reveals sinus rhythm with right bundle branch block. During tachycardia, right bundle branch block persists (B) and eelectrophysiology study confirmed typical slow-fast atrioventricular nodal reentrant tachycardia (C). *CS,* Coronary sinus; *His D,* distal His; *His M,* middle His; *His P,* proximal His; *HRA,* high right atrium; *RVA,* right ventricular apex.

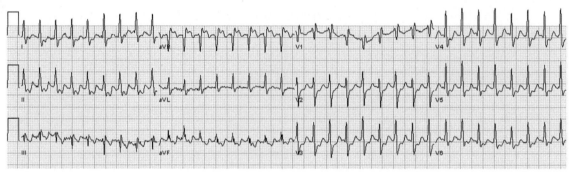

Fig. 5.22 QRS alternans during supraventricular tachycardia. QRS alternans is shown best in leads V2 and V3. The arrhythmia was confirmed to be atrioventricular nodal reentrant tachycardia during electrophysiology study.

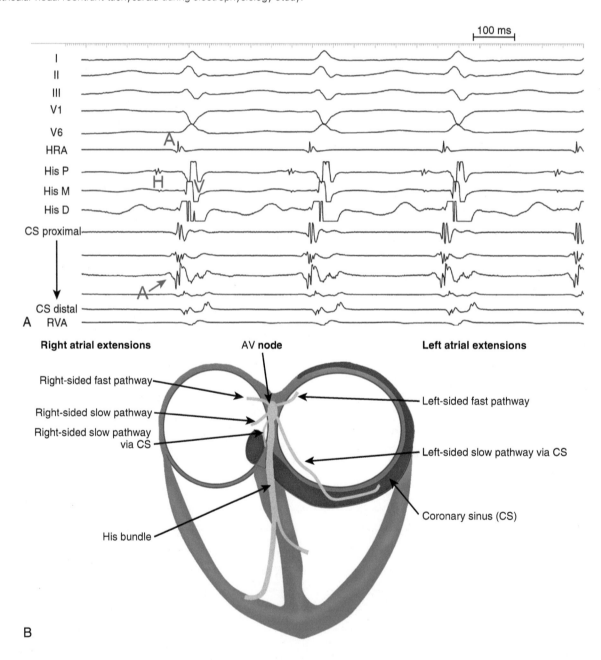

Fig. 5.23 Right- and left-sided atrioventricular (AV) nodal inputs. (A) During AV nodal reentrant tachycardia, the earliest atrial activation was found in the midcoronary sinus catheter located at the posterior mitral annulus (*red arrow*). The tachycardia was proved to be AV nodal reentrant tachycardia by the midline ventriculoatrial conduction, longer ventriculoatrial when pacing from the left ventricle corresponding to the earliest atrial activation. (B) Schematic representations of potential inputs to AV node. Right-sided fast pathway input extends from anterior part of fossa ovalis. The right-sided slow pathway (posterior) input has been demonstrated at the anterior and inside the coronary sinus (CS) musculature. The left-sided fast pathway input has been proposed to reach the AV node via the fossa ovalis. The left-sided slow AV nodal pathway extends to the mid and lateral mitral annulus inside the CS musculature and reaches the AV node via the interventricular septum. *A,* Atrial electrogram; *FP,* fast pathway; *H,* His bundle electrogram; *His D,* distal His; *His M,* middle His; *His P,* proximal His; *HRA,* high right atrium; *RVA,* right ventricular apex; *SP,* slow pathway; *V,* ventricular electrogram.

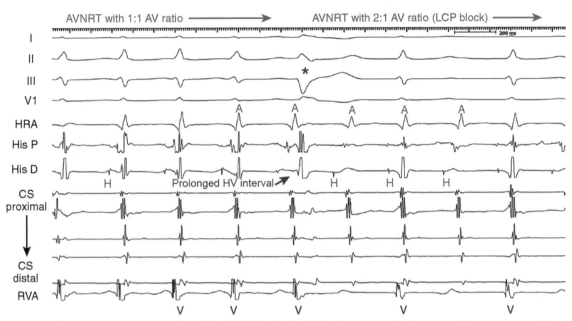

Fig. 5.24 Atrioventricular (AV) nodal reentrant tachycardia (AVNRT) with 2:1 AV block, proving that the ventricle is not a part of the reentry circuit. Intracardiac electrograms show a short R-P' tachycardia (cycle length: 360 ms) with a midline retrograde conduction and inverted P waves in inferior electrocardiogram leads, suggestive of an AVNRT. However, during tachycardia there is slight prolongation of H-V interval with right bundle branch block aberrancy in one beat (*asterisk*) followed by 2:1 AV block, which suggests atrial tachycardia with 2:1 AV conduction. The tachycardia proved to be a typical slow-fast AVNRT during electrophysiologic testing, and 2:1 AV block resulted from lower common pathway (LCP) block during alternate beats. *A*, Atrial electrogram; *CS*, coronary sinus; *H*, His bundle electrogram; *His D*, distal His; *His M*, middle His; *His P*, proximal His; *HRA*, high right atrium; *RVA*, right ventricular apex; *V*, ventricular electrogram.

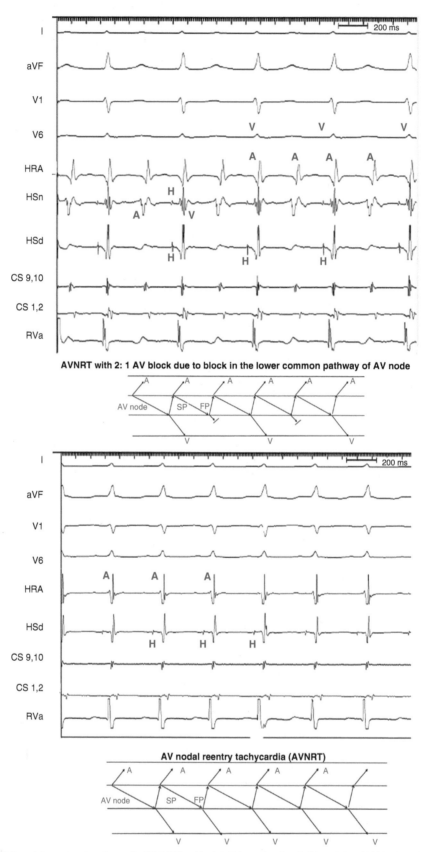

Fig. 5.25 Atrioventricular (AV) nodal reentrant tachycardia (AVNRT) with 1:1 AV conduction (left) and 2:1 AV block (right). Intracardiac electrograms show a short R-P' tachycardia (cycle length: 340 ms) with a midline retrograde atrial activation and inverted P waves in inferior electrocardiogram leads that are more suggestive of an AVNRT. However, during the electrophysiology study 2:1 AV conduction occurs due to block in the lower common pathway of the AV node. *A*, Atrial electrogram; *CS*, coronary sinus; *FP*, fast pathway; *H*, His bundle electrogram; *His D*, distal His; *His M*, middle His; *His P*, proximal His; *HRA*, high right atrium; *RVA*, right ventricular apex; *SP*, slow pathway; *V*, ventricular electrogram.

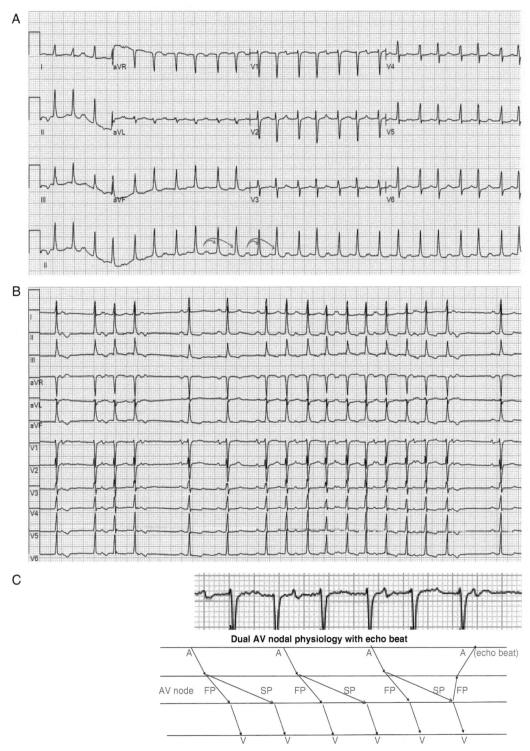

Fig. 5.26 (A) The patient presented with narrow complex tachycardia with heart rate in 150 s. On close inspection, the rhythm is actually sinus rhythm at 75 bpm with alternating long-short cycle length conduction. This results because of double firing due to 1:2 atrioventricular conduction via both the fast and slow atrioventricular nodal pathways (*blue arrows*). This pattern was recorded several times in telemetry. (B) The second electrocardiogram of the same patient shows paroxysms of similar pattern, and the diagram (C) depicts the impulse conduction pattern and one retrograde echo beat. *FP*, fast pathway; *SP*, slow pathway.

REFERENCES

1. Kalbfleisch S, el-Atassi R, Calkins H, Langberg J, Morady F. Differentiation of paroxysmal narrow QRS complex tachycardias using the 12-lead electrocardiogram. *J Am Coll Cardiol.* 1993;21:85–89.

2. Fox DJ, Tischenko A, Krahn AD, et al. Supraventricular tachycardia: diagnosis and management. *Mayo Clin Proc.* 2008;83:1400–1411.

6

Atrioventricular Reentrant Tachycardias

CONCEALED ACCESSORY PATHWAYS AND WOLFF-PARKINSON-WHITE SYNDROME AND VARIANTS

Accessory pathways (APs; bypass tracts) are one or more strands of myocardial fibers that are remnants of atrioventricular (AV) connections caused by incomplete embryologic development of the AV annulus and failure of the fibrous separation between the atria and ventricles. They are capable of conducting electrical impulses across the AV groove when they connect the atrium to the ipsilateral ventricle across the mitral or tricuspid annulus (Fig. 6.1). These APs can conduct impulses bidirectionally; can conduct retrogradely only; or, in rare cases, can conduct anterogradely only. APs that conduct retrogradely only are called *concealed APs* because the presence of conduction cannot be detected on a routine electrocardiogram (ECG). When an AP is capable of conducting retrogradely only (from the ventricles to the atria), the ECG is normal, and no delta wave is seen (concealed AP) (Fig. 6.2). Pathways capable of conducting bidirectionally or, less commonly, anterogradely only are called *manifest APs* or Wolff-Parkinson-White (WPW) or preexcitation pattern because the presence of the pathway can be detected on the routine 12-lead ECG. The terms *WPW syndrome* or *preexcitation syndrome* are usually restricted to patients with a tachyarrhythmia and typical ECG abnormality, whereas the term *WPW pattern* signifies an asymptomatic patient with typical ECG abnormalities of WPW conduction. Normal conduction from the atria to the ventricles occurs by way of the AV node (in which minor physiologic delay occurs) and through the His-Purkinje system, resulting in a normal P-R interval and a narrow QRS complex. In WPW syndrome, because of the physiologic delay of conduction in the AV node, conduction from the atrium reaches the adjacent ventricle earlier by way of the AP, which normally has no conduction delay, and a part of the ventricle is preexcited, resulting in a slurred upstroke at the initiation of the QRS complex known as the delta wave. The QRS complexes in WPW syndrome are the fusion of the normal ventricular depolarization via the AV node and His bundle and the depolarization of a part of the ventricle via the AP. APs can be single or multiple and vary in locations in relation to the valve annulus (Fig. 6.3). The degree of preexcitation depends on the relative contribution of the impulse via the AP versus the AV node in depolarizing the ventricles. Conduction over the AP results in shortening of the P-R interval (<120 ms) and widening of the QRS complex (≥120 ms) with secondary ST-T wave changes. These APs serve as a substrate for reentry and can cause a supraventricular tachycardia (SVT) involving the AV node as one connection between the atrium and the ventricle and the AP as the other. This type of SVT is termed *AV reentrant tachycardia* (AVRT). AVRT is the most common arrhythmia and occurs in approximately 70% to 80% of symptomatic patients with WPW syndrome. The common form of AVRT involves impulse conduction via the AV node and the His-Purkinje system to the ventricles anterogradely and via the AP retrogradely, resulting in rapid atrial activation after ventricular depolarization. This is known as *orthodromic reciprocating tachycardia* (ORT) (Fig. 6.4). Less commonly (in 5%−10% of cases), AVRT results from impulse conduction in a direction opposite to ORT (i.e., conduction from atrium to ventricle via the AP and then from the ventricle to the atrium via the His-Purkinje system and the AV node). Therefore it is a regular wide complex tachycardia because ventricular activation is transmyocardial via the AP insertion rather than via the specialized conduction tissue. This type of AVRT is known as *antidromic reciprocating tachycardia* (ART) (Fig. 6.4). Unlike the AV node, in which conduction slows at faster atrial rates (decremental conduction), approximately 90% of these APs are rapidly conducting, resulting in circus movement tachycardia involving the atrium and ipsilateral ventricle with the AP as one limb and AV node as the other limb of the circuit (AVRT). Approximately 10% of the APs in the WPW syndrome are slowly conducting (AV node−like property). Often a premature atrial complex or a premature ventricular complex can find the AP or the AV node refractory, causing unidirectional block and initiation of reentry and resulting in an ORT (Fig. 6.5) or an ART (Fig. 6.6), respectively. During atrial fibrillation (AF), which occurs in up to one-third of patients with WPW syndrome, the AP can conduct rapidly to the ventricles, rarely causing ventricular fibrillation (VF) and sudden cardiac death (SCD).

LOCALIZATION OF ACCESSORY PATHWAY BASED ON THE ELECTROCARDIOGRAM PATTERNS

Approximately 40% to 60% of APs are located on the left free wall, 25% on the right or left posteroseptal area, 13% to 21% on the right free wall, 2% to 10% on the anteroseptal area, and less than 5% are located on the midseptum area. Multiple APs occur in 5% to 10% of patients. The precise localization of these APs helps in assessing the success rate and risks of catheter ablation and in planning the ablation strategy. It is prudent to recognize that the delta wave vector can be determined with precision only when the ECG shows maximum preexcitation. Several algorithms have been developed, but as a general rule, a positive delta wave (first 40 ms of QRS complex) in lead V1 suggests a left-sided AP and a negative delta wave in V1 suggests a right-sided AP (Figs. 6.7 and 6.8). A positive delta wave in inferior leads with inferior axis represents an anteroseptal AP (Fig. 6.9). A left axis (with a negative delta wave in lead V1) suggests a right lateral AP (Fig. 6.10). If the delta waves in the inferior leads are negative, this denotes a posteroseptal AP in the right (Fig. 6.11) or left (Fig. 6.12) septum, depending on the delta wave vector in lead V1, as described previously. A negative delta wave in lead II (more negative than in lead III) and a positive delta wave in lead aVR suggest a posterior AP involving the coronary sinus or middle cardiac vein (Fig. 6.13). A negative delta wave in lead I, aVL, and V6 (rightward QRS axis) with a positive delta wave in lead V1 suggests a left lateral or anterolateral pathway. Fig. 6.14 shows a left anterolateral AP with ORT.

Collision (fusion) of Wavefronts Down the AV Node and AP

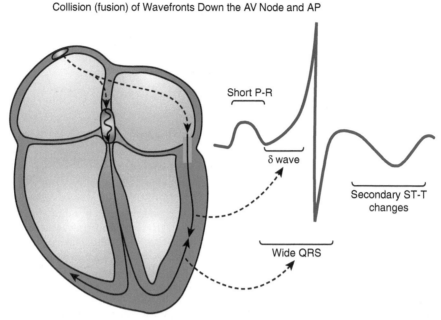

Fig. 6.1 In the Wolff-Parkinson-White syndrome, because of the physiologic delay of conduction in the atrioventricular (AV) node, conduction from the atrium reaches the adjacent ventricle earlier via the *accessory pathway* (AP; depicted as *green rectangle*), which normally has no conduction delay, and a part of ventricle is preexcited, resulting in a slurred upstroke at the initiation of the QRS complex known as the *delta* (δ) *wave*. Degree of preexcitation depends on the distance of the AP from the sinus node and rapidity of the conduction property of the AV node and that of the AP.

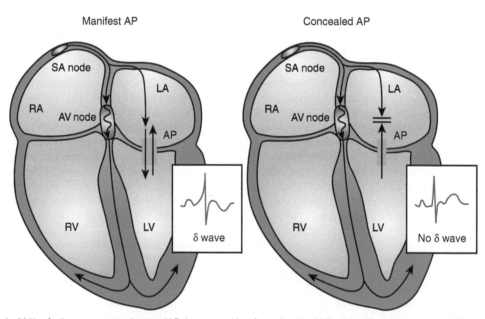

Fig. 6.2 Approximately 60% of all accessory pathways (APs) are capable of conducting bidirectionally (atrium to ventricle and ventricle to atrium, left panel). When an AP is capable of conducting retrogradely only (from the ventricle to the atria), the electrocardiogram is normal and no delta (δ) wave is seen (concealed AP, right panel). Fewer than 5% of all APs in Wolff-Parkinson-White syndrome are capable of anterograde conduction only. *Green* rectangle indicates AP; *arrows* indicate conduction pathways; *AV*, Atrioventricular; *LA*, left atrium; *LV*, left ventricle; *RA*, right atrium; *RV*, right ventricle; *SA*, sinoatrial.

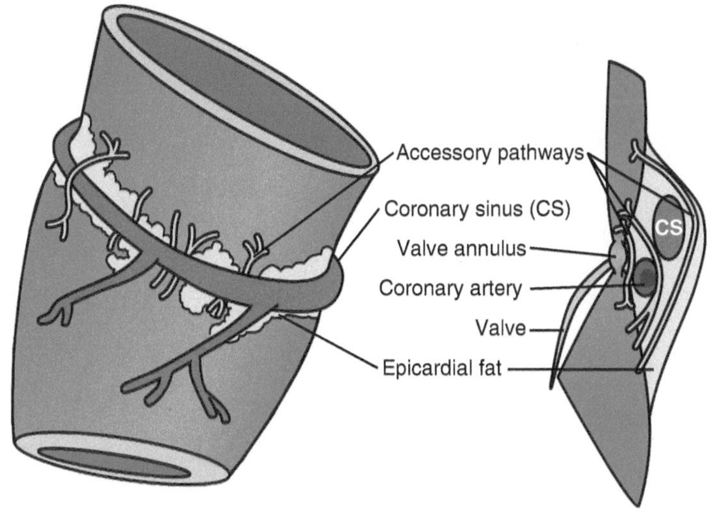

Anatomic Location of Accessory Pathways
Across the Valve Annuli

Accessory pathways

Coronary sinus (CS)

Valve annulus

Coronary artery

Valve

Epicardial fat

Fig. 6.3 Accessory pathways (APs) are usually very thin muscular strands (rarely thicker than 1–2 mm) but can occasionally exist as multiple strands or a broad band of tissue. These APs can run in an oblique course rather than perpendicular to the transverse plane of the atrioventricular groove. As a result, the fibers can have an atrial insertion point that is transversely several centimeters away from the point of ventricular insertion. The figure depicts potential sites of accessory pathways. *Lines* describe the pathway of conduction anterogradely over the atrioventricular node-His bundle to the ventricles and anterogradely over the AP, colliding in the ventricle to produce a QRS fusion beat.

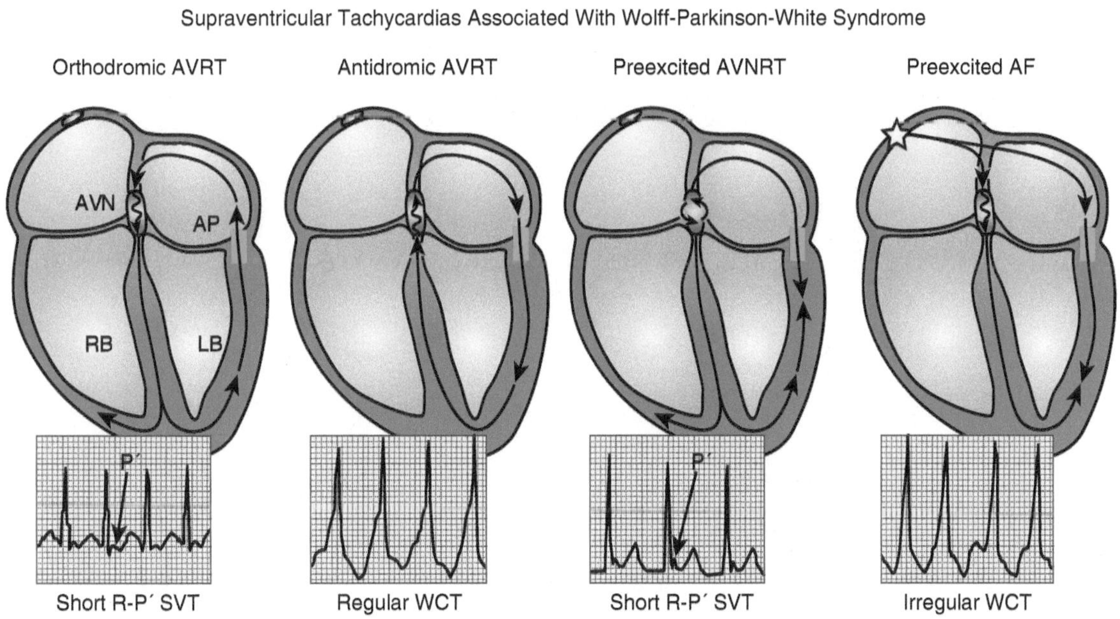

Supraventricular Tachycardias Associated With Wolff-Parkinson-White Syndrome

Orthodromic AVRT	Antidromic AVRT	Preexcited AVNRT	Preexcited AF

Short R-P′ SVT	Regular WCT	Short R-P′ SVT	Irregular WCT

Fig. 6.4 Schematic representation of the reentrant circuit during orthodromic atrioventricular reentrant tachycardia (AVRT), antidromic AVRT, preexcited atrioventricular nodal reentrant tachycardia (AVNRT) using a left-sided accessory pathway (AP), and preexcited atrial tachycardia, or atrial fibrillation (AF). During orthodromic AVRT, anterograde conduction occurs over the AVN-His bundle, with retrograde conduction over the AP. During antidromic AVRT, anterograde conduction occurs over the AP and retrograde conduction over the AVN-His bundle. During preexcited AVNRT, reentry occurs over the AVN slow and fast pathways, with anterograde conduction to the ventricles over the His bundle and AP, resulting in a QRS fusion beat. During preexcited AF, reentry occurs in the atria with anterograde conduction to the ventricles over the His bundle and AP, resulting in a QRS fusion beat. *Green rectangle* depicts the AP; *arrows* demonstrate conduction pathways. *AVN,* Atrioventricular node; *LB,* left bundle branch; *RB,* right bundle branch; *SVT,* supraventricular tachycardia; *WCT,* wide complex tachycardia.

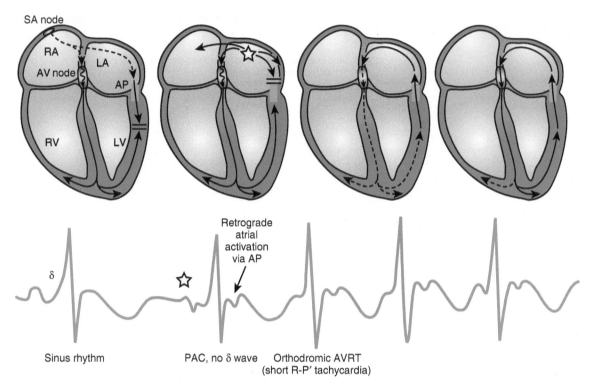

Fig. 6.5 Orthodromic atrioventricular reentrant tachycardia (AVRT) is a macroreentrant tachycardia with an anatomically defined circuit during conduction to the ventricles anterogradely down the normal atrioventricular (AV) conduction system and retrogradely to the atrium via an accessory pathway (AP). Often, an impulse from a premature atrial complex (PAC) or a premature ventricular complex can find the AP refractory, causing unidirectional block and initiation of reentry and resulting in an orthodromic AVRT. The first complex shows preexcitation during the sinus rhythm. It is followed by a PAC, which finds the AP refractory. The impulse reaches the ventricles via the AV node and conduction tissues. It finds the AP recovered retrogradely (third complex), and the circus movement orthodromic tachycardia is initiated (fourth complex). *Green rectangle* represents the AP; *APC,* Atrial premature complex; *LA,* left atrium; *LV,* left ventricle; *RA,* right atrium; *RV,* right ventricle; *SA,* sinoatrial.

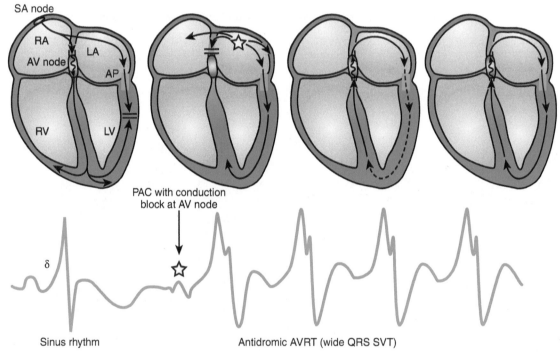

Fig. 6.6 Antidromic atrioventricular reentrant tachycardia (AVRT) or antidromic reciprocating tachycardia is a macroreentrant tachycardia with an anatomically defined circuit during conduction anterogradely to the ventricles down the accessory pathway (AP) and retrogradely to the atrium via the normal atrioventricular (AV) conduction system. Often, a premature atrial or a ventricular impulse finds the AV node refractory, causing unidirectional block and initiation of reentry, resulting in an antidromic reciprocating tachycardia. The first complex shows preexcitation during the sinus rhythm. It is followed by a premature atrial complex, which finds the AV node refractory (second complex). The impulse conducts anterogradely to the ventricles over the AP and retrogradely to the atria via the AV node (third complex), initiating a wide complex circus movement AVRT (fourth complex). *Green rectangle* represents the AP; *APC,* Atrial premature complex; *LA,* left atrium; *LV,* left ventricle; *RA,* right atrium; *RV,* right ventricle; *SA,* sinoatrial; *SVT,* supraventricular tachycardia.

Common Locations of Accessory Pathways Across the Mitral
and Tricuspid Annuli and Their Common Delta Wave Polarity on 12-Lead Electrocardiogram

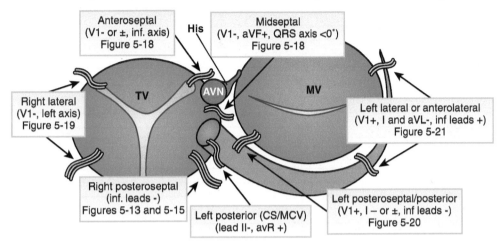

Fig. 6.7 Several algorithms have been developed, but as a general rule, a positive delta wave (first 40 ms of QRS complex) in lead V1 suggests a left-sided accessory pathway (AP), and a negative delta wave in V1 suggests a right-sided AP. A positive delta wave in inferior leads with inferior axis represents an anteroseptal AP. A left axis (with a negative delta wave in lead V1) suggests a right lateral AP. If the delta waves in the inferior leads are negative, it denotes a posteroseptal AP, on right or left side, depending on the delta wave vector in lead V1. A negative delta wave in lead II (more negative than lead III) and a positive delta wave in lead aVR suggest a posterior AP involving coronary sinus (CS) or middle cardiac vein (MCV). A negative delta wave in lead I, aVL, and V6 (rightward QRS axis) with a positive delta wave in lead V1 suggests a left lateral or anterolateral pathway. *AVN,* Atrioventricular node; *MV,* mitral valve; *TV,* tricuspid valve.

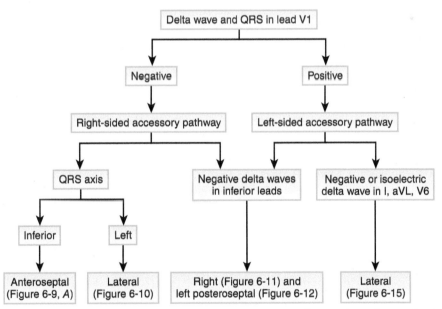

Fig. 6.8 A general guideline for localization of accessory pathway on a 12-lead electrocardiogram depending on the delta wave vector in Wolff-Parkinson-White syndrome.

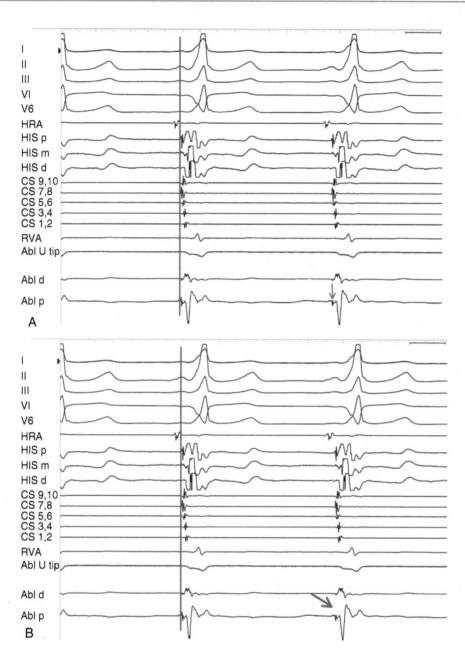

Fig. 6.9 (A) A 12-lead electrocardiogram showing a negative delta wave in lead V1 with inferior axis suggestive of anteroseptal pathway (*red arrow* shows pathway potential). (B) Intracardiac mapping with an ablation catheter revealed an early potential (*red arrow*) in the parahisian area. The potential must be defined, whether it is an atrial, His, or ventricular depolarization. (C) Rapid coronary sinus (CS) pacing separates atrial, His, and ventricular potentials. The pathway potential (*asterisk*) is earlier than the ventricular depolarization. Accessory pathway (AP) is refractory after the second CS paced beat and the His potential is clearly visible on the distal ablation catheter. Red line indicates onset of QRS complex. (D)Ablation catheter is pulled back, but the His potential is still recorded at the site of earliest ventricular depolarization. *Red asterisks* indicate His bundle potential. (E) Cryoablation abolished the delta wave caused by the AP at the parahisian area. *Red asterisk* indicates loss of preexcitation. (F) Right anterior oblique (RAO) view shows the close proximity of the His catheter and the ablation catheter during catheter ablation of the AP in the anteroseptal region. (G) Left anterior oblique (LAO) view shows the close proximity of the His catheter and the ablation catheter during catheter ablation of the AP in the anteroseptal region. *A,* Atrial electrogram; *Ablation,* ablation catheter; *Abl D,* ablation distal; *Abl P,* ablation proximal; *Abl U,* ablation distal unipolar; *CS,* coronary sinus; *H,* His bundle catheter; *HRA,* high right atrium; *His D,* distal His; *His M,* middle His; *His P,* proximal His; *RA,* high right atrial catheter; *RV,* right ventricular catheter; *RVA,* right ventricular apex; *V,* ventricular electrogram.

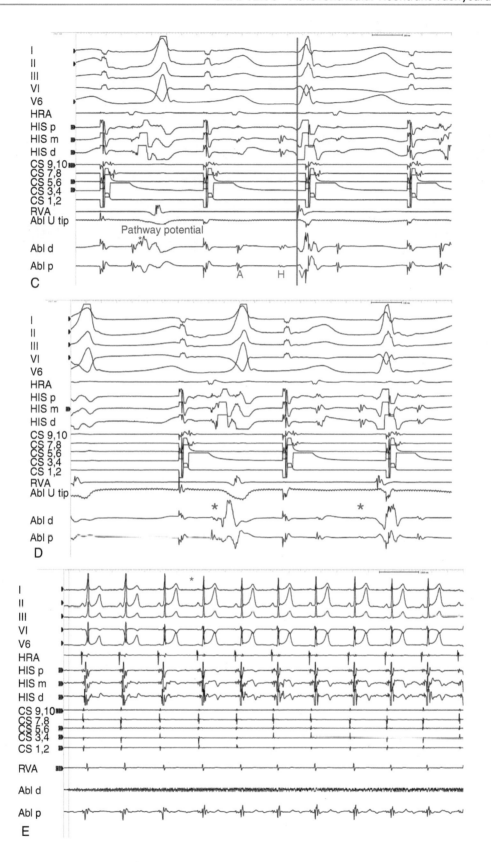

Fig. 6.9 (Continued).

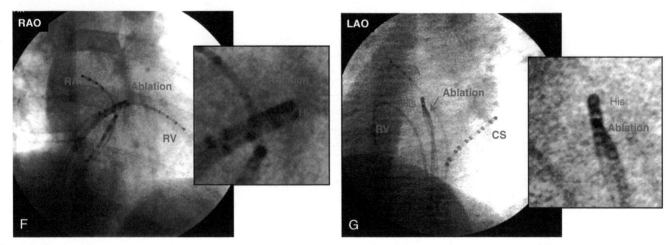

Fig. 6.9 (Continued).

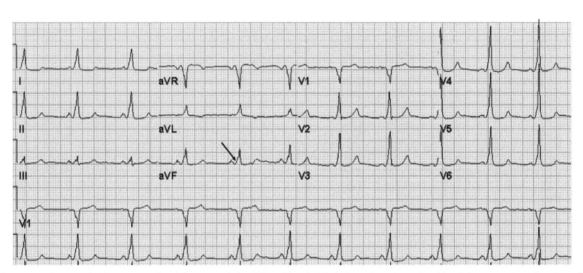

Fig. 6.10 Electrocardiogram depicts a negative delta wave in lead V1 with a left inferior axis suggestive of a right anterolateral or lateral accessory pathway. Accessory pathway was mapped to be in the right lateral tricuspid annulus. The *arrow* indicates delta wave.

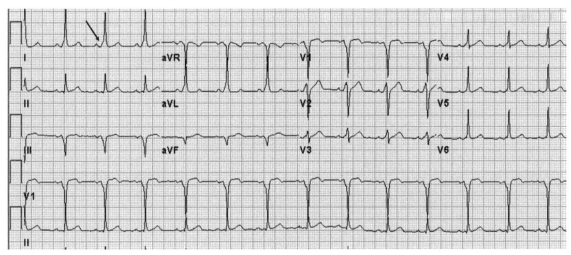

Fig. 6.11 Electrocardiogram reveals a negative delta wave in lead V1 suggesting a right-sided accessory pathway. Negative delta waves in leads III and aVF suggest posteroseptal or posterior location. The *arrow* indicates delta wave.

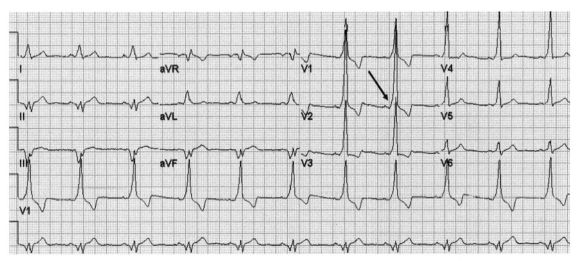

Fig. 6.12 Electrocardiogram shows a positive delta wave in lead V1 and negative delta waves in inferior leads, suggesting a left posteroseptal accessory pathway. The *arrow* indicates delta wave.

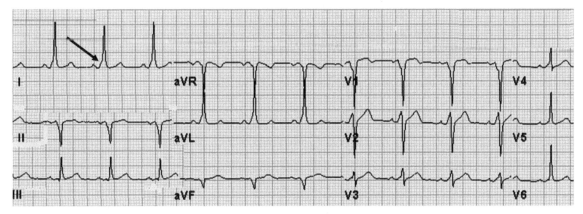

Fig. 6.13 Electrocardiogram depicts a more negative delta wave in lead II than in lead III, which suggests a pathway location in coronary sinus or middle cardiac vein. The *arrow* indicates delta wave.

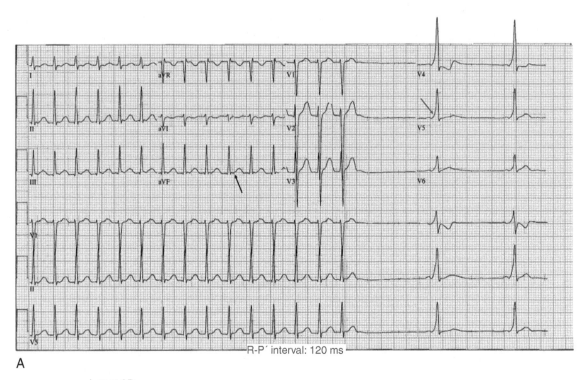

R-P′ interval: 120 ms

A

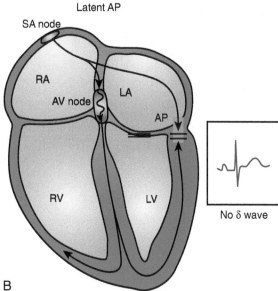

Latent AP

No δ wave

B

Fig. 6.14 (A) Electrocardiogram shows a short R-P′ tachycardia that terminates spontaneously. R-P′ interval is greater than 70 ms, suggesting an atrioventricular (AV) reentrant tachycardia rather than an AV nodal reentrant tachycardia. The *black arrow* indicates retrograde P waves. The last two beats show sinus rhythm with a positive delta (δ) wave in lead V1 and negative δ waves in lead I, aVL, and V6 (rightward QRS axis), suggesting a left lateral or anterolateral pathway. The *red arrow* indicates delta wave. (B) Latent pathway: Left lateral pathway is farther from the sinus node and, by the time the sinus impulse reaches the accessory pathway (AP), impulse via the AV node can reach the ventricular myocardium adjacent to the insertion of the AP, prohibiting preexcitation in some patients. However, these pathways are capable of initiating an orthodromic reciprocating tachycardia or antidromic reciprocating tachycardia by a premature atrial or ventricular complex. *Lines* indicate conduction pathways. *Green rectangle* indicates AP; *LA,* Left atrium; *LV,* left ventricle; *RA,* right atrium; *RV,* right ventricle; *SA,* sinoatrial.

LATENT ACCESSORY PATHWAYS

It is also important to note that left lateral APs may not be able to preexcite the left ventricle earlier than the arrival of the impulse via the normal route because of its distance from the sinus node. Alternatively, AV nodal conduction can be fast enough to excite the entire ventricular myocardium before the impulse reaches the ventricle by way of the more distant left lateral AP (Fig. 6.14B). Therefore the baseline ECG can be unremarkable or show minimal preexcitation with a normal PR interval and no delta wave on the ECG. These pathways can become manifest only when AV nodal conduction is relatively slow as a result of altered autonomic tone or a rapid atrial rate caused by sinus tachycardia (e.g., during exercise) or during atrial arrhythmias. This is known as a *latent WPW syndrome*. Fig. 6.15 shows the ECG of a patient with minimal preexcitation who developed an AVRT. Fig. 6.16 shows the ECG of a patient with minimal preexcitation who developed an ORT (Fig. 6.16B). The intracardiac recording shows earliest atrial activation at the lateral mitral annulus during the SVT (Fig. 6.16C). The patient developed ART (Fig. 6.16D) on a different occasion. Fig. 6.17 shows a right-sided AP with minimal preexcitation, but its posteroseptal location cannot be determined with a high probability until the ART occurs.

EFFECT OF BUNDLE BRANCH BLOCK ON THE TACHYCARDIA CYCLE LENGTH DURING ORTHODROMIC RECIPROCATING TACHYCARDIA

When a patient develops bundle branch block (BBB) (aberrancy) ipsilateral (same side) to the AP during an ORT, the tachycardia usually slows because the anterograde impulse from the His bundle to the ventricle must travel over the contralateral bundle branch and ventricle, and then transseptally to the ipsilateral ventricle and atrium via the AP. This prolongs the impulse transit time from the AV node to the AP by

30 to 50 ms, and therefore the tachycardia cycle length (CL) prolongs during the ipsilateral BBB (Fig. 6.18). However, if the same patient develops bundle branch aberrancy on the side contralateral to the location of the AP, the tachycardia CL does not change because that bundle branch does not take part in the anterograde conduction during the ORT.

ATRIAL ARRHYTHMIAS IN WOLFF-PARKINSON-WHITE SYNDROME AND RISK FOR SUDDEN CARDIAC DEATH

SCD resulting from VF is a rare manifestation of WPW syndrome, with an incidence of 0.09% to 0.13%. High-risk patients include those with rapidly conducting APs (1:1 AV conduction usually at >250 bpm) and multiple APs. SCD can be the first manifestation of the WPW syndrome in approximately half of these patients. Fig. 6.19 shows the ECG of a previously asymptomatic patient who presented with AF and a rapid ventricular response that later degenerated to VF. The artifacts on the ECG suggest generalized convulsions resulting from cerebral anoxia caused by hypoperfusion during the tachyarrhythmia. The ECG after defibrillation (Fig. 6.12) revealed a left posteroseptal AP that was ablated successfully. Careful examination of the ECG is necessary to recognize preexcitation in a relatively regular wide complex tachycardia because it can mimic a ventricular tachycardia. Fig. 6.20A shows a subtle variation in the ventricular rate with a slurred upstroke in QRS complexes during AF and atrial flutter. ECG repeated after a few minutes revealed a preexcited rhythm during AF (Fig. 6.20B). The ECG revealed sinus rhythm after chemical cardioversion with ibutilide with a positive delta wave in lead V1 and negative delta wave in lead III and aVF (Fig. 6.20C). The AP was mapped at the posteroseptal mitral annulus. Atrial flutter or atrial tachycardia can also conduct rapidly via the AP (Fig. 6.21).

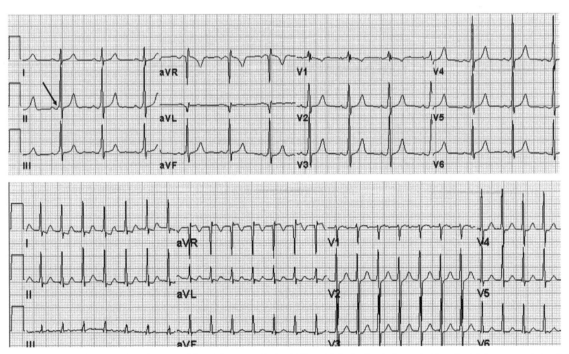

Fig. 6.15 Baseline electrocardiogram showing a positive delta wave in lead V1 and inferior leads (*arrow*). Negative delta waves in lead aVR and aVL suggest a more midline location. The patient presented with an orthodromic reciprocating tachycardia (*lower* electrocardiogram). The accessory pathway was mapped in the anterolateral mitral annulus.

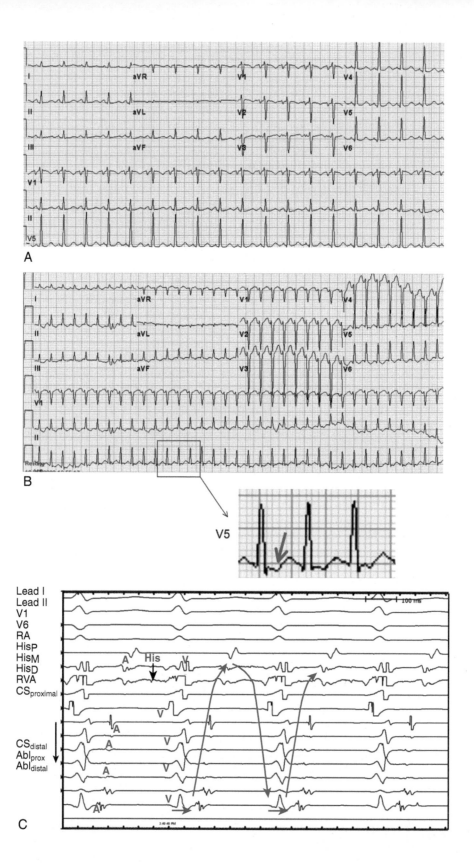

Fig. 6.16 Latent Wolff-Parkinson-White syndrome. Baseline electrocardiograms (ECGs) of a patient with Wolff-Parkinson-White syndrome do not show any evidence of preexcitation. (A) Delta wave was demonstrated during rapid atrial pacing during the electrophysiology study. (B) ECG of the same patient who presented with an orthodromic reciprocating tachycardia. The retrograde P waves are not clearly visible, except in lead V5. Negative P waves suggest a possible left lateral accessory pathway (AP). (C) Intracardiac recording during the orthodromic reciprocating tachycardia revealed earliest atrial activation in the ablation catheter placed in the lateral mitral annulus. *Red arrows* show the pathway of impulses traveling from the left atrium (A) anterogradely via the atrioventricular node to the His bundle (His) to the ventricles (V) and retrogradely via the AP in the lateral mitral annulus back to the atrium. (D) ECG of same patient reveals an antidromic reciprocating tachycardia with slurred upstrokes in lead V1 with isoelectric delta waves in lead I and aVL. Inferior leads show positive delta waves (*arrow*). AP was mapped at the lateral mitral annulus. *Abl*, Ablation catheter; *CS*, coronary sinus; *His D*, distal His; *His M*, middle His; *His P*, proximal His; *RA*, right atrium; *RVA*, right ventricular apex.

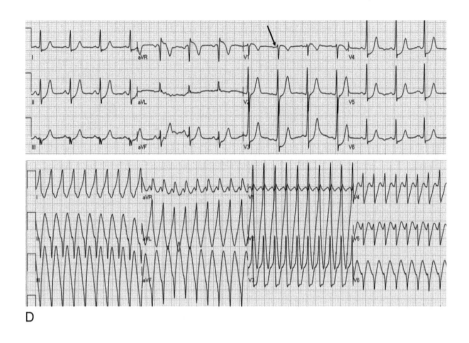

D

Fig. 6.16 (Continued).

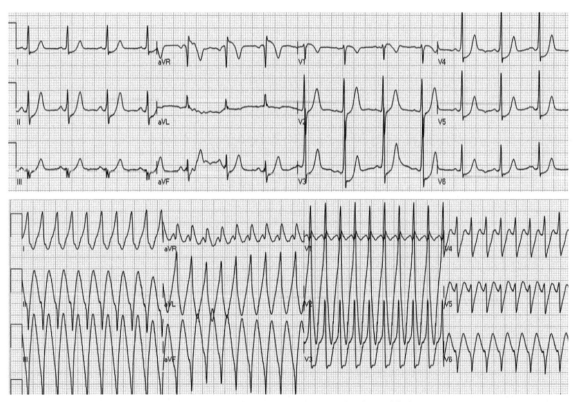

Fig. 6.17 Baseline electrocardiogram showing sinus rhythm with a minimal preexcitation in lead II. *Lower* electrocardiogram revealed an antidromic reciprocating tachycardia with a positive delta wave in lead V1 and negative delta wave in the inferior leads.

Effect of Bundle Branch Block on Tachycardia Rate

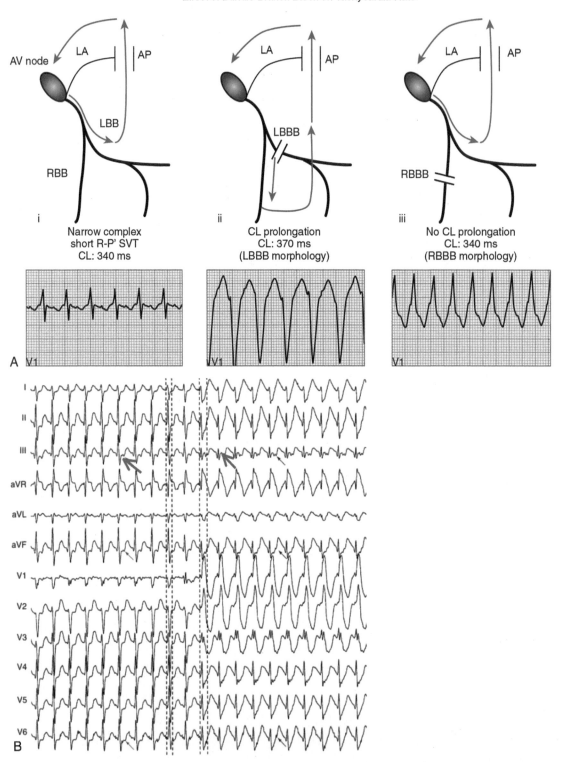

Fig. 6.18 (A) (i) Short R-P' orthodromic reciprocating tachycardia (ORT) at cycle length (CL) 340 ms in patient with left lateral accessory pathway (AP). Impulse from the left atrium travels anterogradely down the atrioventricular (AV) node, His bundle, and left bundle branch (LBB) to the AP (parallel vertical lines) to reach the left atrium. (ii) Tachycardia slows during left bundle branch block (LBBB) aberrancy because the impulse from the His bundle travels to the right bundle branch (RBB) and then transmyocardially from the right ventricle to the left ventricle to left atrium via the AP. This prolongs the impulse transit time from the AV node to the AP by 30 to 50 ms, and therefore the tachycardia CL prolongs during the ipsilateral bundle branch block. (iii) Same patient developed RBB aberrancy, but the tachycardia CL did not change because the pathway of impulse is unaffected insofar as the RBB does not take part in the ORT. Therefore the tachycardia rate essentially remains similar to the *narrow* complex ORT. (B) Electrocardiogram of ORT using a concealed right-sided paraseptal AP. Note the P waves (*arrows*) inscribed within the ST-T wave segment (short R-P' interval). Ischemic-appearing ST segment depression is also observed. Functional right bundle branch block (RBBB) occurs in the right side of the tracing, with prolongation of the R-P' (ventriculoatrial) interval, suggesting that retrograde ventriculoatrial conduction during the supraventricular tachycardia (SVT) is mediated by a right-sided AP. *Dashed lines* denote the QRS onset and P wave onset.[3]

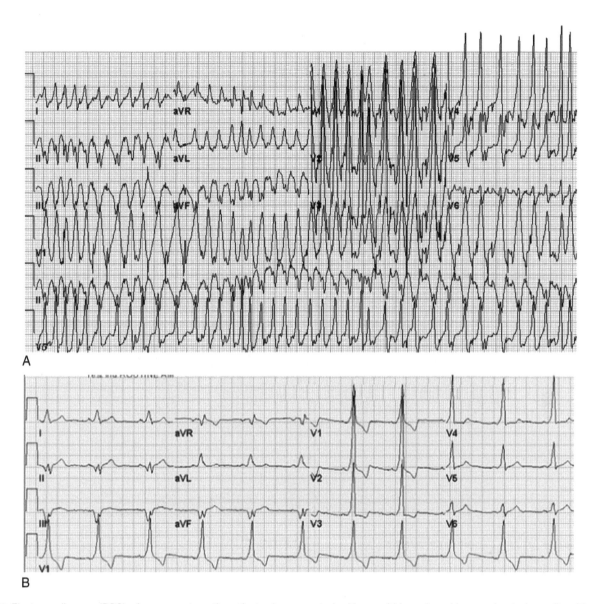

Fig. 6.19 Electrocardiogram (ECG) of an asymptomatic patient who presented with a rapid irregular wide complex tachycardia with a slurred upstroke in leads V1 through V5 with changing amplitude and duration of QRS. However, the QRS vector remains the same in each lead. This is suggestive of atrial fibrillation and a rapid ventricular response caused by rapid conduction via the accessory pathway. Rhythm later degenerated to ventricular fibrillation. Patient was resuscitated with two successive biphasic direct current shocks of 360 joules. ECG after resuscitation (Fig. 6.12) revealed a left posteroseptal accessory pathway that was ablated successfully.

INTERMITTENT PREEXCITATION

Signs of preexcitation are absent in the initial ECG in 22% of subjects with WPW pattern, and 40% of these may lose preexcitation in subsequent ECG recordings. Intermittent preexcitation results from age-related degeneration of the APs, and usually these pathways have a longer refractory period. Intermittent preexcitation indicates that the AP is incapable of conduction to the ventricle fast enough to pose a risk for VF during rapid atrial arrhythmias, such as AF or atrial flutter (Fig. 6.22). An important indicator of a low risk is the disappearance of preexcitation during exercise owing to a long anterograde refractory period of the AP (Fig. 6.23).

MULTIPLE ACCESSORY PATHWAYS

Multiple APs are present in 5% to 10% of patients and are higher in patients with Ebstein anomaly (10%–38%). It can involve an AP as one limb and the AV node or another AP as the other limb during SVT. If pathways are anatomically close, the tachycardia rate may not vary much and is difficult to diagnose on a 12-lead ECG. Antidromic tachycardia involving two different pathways may be present if there is a change in the morphology of QRS complexes and a change in the tachycardia rate when the impulse switches from one AP to the other during an ART (Figs. 6.24 and 6.25). When tachycardia involves APs only for the circuit, then the SVT can be fast and can induce ventricular tachycardia and pose a risk for SCD. Fig. 6.25A and B show ECGs of one patient with two APs.

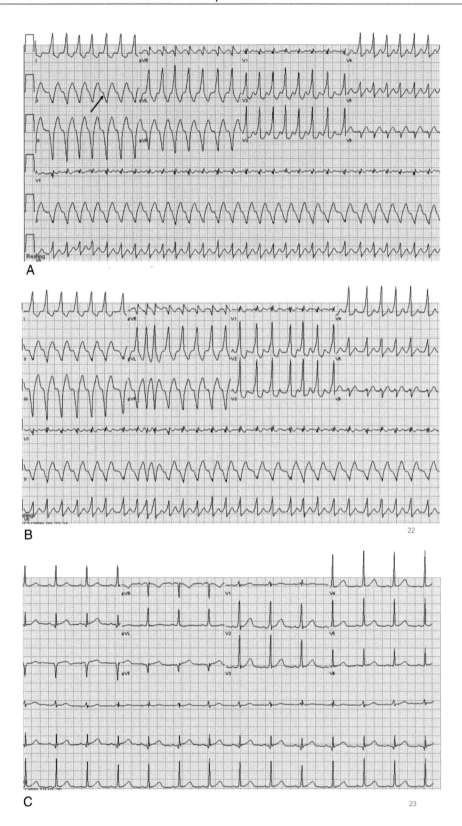

Fig. 6.20 (A) Electrocardiogram (ECG) shows a wide complex tachycardia with slurred upstrokes in precordial leads (V2–V5) and slurred downstroke in inferior lead (*arrow*). Tachycardia appears regular, mimicking a monomorphic ventricular tachycardia. However, on careful measurement the tachycardia cycle length variation is evident. (B) After a few minutes, ECG reveals an irregular wide complex tachycardia with slurred upstrokes in precordial leads (V2–V5) and slurred downstroke in inferior lead. This is atrial fibrillation with antidromic conduction via the accessory pathway. Tachycardia terminated with intravenous ibutilide. (C) ECG depicts sinus rhythm after chemical cardioversion with a positive delta wave in lead V1 and negative delta wave in lead III and aVF. Accessory pathway was mapped at the posteroseptal mitral annulus.

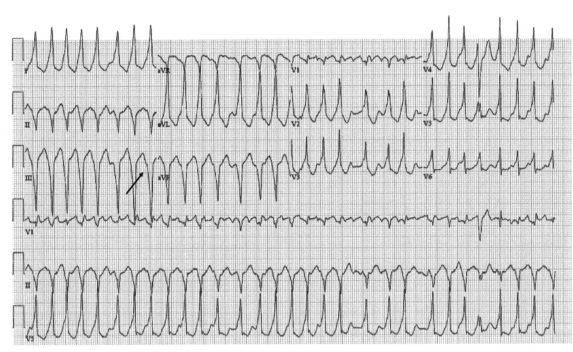

Fig. 6.21 Electrocardiogram shows atypical atrial flutter with negative delta waves in inferior leads (*arrow*). The delta wave polarity is not clear in lead V1 owing to flutter waves. The accessory pathway could not be ablated at the right posteroseptal tricuspid annulus or left posteroseptal mitral annulus via a transseptal approach. Accessory pathway was abolished by retrograde aortic approach in the posteroseptal mitral annulus.

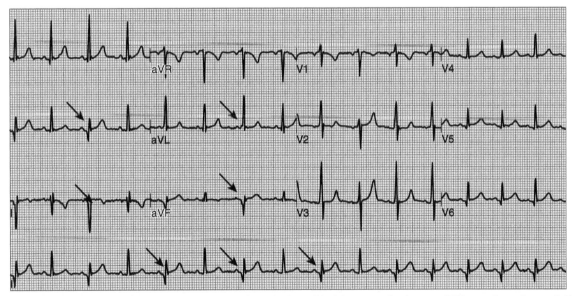

Fig. 6.22 Intermittent preexcitation. Electrocardiogram shows sinus rhythm with delta waves in alternate QRS complexes (*arrows*). This pathway is unlikely to conduct to the ventricle to initiate an antidromic reciprocating tachycardia or cause rapid ventricular rates during atrial tachycardia, atrial flutter, or atrial fibrillation.

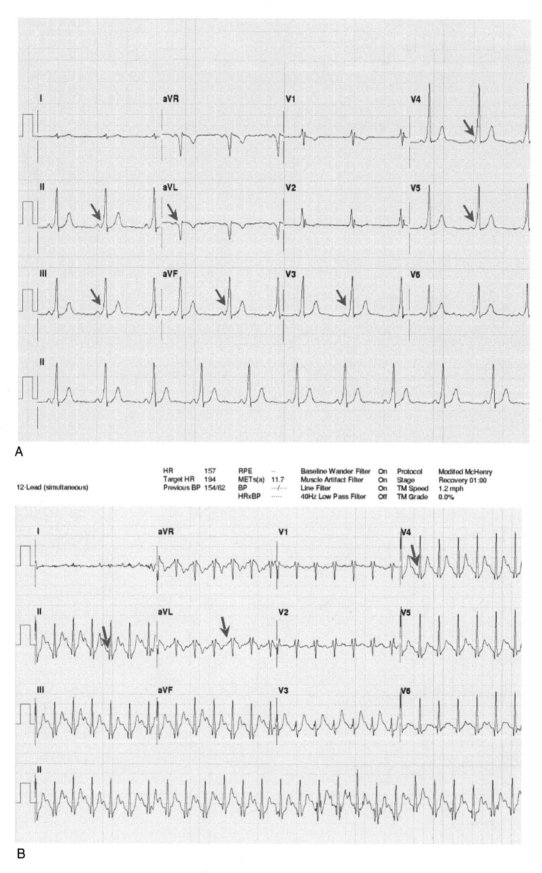

Fig. 6.23 (A) Resting 12-lead electrocardiogram (ECG) before exercise stress test shows positive delta waves in lead V1 and inferior leads (*red arrows*) suggestive of a left lateral or, most likely, an anterolateral pathway (negative delta waves in lead aVR and aVL suggest the pathway location toward midline). (B) ECG during treadmill exercise at 157 bpm shows loss of delta waves in all ECG leads (*red arrows*). It is suggestive of a relatively longer anterograde refractory period of the accessory pathway with almost no risk of atrial fibrillation with a rapid ventricular response causing ventricular fibrillation and sudden cardiac death.

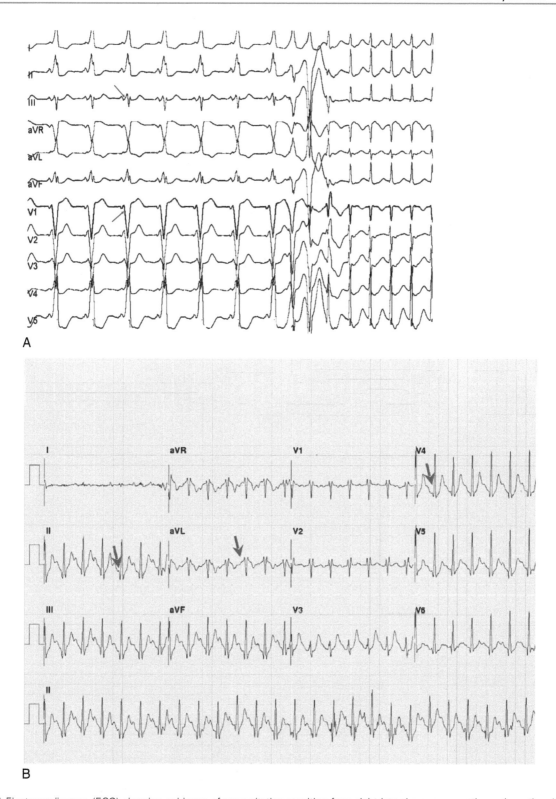

Fig. 6.24 (A) Electrocardiogram (ECG) showing evidence of preexcitation resulting from right lateral accessory pathway (negative delta waves in lead V1 and positive delta waves in inferior leads (*arrows*). The orthodromic reciprocating tachycardia (ORT) was induced following ventricular couplets during an electrophysiology study. (B) ECG depicts the ORT with a R-P′ (*red arrow*) interval greater than 80 ms, suggesting an atrioventricular reentrant tachycardia. (C) Another short R-P′ tachycardia was induced with a slightly longer R-P′ interval during the electrophysiology study in the same patient. (D) ECG reveals evidence of preexcitation owing to right lateral accessory pathway with negative delta waves in lead V1 and positive delta waves in inferior leads (*black arrow*) and left lateral pathway during coronary sinus pacing (*red arrow*) in the same patient. (E) Intracardiac recordings show an ORT involving left lateral pathway demonstrated by the earliest atrial excitation in the distal coronary sinus (*red arrow*). Blue arrow shows atrial electrogram recording at His-bundle catheter. The activation changes spontaneously with earliest atrial activation in the high right atrium/His bundle (*blue arrow*), suggesting that ORT now involves a right-sided accessory pathway. In summary, this patient had two accessory pathways (right lateral and left lateral). *His D,* Distal His; *His M,* middle His; *His P,* proximal His; *HRA,* high right atrium; *RV,* right ventricle.

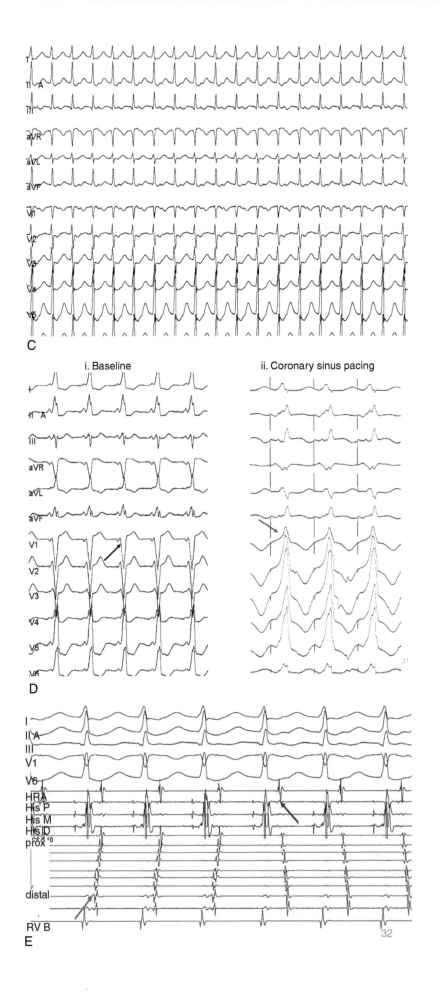

Fig. 6.24 (Continued).

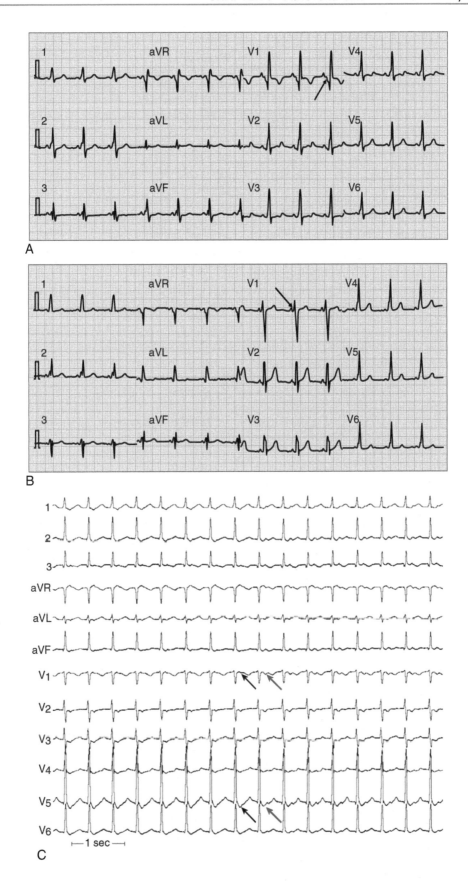

Fig. 6.25 (A) Electrocardiogram showing negative delta waves in lead V1 suggestive of a right-sided accessory pathway (AP) (*arrow*). (B) Another electrocardiogram of the same patient reveals positive delta waves in lead V1 suggestive of a left-sided AP (*arrow*). (C) During the orthodromic reciprocating tachycardia in the same patient, retrograde P wave morphology (*black arrows*) switches after the ninth QRS complex (*red arrows*), indicating the presence of two retrogradely conducting APs. Retrograde limb switches from one pathway to the other during tachycardia.

CONGENITAL ANOMALY AND INHERITED WOLFF-PARKINSON-WHITE SYNDROME

WPW syndrome can be familial, occur in congenital heart diseases, such as Ebstein anomaly (Fig. 6.26), and be associated with multiple APs. Inherited cardiomyopathies, such as hypertrophic cardiomyopathy, resulting from γ2 regulatory subunit of adenosine monophosphate—activated protein kinase (*PRKAG2*) and (*PRKAG3*) gene mutations can also be associated with an AP (Fig. 6.27).

VARIANTS OF PREEXCITATION

Atypical APs are a group of rare APs with uncommon connections known as *Mahaim fibers*. These were described by Mahaim and Bennett[1] during pathologic examination of the heart (Fig. 6.28). They include atriofascicular, nodoventricular, and nodofascicular pathways. Although these APs are sometimes collectively referred to as Mahaim fibers, the use of this term is discouraged because it is more illuminating to name the precise AP according to its connections. Therefore these APs are often collectively called *atypical* APs to differentiate them from the more common (*typical*) rapidly conducting APs that result in the WPW syndrome. The role of these connections in initiating a tachycardia is not proved in many instances. The most common atypical AP is the atriofascicular pathway. The tissue of these APs appears structurally similar to that of the normal AV node, with an AV node—like structure leading to a His bundle—like structure, and has decremental conduction properties (i.e., conduction slows at faster heart rates) and can be blocked by adenosine. In contrast to WPW syndrome, there is no delta wave with atriofascicular fiber conduction because these fibers connect to the distal right bundle branch. In addition, the atriofascicular pathways have decremental properties, and therefore the baseline ECG is narrow or minimally preexcited and the AV interval prolongs with rapid atrial pacing. These fibers conduct anterogradely only. ART associated with an atriofascicular pathway has a left BBB and left superior axis QRS morphology resulting from anterograde conduction over the atriofascicular pathway, and its common anatomic location is in the right ventricle (Fig. 6.29).

Enhanced AV nodal conduction is described as a short P-R interval (<120 ms) and a normal QRS complex on ECG (Fig. 6.30). A perinodal structure described by Lown et al.[2] was suggested as the anatomic substrate. However, the existence of such a pathway is doubtful, and the entity may simply represent patients who have enhanced AV nodal conduction and also happen to have tachycardias, possibly caused by a coexisting AP or dual AV nodal physiology. The term "LGL syndrome" is catchy for this because its phrasing is similar to "WPW," but it probably does not exist as a distinct entity. AF and atrial tachycardia can conduct to the ventricles rapidly in patients with a short P-R interval. The short P-R interval can have different mechanisms, such as a low atrial ectopic rhythm with differential input into the AV node and isorhythmic AV dissociation, in which case the short P-R interval is not caused by a conducted P wave (Fig. 6.31).

ELECTROCARDIOGRAM CHARACTERISTICS OF ORTHODROMIC RECIPROCATING TACHYCARDIA CAUSED BY CONCEALED ACCESSORY PATHWAYS

ECG during a short R-P′ tachycardia can help in differentiating an ORT resulting from a concealed AP from an AV nodal reentrant tachycardia (AVNRT) or atrial tachycardia.

1. A 1:1 A-V relationship is a prerequisite for maintenance of an orthodromic or antidromic AVRT because parts of both the atrium and ventricle are essential components of the reentrant circuit. Therefore an orthodromic AVRT is excluded if a tachycardia persists in the presence of AV block or if there are more QRS complexes than P waves (likely a ventricular tachycardia) or more P waves than QRS complexes (likely an atrial tachycardia) present during the tachycardia.
2. R-P interval during SVT:
   a. Orthodromic AVRT is a short R-P′ tachycardia because the conduction time over the AP is commonly 40 to 120 ms (except for those APs that are slowly conducting). Therefore the R-P interval is short but still longer than that during typical AVNRT because the wavefront has to activate a part of the ipsilateral ventricle before it reaches the atrium by way of

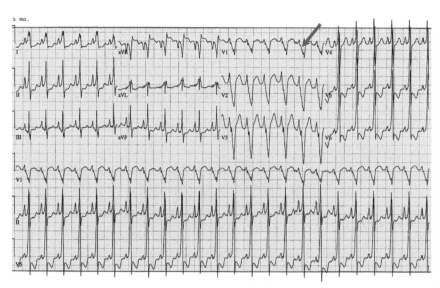

Fig. 6.26 Electrocardiogram of a patient with Ebstein anomaly with a right-sided accessory pathway. Peaked P wave (>0.5 mV) with an inferior axis is suggestive of right atrial enlargement. Negative delta wave in lead V1 (*arrow*) and positive delta wave in II and aVF suggest a possible right lateral accessory pathway. Up to 10% of these patients may have multiple accessory pathways.

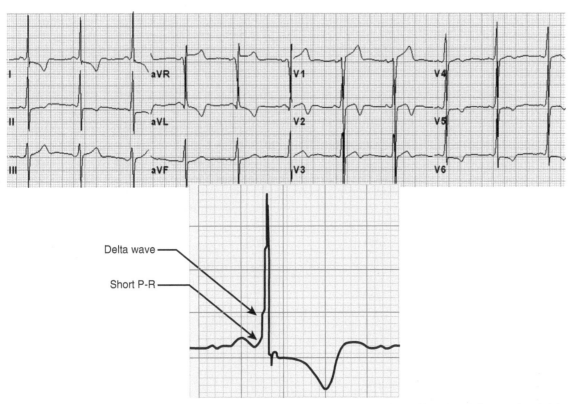

Fig. 6.27 Electrocardiogram of a patient with hypertrophic cardiomyopathy showing sinus rhythm with a short P-R interval and delta waves with evidence of left ventricular hypertrophy (R wave amplitude 1.7 mV and T wave inversion in precordial and lateral leads).

Atypical and Rare Accessory Pathway Location

Atriofasciular

Atrioventricular

Nodoventricular

Atriohisian

Nodofascicular

Fasciculoventricular

Fig. 6.28 Atypical accessory pathways (APs). APs commonly connects atrium to the ventricle (*purple*). Rarely, APs involve atypical anatomy. The most common atypical AP is *atriofascicular* (*green*), which connects the right atrium to the right ventricle (RV). The AP usually crosses the lateral RV and reaches the right ventricular apex subendocardially. It inserts into the distal right bundle branch. The pathway is slowly conducting and has decremental property, and therefore does not show preexcitation or has a minimal preexcitation at normal heart rates. The antidromic tachycardia results in left bundle branch block, left superior axis morphology. *Nodoventricular* (*blue*) AP connects the atrioventricular (AV) node to the ventricles (usually the RV). Electrocardiogram reveals evidence of preexcitation, but the AP does not cause tachycardia. *Nodofascicular* (*red*) AP connects the AV node to one of the bundle branches, and therefore there is no evidence of preexcitation on the electrocardiogram. AV pathways usually connect the atrium to the ipsilateral ventricle across the valve annulus and usually inserts in close proximity to the valve annulus. These APs may be oblique. Sometimes these pathways may insert farther away from the valve annulus in the atrium or the ventricle. Rarely, these pathways may connect the atrial appendage to the ventricle. The *atriohisian* (*dark green*) AP connects the atrium to the His bundle and is associated with a short P-R interval. The existence of this type of AP is controversial, and most of these APs are thought to be just an enhanced AV nodal conduction. *Fasciculoventricular* (*light blue*) APs connect one of the bundles to the ventricular myocardium.

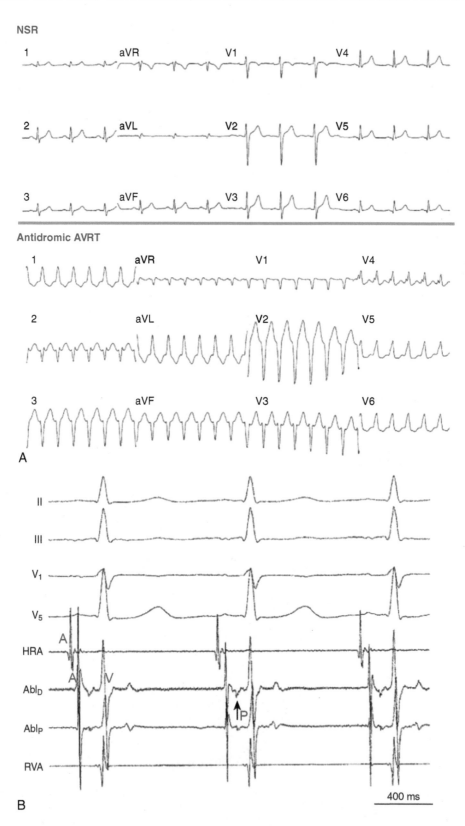

Fig. 6.29 (A) Because the accessory pathway (AP) conducts slowly, sinus rhythm electrocardiogram of a patient with atriohisian AP is usually unremarkable owing to ventricular depolarization via the normal conduction tissue via the atrioventricular node, His bundle, and the bundle branches. However, during the antidromic reciprocating tachycardia, conduction anterogradely down the AP to the right ventricle near the apex and then to both the ventricles results in a left bundle branch block and left superior axis morphology. (B) Intracardiac mapping at the lateral tricuspid annulus shows a pathway potential (P, *arrow*) at the ablation catheter. *A,* Atrial electrogram; *Abl D,* ablation distal; *Abl P,* ablation proximal; *AVRT,* atrioventricular reentrant tachycardia, *HRA,* high right atrium; *NSR,* normal sinus rhythm; *RVA,* right ventricular apex; *V,* right ventricular electrogram.

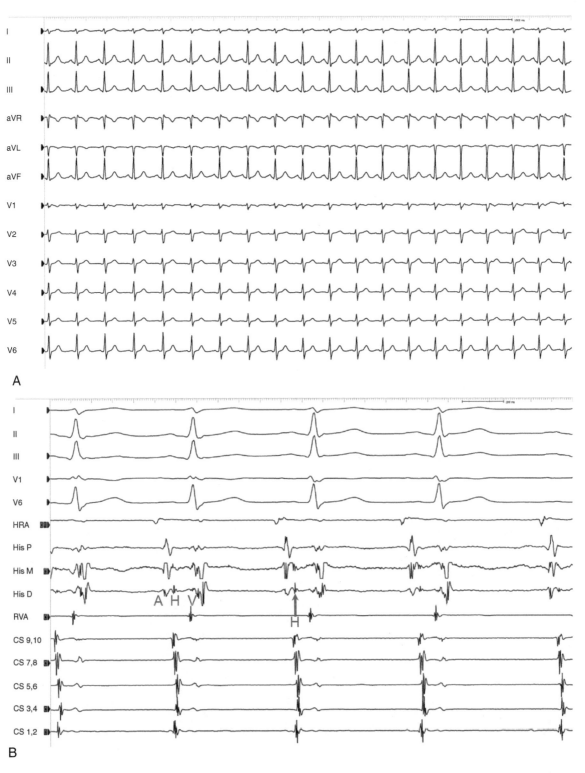

Fig. 6.30 (A) Scalar electrocardiogram (ECG) of an asymptomatic patient with short P-R interval due to rapid AVN conduction and no accessory pathway found. (B) Intracardiac ECGs revealed an A-H interval of 48 ms and H-V of 50 ms. (C) Intracardiac ECGs revealed an A-H interval of 60 ms and H-V of 50 ms during 200 bpm with 1:1 atrioventricular conduction with right bundle branch block pattern. *A*, Atrial electrogram; *CS*, coronary sinus; *H*, His bundle electrograms; *His D*, distal His; *His M*, middle His; *His P*, proximal His; *HRA*, high right atrium; *RVA*, right ventricular apex; *V*, ventricular electrogram.

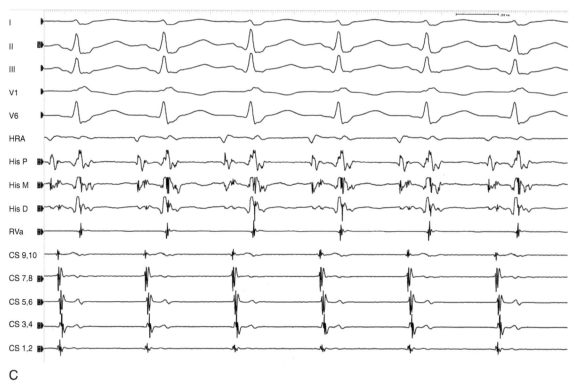

C

Fig. 6.30 (Continued).

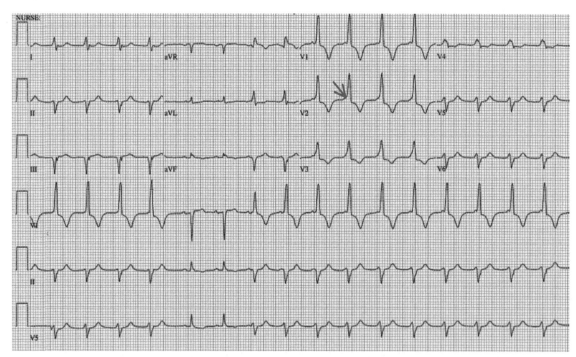

Fig. 6.31 Electrocardiogram shows slurred upstroke in leads V2 through V4 (*arrow*) due to fusion beats mimicking Wolff-Parkinson-White syndrome. Electrocardiogram reveals sinus rhythm with a four-beat run of narrow ventricular tachycardia followed by two beats of normal sinus rhythm with a normal P-R interval. The ventricular tachycardia initiated again at a cycle length nearly identical to the sinus rate resulting in isorhythmic atrioventricular dissociation and a short P-R interval, which is more clearly seen in the rhythm strip (leads V1 and II).

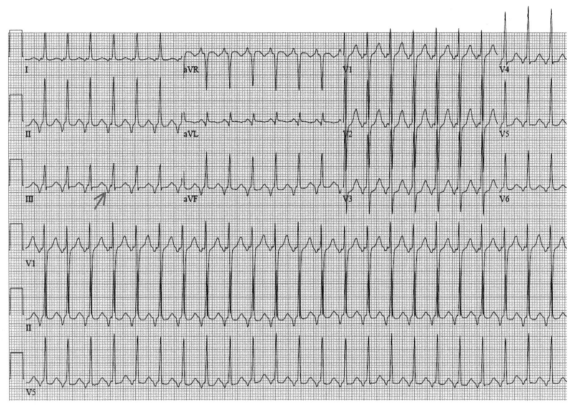

Fig. 6.32 Electrocardiogram of a patient with incessant atrioventricular reentrant tachycardia and tachycardia-induced cardiomyopathy depicts a long R-P′ tachycardia with narrow and inverted P waves in inferior leads (*arrow*) suggestive of posteroseptal pathways. The tachycardia should be differentiated from atypical atrioventricular nodal reentrant tachycardia, which has similar P wave morphology.

the AP at the AV groove. An R-P′ interval of less than 70 ms during tachycardia practically excludes an orthodromic AVRT and is consistent with AVNRT.

b. Slow-slow AVNRT versus AVRT using a posteroseptal AP: A slow-slow AVNRT is associated with an R-P′ interval greater than 70 ms and P wave morphology similar to that during orthodromic AVRT using a posteroseptal AP. Although both SVTs have the earliest atrial activation in the posteroseptal region, conduction time from that site to the His bundle region is significantly longer in AVNRT than in AVRT, resulting in a significantly longer R-P interval in lead V1 and a larger difference in the R-P interval between V1 and the inferior leads. Therefore ΔR-P′ interval (lead V1−III) greater than 20 ms suggests slow-slow AVNRT rather than an AVRT using a posteroseptal AP.

c. Slowly conducting concealed APs, such as permanent junctional reciprocating tachycardia, are usually a long R-P′ tachycardia that can be incessant and can cause tachycardia-induced cardiomyopathy (Fig. 6.32).

3. Tachycardia CL changes:

a. Tachycardia CL variation or oscillation: The R-P intervals during orthodromic AVRT remain constant regardless of oscillations in tachycardia CL. The tachycardia CL usually

changes as a result of changes in AV nodal conduction properties mostly owing to changes in autonomic tone.

b. Tachycardia CL can also change if the patient has dual AV nodal pathways and the conduction via the AV node alternates between slow and fast AV nodal pathways. Alternatively, AVRT can change to AVNRT.

c. Tachycardia CL changes can occur if the patient has more than one AP.

4. BBB during SVT: Ipsilateral BBB can prolong the tachycardia CL, as described previously (Fig. 6.18).

REFERENCES

1. Mahaim I, Bennett A. Nouvelle recherches sur les connexions sup'erieures de la branche gauche du faisceau de His-Tawara avec cloison interventriculaire. *Cardiologia.* 1938;1:61−76.
2. Lown B, Canong WF, Levine SA. The syndrome of short P-R interval, normal QRS complex and paroxysmal rapid heart action. *Circulation.* 1952;5:693.
3. Issa ZF, Miller JM, Zipes DP. *Clinical Arrhythmology and Electrophysiology.* 3rd ed. Philadelphia, PA: WB Saunders; 2019:599−677.

7

Atrial Tachycardia

Atrial tachycardia (AT) is defined as a usually regular atrial rhythm originating from the atrium at 100 to 240 bpm. The presence of an atrial rate above 100 bpm with three different P wave morphologies signifies different foci of atrial depolarization and is called a *multifocal atrial tachycardia*. It is often irregular. Previous classifications of AT had been based exclusively on the scalar electrocardiogram (ECG) with a constant rate and an isoelectric line between the two consecutive P waves. Atrial flutter (AFL) is typically a reentrant arrhythmia defined as having a pattern of regular tachycardia with a rate above 240 bpm without an isoelectric baseline between deflections. The typical (cavotricuspid dependent; see Chapter 8) AFL usually shows sawtooth pattern in inferior ECG leads. ATs can also have a reentrant mechanism, usually seen around a scar in the atrium. The ECG pattern can mimic an atypical (noncavotricuspid dependent) AFL. However, neither rate nor lack of isoelectric baseline is specific for any tachycardia mechanism. A rapid AT in a scarred atrium can mimic AFL; however, a typical AFL can show distinct isoelectric intervals between flutter waves in diseased atria, or in the presence of antiarrhythmic drug therapy. Therefore it becomes a matter of semantics to define an AT or an atypical AFL. AT can result from a focal mechanism, such as abnormal automaticity or triggered activity. Unlike prior definitions stating that focal ATs have a constant rate, a focal AT can show a significant cycle length ($>15\%$) variation, more than that seen in a reentrant AT, and can also occur in diseased atria. Table 7.1 shows the classification of AT/AFL. Focal automatic ATs occur mostly in children and young adults. Focal automatic ATs begin with a P wave identical to the P wave during the arrhythmia, and the rate generally increases gradually (warms up) over the first few seconds. Automatic ATs are catecholamine sensitive and cannot be induced or terminated by programmed electrical stimulation (PES). ATs resulting from triggered activity can arise anywhere in the atria but most commonly originate from the crista terminalis, tricuspid annulus, and mitral annulus. These ATs can be induced and terminated with PES. The majority of focal ATs caused by triggered activity are adenosine sensitive. Rarely, a microreentrant AT can appear to be focal in origin during mapping, but its reentrant mechanism can be elucidated after a careful electrophysiology study including entrainment. Macroreentrant AT and AFL are discussed in detail in Chapter 8.

The location of the focal source of an AT is determined by P wave morphology and vector on 12-lead ECG (Figs. 7.1 and 7.2). Focal AT can arise anywhere in the atrium, pulmonary veins (PVs), and venae cavae (Figs. 7.3 through 7.9). Focal ATs usually have discrete P waves at rates of 110 to 240 bpm, but AT/AFL arising from PVs can be as fast as 300 bpm. Antiarrhythmic drugs can slow the AT/AFL rate by decreasing the conduction velocity or increasing the refractory period of the reentrant circuit, and an isoelectric line between two P waves can be seen. Shorter atrial activation with a shorter P wave duration and longer diastolic intervals on the ECG distinguishes a focal from a macroreentrant AT with 90% sensitivity and specificity. Careful analysis of the 12-lead ECG and rhythm strips, as well as vagal maneuvers and

drug interventions (adenosine and atrioventricular [AV] nodal blockers), help in determining the mechanism of an AT. An electrophysiology study is helpful in determining the focus of an AT or the isthmus of a reentrant AT (Figs. 7.10 through 7.18).

P AND QRS RELATIONSHIP DURING ATRIAL TACHYCARDIA

1. ATs usually have a long R-P′ interval but can have a short R-P′ interval in the presence of significant first-degree AV block at baseline or in the presence of dual AV nodal physiology with AV conduction via the slow pathway.
2. The atrial to ventricular relationship depends on the ability of AV nodal conduction during the tachycardia. It is usually 1:1 conduction during ATs; however, Wenckebach pattern or 2:1 AV block can occur. The presence of AV block during supraventricular tachycardia strongly suggests AT and excludes an AV reentrant tachycardia (AVRT) (see Chapter 6). Rarely, an AV nodal reentrant tachycardia (AVNRT) with lower common pathway block or His-Purkinje disease can show AV block and variable relation of P waves with QRS.
3. Termination of a supraventricular tachycardia without a following QRS practically rules out an AT.

EFFECT OF DRUG THERAPY ON ATRIAL TACHYCARDIA AND ATRIAL FLUTTER

With AV nodal disease or AV nodal drug therapy, 4:1 or variable AV block can occur. In the presence of antiarrhythmic drug therapy, the cycle length of AFL can prolong or atrial fibrillation can organize to a relatively slower flutter that allows the AV node to conduct 1:1 to the ventricles resulting in a rapid ventricular response and increased risk for life-threatening ventricular arrhythmia. Adenosine can terminate focal ATs resulting from triggered activity.

LOCALIZATION OF FOCAL ATRIAL TACHYCARDIAS

Several algorithms have been proposed for ECG localization of focal AT using the P wave morphology and axis on a 12-lead ECG (Figs. 7.1 and 7.2). However, sometimes P wave morphology can be difficult to determine because of partial masking by the ST segment/T wave. Simple vagal maneuvers or intravenous adenosine administration during 12-lead ECG rhythm strip recording can separate the P wave from T wave. Alternatively, a post−premature ventricular complex compensatory pause can separate the P wave from the T wave and delineate P wave morphology. ECG lead V1 is the most useful in identifying the likely anatomic site of origin for a focal AT. The right atrium (RA) is an anterior structure, and the left atrium (LA) is a posterior structure. The lead V1 is located to the right and anteriorly in relation to the atria.

TABLE 7.1 Classification of Atrial Tachycardia and Atrial Flutter

Type	Mechanism	Mapping Properties	Induction	Termination
Focal	Abnormal automaticity	A focal in origin	Spontaneous, catecholamine	Beta blockers
	Triggered activity	A focal in origin	PES	Adenosine, calcium blocker
	Microreentry	A focal in origin but careful mapping shows an area of continuous or mid-diastolic potential	PAC, PES	PES
Macroreentrant AT and AFL	Cavotricuspid isthmus–dependent right AFL	Typical counterclockwise	PES, PAC, PVC (rarely)	PES
		Typical clockwise		
		Lower-loop reentry		
		Double-loop reentry		
		Intraisthmus reentry		
	Noncavotricuspid isthmus—dependent	Upper-loop reentry (see Chapter 8)		PES
		Lesional (incision related)		
		Scar related (congenital heart disease, cardiac surgery, cardiomyopathy)		
	Left atrial or biatrial	Postablation	Postatrial fibrillation catheter ablation or maze procedure	PES
		Around scar or anatomic structures	Perimitral, peripulmonary vein posttransplant, septal reentry	PES

AFL, Atrial flutter; *AT,* atrial tachycardia; *PAC,* premature atrial complex; *PES,* programmed electrical stimulation; *PVC,* premature ventricular complex.

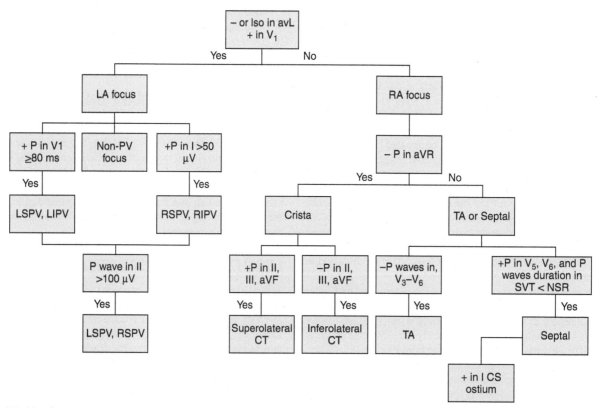

Fig. 7.1 Algorithm for localization of atrial tachycardia origin based on P wave morphology on the surface electrocardiogram. *+ P,* Positive P wave; *− P,* negative P wave; *0,* isoelectric P wave; *−/+ P,* biphasic P wave; *CS,* coronary sinus; *CT,* crista terminalis; *LA,* left atrium; *LSPV,* left superior pulmonary vein; *LIPV,* left inferior pulmonary vein; *NRS,* normal sinus rhythm; *RA,* right atrium; *RSPV,* right superior pulmonary vein; *RIPV,* right inferior pulmonary vein; *SR,* sinus rhythm; *SVT,* supraventricular tachycardia; *TA,* tricuspid annulus. (From Ellenbogen KA, Koneru JN. Atrial tachycardia. In: Zipes DP, Jalife J, Stevenson WG, eds. *Cardiac Electrophysiology: From Cell to Bedside.* 7th ed. Philadelphia, PA: WB Saunders; 2018:681-699).

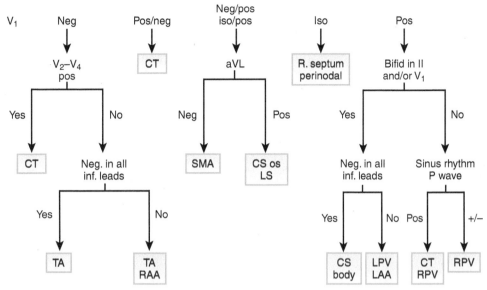

Fig. 7.2 Another P wave algorithm constructed on the basis of findings from 130 atrial tachycardias correctly localized the focus in 93% of patients.[1] *CS*, Coronary sinus; *CT*, crista terminalis; *LAA*, left atrial appendage; *LPV*, left pulmonary vein; *LS*, left superior; *RAA*, right atrial appendage; *RPV*, right pulmonary vein; *SMA*, superior mitral annulus; *TA*, tricuspid annulus.

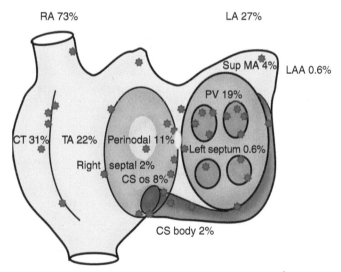

Fig. 7.3 A schematic representation of the anatomic distribution of focal atrial tachycardias.[1] The atrioventricular valvular annuli have been removed. *CS*, Coronary sinus; *CS os*, coronary sinus ostium; *CT*, crista terminalis; *LA*, left atrium; *LAA*, left atrial appendage; *MA*, mitral annulus; *PV*, pulmonary vein; *RA*, right atrium; *RAA*, right atrial appendage; *TA*, tricuspid annulus.

Therefore P wave morphology in lead V1 plays a vital role in determining the origin of focal ATs. A right AT originating from the tricuspid annulus or crista terminalis has negative P waves in lead V1 because the atrial activation travels away from lead V1.[1,2] P waves in lead V1 are positive for ATs originating from the PVs because of the posterior location in the chest and conduction traveling anteriorly toward V1. In general, negative P waves in the anterior precordial leads suggest an anterior RA or LA free wall location. Negative P waves in the inferior leads suggest a low (inferior) atrial origin. One study showed that ATs originating from PVs are significantly faster (mean cycle lengths: 289 ± 45 ms and 280 ± 48 ms in patients without and with PV ablation for atrial fibrillation, respectively) compared with left ATs (mean cycle lengths: 392 ± 106 ms and 407 ± 87 ms, patients without and with PV ablation for atrial fibrillation, respectively).[3] P waves in focal PV ATs usually have longer duration (≥110 ms). A prior catheter ablation of atrial fibrillation or reentrant AT, maze procedure, and surgery for congenital heart disease can affect the localization of the AT/AFL focus or circuit.

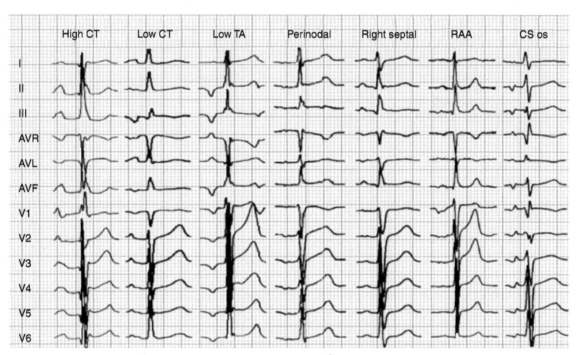

Fig. 7.4 Representative examples of the tachycardia P wave from left atrial sites.[1] *CS os*, Coronary sinus ostium; *CT*, crista terminalis; *RAA*, right atrial appendage; *TA*, tricuspid annulus.

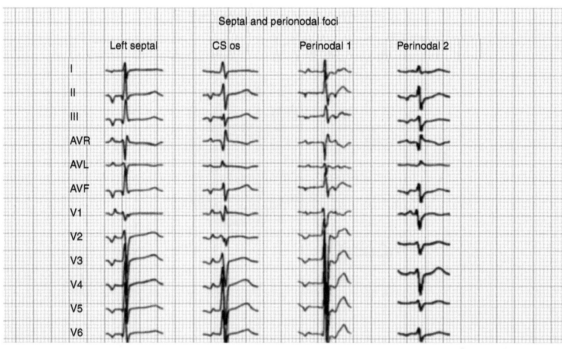

Fig. 7.5 Representative examples of the P wave morphology during atrial tachycardia for septal and midline foci.[2] *CS os*, Coronary sinus ostium.

RIGHT ATRIAL TACHYCARDIA

A negative or biphasic (positive, then negative) P wave in lead V1 has a 100% specificity and positive predictive value for ATs arising from the RA (Figs. 7.19 through 7.30; see also Figs. 7.9 through 7.18). P waves during ATs arising near the septum are generally narrower than those arising in the RA or LA free wall because of a relatively rapid activation from the midline to both atria, whereas the impulse from ATs with a right or left lateral atrial origin has to travel a longer distance to excite the entire contralateral atria.

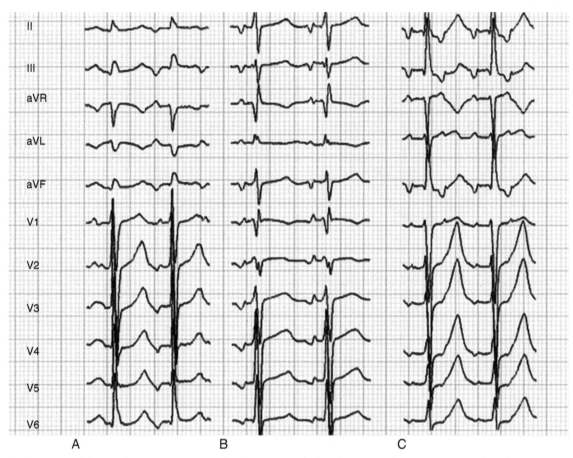

Fig. 7.6 Atrial tachycardia originating from coronary sinus. The P wave morphology from 13 patients is presented. The characteristic findings were as follows: a deeply inverted P wave in the inferior leads with 4 of 13 patients having a secondary upright component (B and C). Lead V1 was inverted (B and C) or isoelectric (A) then upright. Leads aVL and aVR were positive in all 13 patients in case series.[5]

Sinus Node Reentry Tachycardia

Sinus node reentry is defined as a reentrant tachycardia involving the sinus node and perinodal tissue that can be induced and terminated with PES and is adenosine sensitive. However, there has not been recent confirmation of this entity in the literature. It is possible that sinus node reentry tachycardia represents a high cristal AT originating near the sinus node that is adenosine sensitive if the mechanism of the tachycardia is triggered activity. Alternatively, it is an AT owing to microreentry in tissue near the sinus node or perinodal region (superior crista terminalis) that is responsive to adenosine because of involvement of sinus nodal tissue. The P wave morphology during the tachycardia is identical to that seen during sinus rhythm.

Inappropriate Sinus Tachycardia

Inappropriate sinus tachycardia (Fig. 7.12) is defined as a persistent increase in the resting sinus rate (usually >80–90 bpm) unrelated to, or out of proportion with, the level of physical, emotional, pathologic, or pharmacologic stress, or an exaggerated heart rate response to minimal exertion or a change in body posture. It occurs in a disproportionately high number among health care professionals. The tachycardia originates at the superior part of the sinus node and is refractory to medical therapy. During electrophysiology study it is mapped at the sinus node at the superior part of the crista terminalis.

Cristal Atrial Tachycardia

In cristal AT (Figs. 7.4 and 7.18 through 7.22), P waves are biphasic in lead V1 and negative in lead aVR. The presence of negative P waves in aVR identifies cristal ATs with 100% sensitivity and 93% specificity. P waves are positive and broad in leads I and II, as well as positive in lead aVL, owing to right-to-left activation. High, mid, or low cristal ATs can be identified according to the P wave polarity in the inferior leads.

Tricuspid Annular and Lateral Right Atrial Tachycardia

Tricuspid annular and lateral right ATs (Figs. 7.4 and 7.22 through 7.26) have negative P waves in lead V1. The P wave polarity in inferior leads helps to differentiate the inferior from the superior location of the AT. ATs originating from superior sites closer to the interatrial septum have transition from negative in lead V1 through biphasic to upright in the lateral precordial leads. An anteroinferior AT usually has inverted P waves across the precordial leads and in inferior leads.

SEPTAL ATRIAL TACHYCARDIA AND ATRIAL TACHYCARDIAS ORIGINATING FROM CORONARY SINUS

The predictive value of P wave morphology for localizing the atrium of origin is more limited because of a variation of activation of atrial pattern

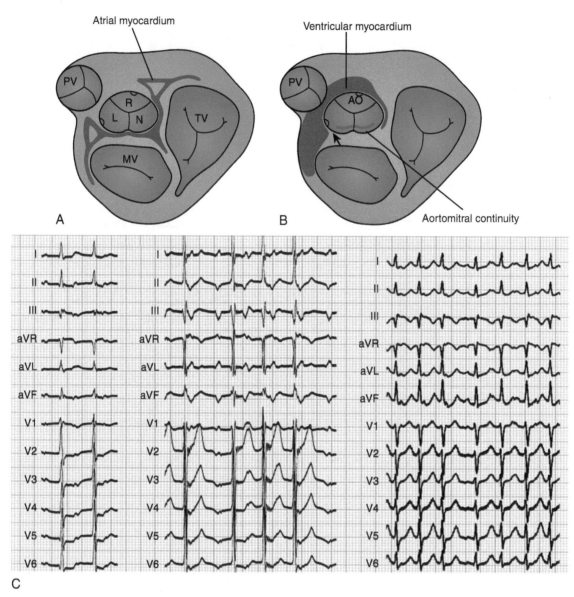

Fig. 7.7 Atrial tachycardia arising from the noncoronary aortic cusp. Noncoronary and, to some extent, left aortic cusps are in close relation with atrial myocardium (A), whereas right and left coronary cusps are in close relationship with ventricular myocardium (B). Atrial and ventricular tachycardias can be mapped from these coronary cusps, depending on the relationship of muscular bands (atrial or ventricle). Examples of P wave morphology in three patients with noncoronary cusp atrial tachycardia are shown in (C). *AO,* Aortic root; *L,* left coronary cusp; *MV,* mitral valve; *N,* noncoronary cusp; *PV,* pulmonary valve; *R,* right coronary cusp; *TV,* tricuspid valves.

of both atria. Those ATs are associated with variable P wave morphology, with considerable overlap for tachycardias located on the left and right sides of the septum. The P wave during the AT is approximately 20 ms narrower than the sinus P wave and is negative or biphasic in lead V1. These ATs can mimic AVNRT or orthodromic AVRT associated with a septal bypass tract, depending on the site of origin. ATs originating above the membranous septum, between the membranous septum and coronary sinus, and below and around the coronary sinus ostium are designated as high, mid, and low septal ATs, respectively (Fig. 7.31; see also Figs. 7.4 through 7.6 and 7.27 through 7.29).

High Septal Atrial Tachycardia

High septal ATs with a relatively long P-R interval can mimic slow-fast AVNRT or orthodromic AVRT with superoparaseptal accessory pathways.

Midseptal Atrial Tachycardia

Midseptal ATs can mimic fast-intermediate AVNRT or orthodromic AVRT with midseptal accessory pathway.

Posteroseptal Atrial Tachycardia

Posteroseptal ATs have P waves positive in lead V1, negative in the inferior leads, and positive in leads aVL and aVR. These ATs can mimic fast-slow AVNRT or orthodromic AVRT using a posteroseptal accessory pathway or persistent form of junctional reciprocating tachycardia.

Anteroseptal and midseptal right ATs have a biphasic or negative P wave morphology in lead V1. The combination of a negative or biphasic P wave in V1 and a positive or biphasic P wave in all inferior leads favors an anteroseptal AT, whereas the presence of a negative or biphasic P wave in V1 and a negative

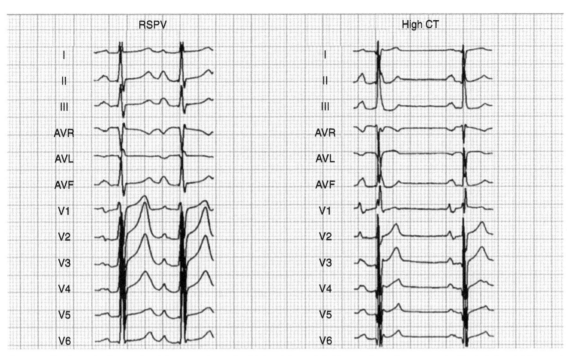

Fig. 7.8 The P waves in sinus rhythm and atrial ectopy from the high crista and right superior pulmonary vein. Foci at the right superior pulmonary vein (RSPV) show a change in configuration in lead V1 from biphasic in sinus rhythm to upright during tachycardia, a change not observed for right-sided tachycardias.[1] *CT*, Crista terminalis.

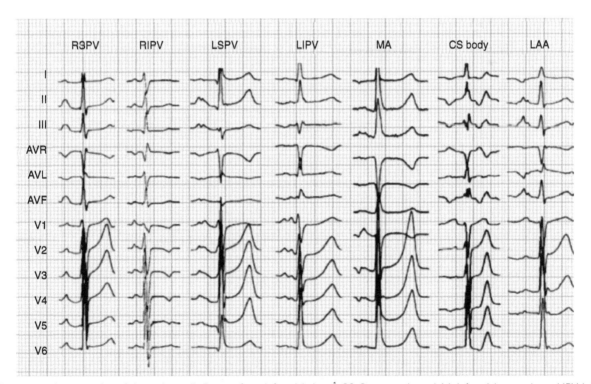

Fig. 7.9 Representative examples of the tachycardia P wave from left atrial sites.[1] *CS*, Coronary sinus; *LAA*, left atrial appendage; *LIPV*, left inferior pulmonary vein; *LSPV*, left superior pulmonary vein; *MA*, mitral annulus; *RIPV*, right inferior pulmonary vein; *RSPV*, right superior pulmonary vein.

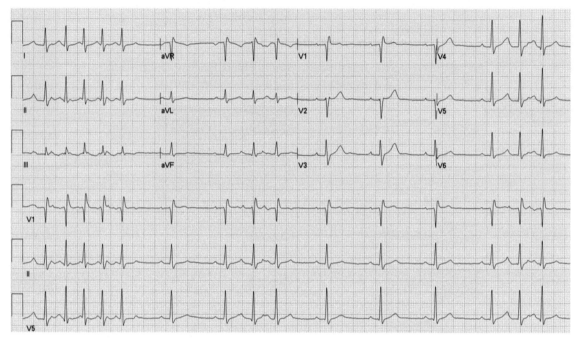

Fig. 7.10 Focal atrial tachycardia: The frequent bursts of atrial tachycardia may represent a focal source.

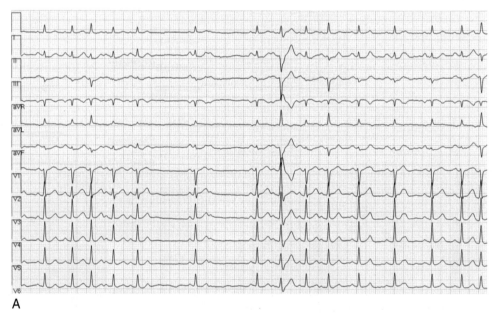

A

Fig. 7.11 Automatic atrial tachycardia (AT). Automatic ATs (focal) may present in repetitive bursts with acceleration and deceleration of tachycardia rate (warm-up and cool-down phenomenon). (A) Cycle length variation greater than 15% suggests a focal source of the AT. (B) Negative P waves in lead aVL and positive P wave in lead V1 suggest a left atrial origin. P wave duration greater than 80 ms and P wave voltage greater than 0.1 mV suggest a left superior pulmonary vein focus. This focal AT was mapped at the posterior left superior pulmonary vein (C).

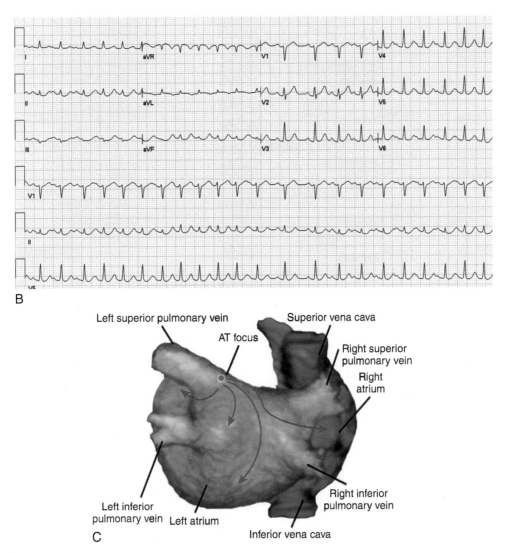

B

Left superior pulmonary vein

AT focus

Superior vena cava

Right superior pulmonary vein

Right atrium

Left inferior pulmonary vein   Left atrium

Right inferior pulmonary vein

Inferior vena cava

C

Fig. 7.11 (Continued).

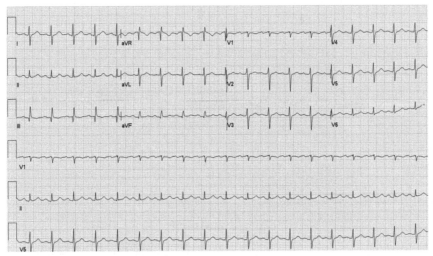

Fig. 7.12 Resting electrocardiogram of a 47-year-old woman without any structural heart disease, anxiety, or thyroid disorder. Electrocardiogram shows sinus tachycardia at 117 bpm. Her baseline heart rate fluctuated between 85 and 120 bpm, and the heart rate increased disproportionately with minimal exertion. She was very symptomatic with this heart rate. Partial success was achieved with catheter ablation of the upper part of the sinus node.

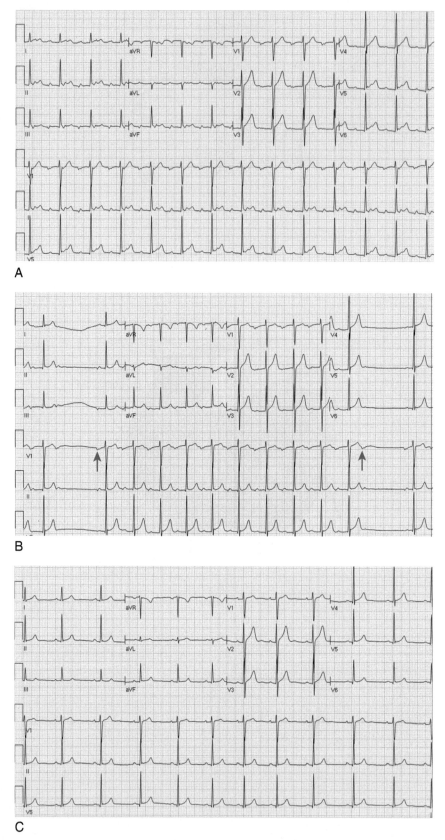

A

B

C

Fig. 7.13 (A) Electrocardiogram depicts atrial tachycardia (AT) with 2:1 atrioventricular (AV) block. (B) AT reinitiates (*red arrow*) after spontaneous termination during AV nodal–blocking drug therapy, and later showed type 1 second-degree AV block (Wenckebach pattern) with termination after the nonconducted P waves (*blue arrow*). AT also terminates and reinitiates. (C) Morphology of sinus P waves. Negative P waves in leads V1 and aVR suggest a cristal source of the AT. Negative P waves and positive P waves in inferior leads suggest an inferolateral source and cristal source, respectively. AT was mapped at the low lateral right atrium. (D) Diagram showing the focus of AT, the lower right lateral atrium, and possible activation pattern of the right atrium (*white arrows*). *AAo,* Ascending aorta; *CS/ThV,* coronary sinus/Thebesian valve; *CT,* crista terminalis; *CTI,* cavotricuspid isthmus; *ER/EV,* eustachian ridge/eustachian valve; *IVC,* inferior vena cava; *OF,* foramen ovale; *RA,* right atrium; *RAA,* right atrial appendage; *RCA,* right coronary artery; *RV,* right ventricle; *SI,* inferior septum; *STV,* septal tricuspid valve leaflet; *SVC,* superior vena cava; *TT,* tendon of Todaro.

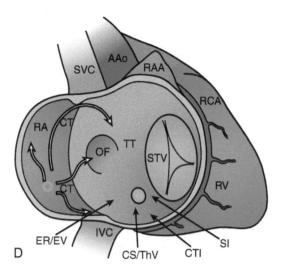

Fig. 7.13 (Continued).

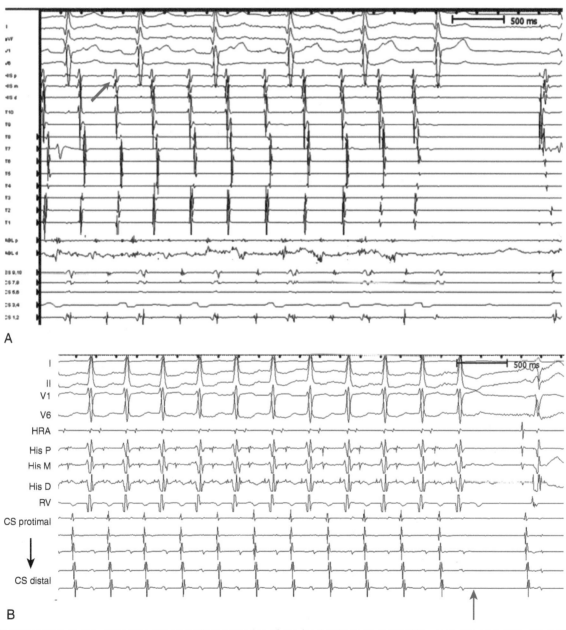

Fig. 7.14 (A) Intracardiac electrocardiogram shows earliest activation of the focal atrial tachycardia (AT) was in the high right atrium (HRA) (*arrow*) anterior to the His bundle. (B) AT terminated (*red arrow*) with intravenous adenosine, which is one of the characteristics of focal ATs resulting from a triggered mechanism. The reentrant and automatic focal ATs do not terminate with adenosine. *CS*, Coronary sinus; *His D*, distal His; *His M*, middle His; *His P*, proximal His; *RV*, right ventricle.

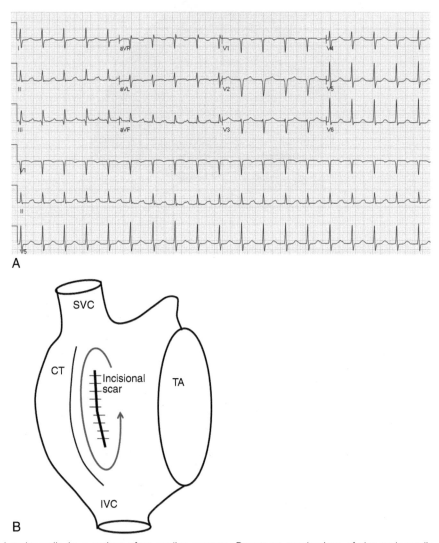

Fig. 7.15 Persistent atrial tachycardia in a patient after cardiac surgery. Reentrant mechanism of the tachycardia was demonstrated in the electrophysiology laboratory during entrainment mapping (A). Atrial tachycardia circuit was mapped around the atriotomy scar in the lateral right atrium (*red arrow*) (B). *CT*, Crista terminalis; *IVC*, inferior vena cava; *SVC*, superior vena cava; *TA*, tricuspid annulus.

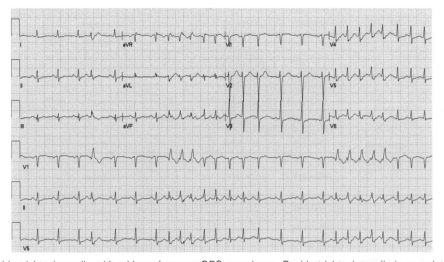

Fig. 7.16 Paroxysmal rapid atrial tachycardia with wide and narrow QRS complexes. Rapid atrial tachycardia is associated with intermittent right bundle branch block aberrancy (Ashman phenomenon).

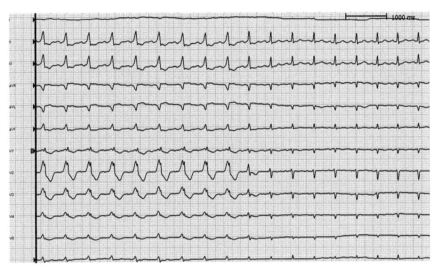

Fig. 7.17 Atrial tachycardia with wide and narrow QRS complexes. Atrial tachycardia initially conducts antidromically over the parahisian accessory pathway (wide QRS complexes) but later blocks, and conduction to the ventricle is entirely via the atrioventricular node.

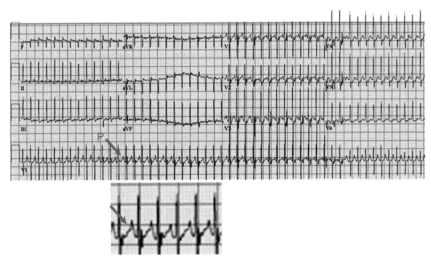

Fig. 7.18 Rapid atrial tachycardia (AT) in a 6-month-old child with sepsis and a structurally normal heart. AT rate is 300 bpm, which was associated with a left atrial thrombus. Usually, a left atrial thrombus is seen in patients with atrial fibrillation and atrial flutter; however, rapid AT can also result in left atrial thrombus.

P wave in at least two of the three inferior leads favors a midseptal AT. The presence of a positive P wave in V1 and a negative P wave in all three inferior leads favors a posteroseptal AT. The electrophysiology study is critical for differentiating these tachycardias from atypical AV node reentry or a septal accessory pathway. In several series, 27% to 35% of patients had ATs originating from septal tricuspid annulus and coronary sinus ostium.

Aortic Cusp

Atrial musculature has not been demonstrated to extend into the aortic coronary cusps of the sinus of Valsalva (Fig. 7.32; see also Fig. 7.7). However, the origin of focal ATs can be mapped from the aortic sinus of Valsalva because of its close relation with right and left atrial myocardium behind the thin aortic wall at the level of the sinotubular junction. Most of the ATs reported are from the

noncoronary cusp but rarely can arise from the left or the right coronary cusp. P wave morphology in ATs originating from the noncoronary cusp of the aorta is negative-positive in leads V1 and V2, predominantly upright or biphasic in inferior leads and lead aVL, and negative in aVR.[4] The precordial leads are negative-positive in V1 and V2, negative-positive or positive in leads V3-V5, and positive in lead V6.

LEFT ATRIAL TACHYCARDIA

Left-sided ATs can arise anywhere from the LA, but PVs and the mitral valve annulus are the main sources. A positive or biphasic (negative, then positive) P wave in lead V1 is associated with a 100% sensitivity and negative predictive value for ATs originating in the LA (Figs. 7.33 through 7.42; see also Figs. 7.8 and 7.9).

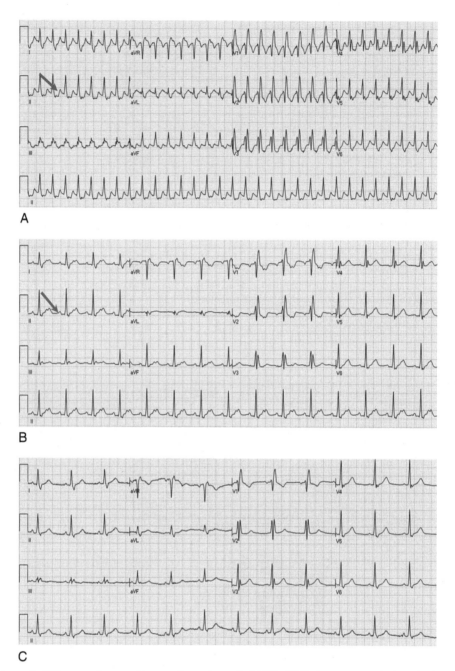

Fig. 7.19 Focal atrial tachycardia (AT) presenting as wide complex tachycardia (WCT). (A) Patient presented with a WCT with a right bundle branch block morphology. QRS complexes during the WCT have a typical right bundle branch block morphology, suggesting aberrancy. Presence of upright P waves in inferior leads (*arrow*) practically rules out a ventricular tachycardia with 1:1 retrograde conduction. (B) During intravenous diltiazem therapy, AT with 2:1 atrioventricular block developed. (C) Morphology of P waves during the sinus rhythm. P waves during AT are negative in leads V1 and aVR and positive in the inferior leads. AT was focal and was mapped at the high crista terminalis region (D). Arrows show centrifugal impulse propagation from the focal source.

Atrial Tachycardias Arising From Mitral Annulus, Left Atrial Appendage, and Coronary Sinus[1]

Mitral annular ATs mostly originate from the superior aspect of the mitral annulus in close proximity to the aortomitral continuity. P waves of AT originating from this area have an initial narrow negative deflection followed by a positive deflection in lead V1, negative/isoelectric in lead aVL, negative in lead I, and isoelectric or slightly positive in the inferior leads. The positivity of the P wave becomes progressively less from V1 through V6. ATs originating from anterolateral mitral annulus and LA appendage have P wave positive in lead V1 and inferior leads (lead III >II), and negative in lateral leads (I and aVL) with a deeply negative P wave in lead I. ATs arising from coronary sinus or posterior mitral annulus have bifid-positive P waves in leads V1, aVL, and negative P waves in the inferior leads (Figs. 7.43 and 7.44; see also Figs. 7.36 through 7.42).

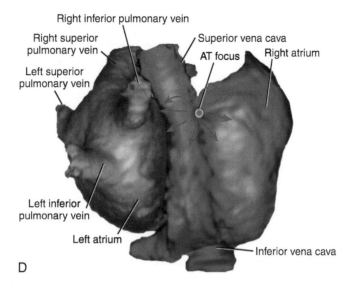

Fig. 7.19 (Continued).

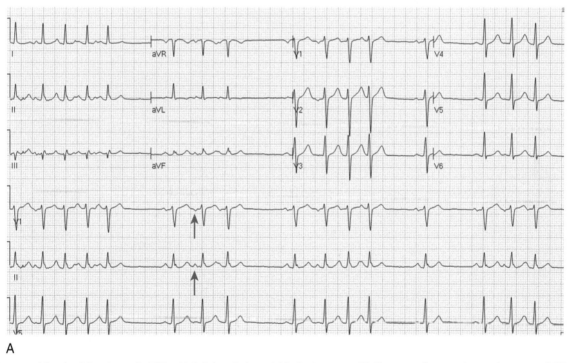

Fig. 7.20 Paraseptal focal atrial tachycardia (AT) with left bundle branch block aberrancy. (A) Electrocardiogram shows short runs of AT that started after a single sinus beat (*arrow*) and terminated spontaneously. AT conducted with left bundle branch block aberrancy (B and C) and with a slight change in QRS axis in alternate beats. AT terminated spontaneously and reinitiated without aberrancy (B). P wave is negative in leads V1 and positive-negative in aVR, suggesting a right atrial source at tricuspid annulus or septum. P waves are positive in leads V5 and V6. More commonly, P waves in supraventricular tachycardia are narrower than P waves in sinus rhythm. Findings suggest a septal focus of AT. Positive P waves in inferior leads suggest a high septal source. AT was mapped at the paraseptal area above the proximal His bundle (D). *AAo*, Ascending aorta; *AVN*, atrioventricular node; *CS/ThV*, coronary sinus/Thebesian valve; *CT*, crista terminalis; *CTI*, cavotricuspid isthmus; *ER/EV*, eustachian ridge/eustachian valve; *IVC*, inferior vena cava; *OF*, fossa ovalis; *RAA*, right atrial appendage; *RCA*, right coronary artery; *RV*, right ventricle; *SI*, inferior septum; *STV*, septal tricuspid valve; *SVC*, superior vena cava; *TT*, tendon of Todaro. Arrows show centrifugal impulse propagation from the focal source.

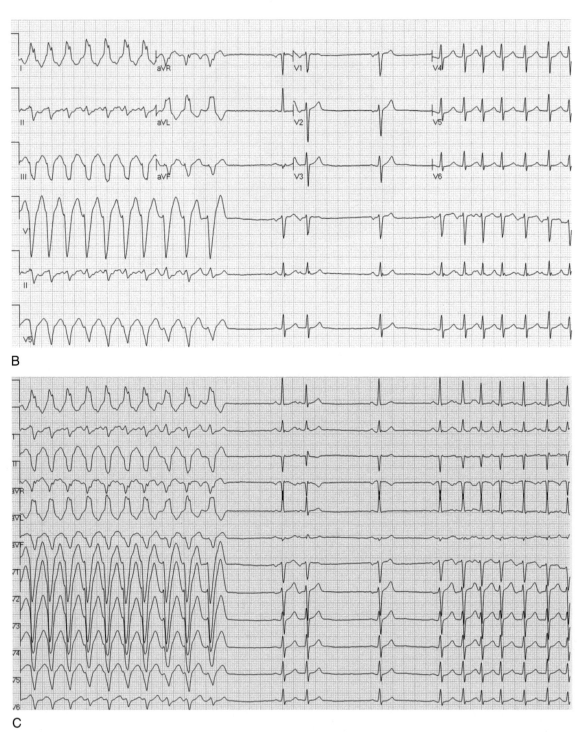

Fig. 7.20 (Continued).

Atrial Tachycardias Arising From Pulmonary Veins

ATs arising from PVs (Table 7.2; see also Figs. 7.8, 7.9, 7.37 through 7.46) are characterized by entirely positive P waves in lead V1 in 100%, isoelectric or negative in lead aVL in 86%, and negative in lead aVR in 96% of cases. ATs originating from the superior PVs have larger amplitude P waves in the inferior leads than those in ATs arising from the inferior PVs. P wave morphology and polarity of ATs originating from right superior PVs can mimic ATs from the superior region of the RA, except that it is positive in V1. It is unlike negative P waves in lead V1 in right ATs or a biphasic (positive-negative) P wave in ATs originating from posterior RA. P wave morphology generally is of greater accuracy in distinguishing right-sided from left-sided PVs in contrast to superior from inferior PVs. ATs arising from inferior PVs generally show lesser amplitude (or negative P waves in inferior leads) than ATs arising from superior PVs.

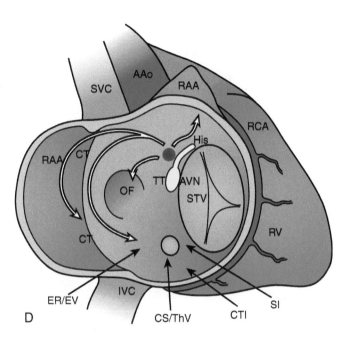

Fig. 7.20 (Continued).

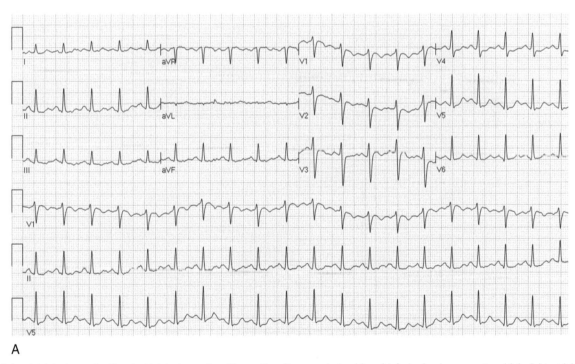

Fig. 7.21 High cristal tachycardia. Focal atrial tachycardia with positive P waves in lead I and inferior leads suggests a high right atrial source (A). Negative P waves in lead V1 suggest right atrial source. Negative P waves suggest a cristal rather than lateral or tricuspid annular source. Focal atrial tachycardia was mapped at the high cristal area (B). *AAo,* Ascending aorta; *AVN,* atrioventricular node; *CS/ThV,* coronary sinus/Thebesian valve; *CT,* crista terminalis; *CTI,* cavotricuspid isthmus; *ER/EV,* eustachian ridge/eustachian valve; *IVC,* inferior vena cava; *OF,* fossa ovalis; *RAA,* right atrial appendage; *RCA,* right coronary artery; *RV,* right ventricle; *SI,* inferior septum; *STV,* septal tricuspid valve; *SVC,* superior vena cava; *TT,* tendon of Todaro.

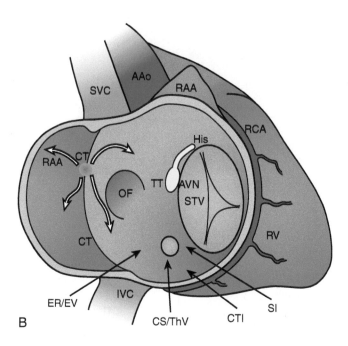

B

Fig. 7.21 (Continued).

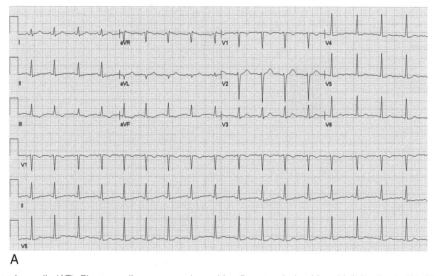

A

Fig. 7.22 Midcristal atrial tachycardia (AT). Electrocardiogram reveals positive P waves in lead I and inferior leads (A). However, P wave amplitude in inferior lead is less than that in sinus rhythm or compared with sinus tachycardia (B) or a high cristal AT (see Fig. 7.21). This suggests the focus of AT in the midcristal region. Tachycardia was mapped in this region 2 cm below the superior vena cava (C). Arrows show centrifugal impulse propagation from the focal source.

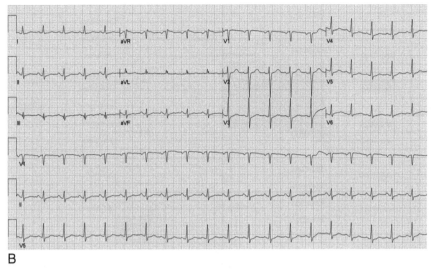

B

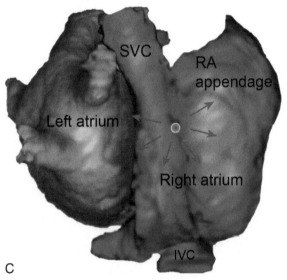

C

Fig. 7.22 (Continued).

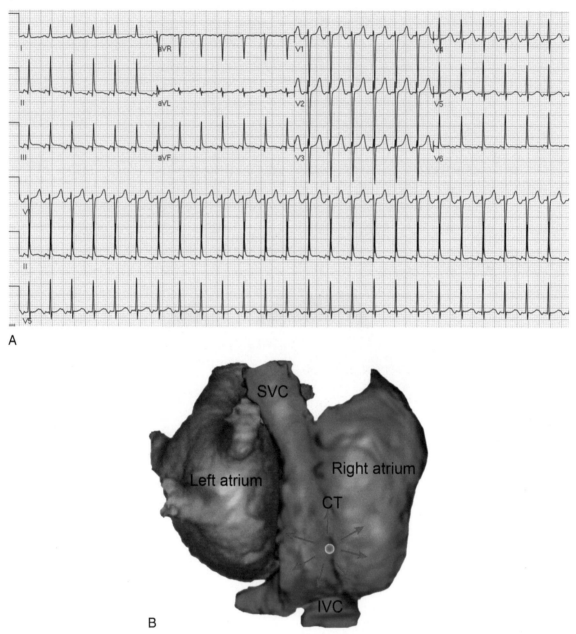

Fig. 7.23 Low cristal atrial tachycardia (AT). Electrocardiogram depicts positive P waves in lead I and negative in the inferior leads (A). This suggests the focus of AT in the midcristal region. Negative P waves in lead V1 and aVR suggest cristal or posterior focus of AT. Negative P waves in inferior leads suggest inferior focus in the right atrium. The focus of the AT was mapped at the low crista terminalis (B). Arrows show centrifugal impulse propagation from the focal source.

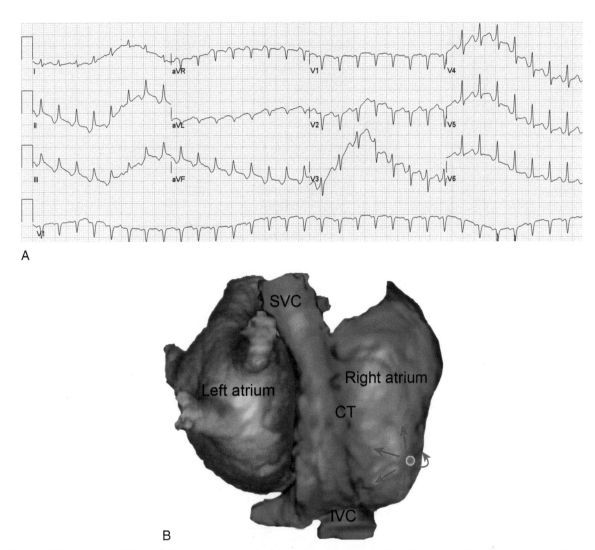

Fig. 7.24 Focal atrial tachycardia (AT) originating from the inferior lateral right atrial atrium. The AT has negative P waves in lead V1 and positive P waves in lead aVR, which suggest a relatively anterior or annular focus of AT in the right atrium. (A) Negative P waves in inferior leads suggest inferior focus in the right atrium. (B) AT focus was mapped at the low lateral right atrium. Arrows show centrifugal impulse propagation from the focal source.

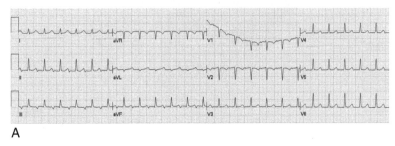

Fig. 7.25 Atrial tachycardia (AT) originating from the low lateral tricuspid annulus (A). Later ventricular rate slowed down following the development of 2:1 atrioventricular (AV) block with antiarrhythmic therapy (B). (C) P wave morphology during sinus rhythm in the same patient. The AT has negative P waves in lead V1 and positive P waves in lead aVR, which suggest a relatively anterior or annular focus of AT in the right atrium. Negative P waves in the inferior leads suggest an inferior focus in the right atrium. Negative P waves in leads V3 to V6 (≥3 precordial leads) suggest an annular focus. AT focus was mapped at the low lateral tricuspid annulus (D).

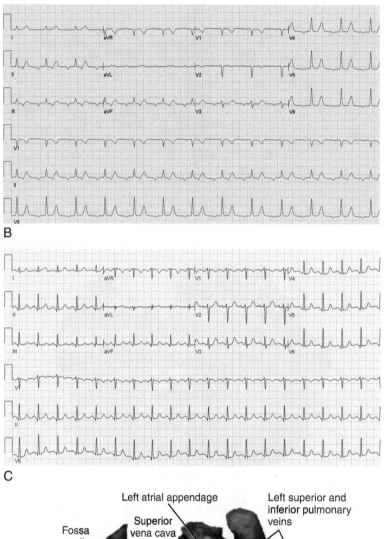

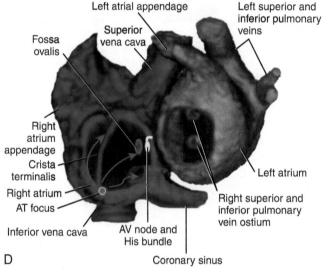

Fig. 7.25 (Continued).

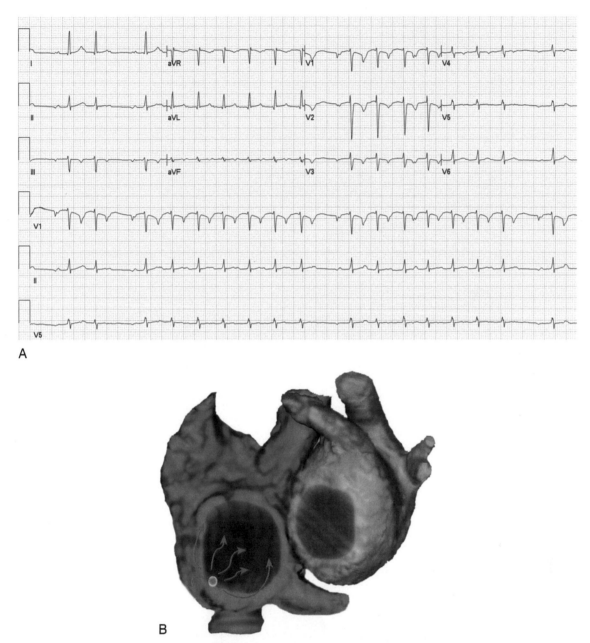

Fig. 7.26 Focal atrial tachycardia (AT) in an 18-year-old woman with postpartum cardiomyopathy. AT has negative P waves in lead V1 and positive P waves in lead aVR, which suggest a relatively anterior or annular focus of AT in the right atrium (A). Negative P waves in inferior leads suggest an inferior focus in the right atrium. Negative P waves in leads V3 to V6 (≥3 precordial leads) suggest an annular focus. AT shows type 1 second-degree atrioventricular block. AT focus was mapped at the low lateral tricuspid annulus. Tachycardia originated from the inferolateral tricuspid annulus (B). Anatomic structures as labeled in Fig. 7.25D. Arrows show centrifugal impulse propagation from the focal source.

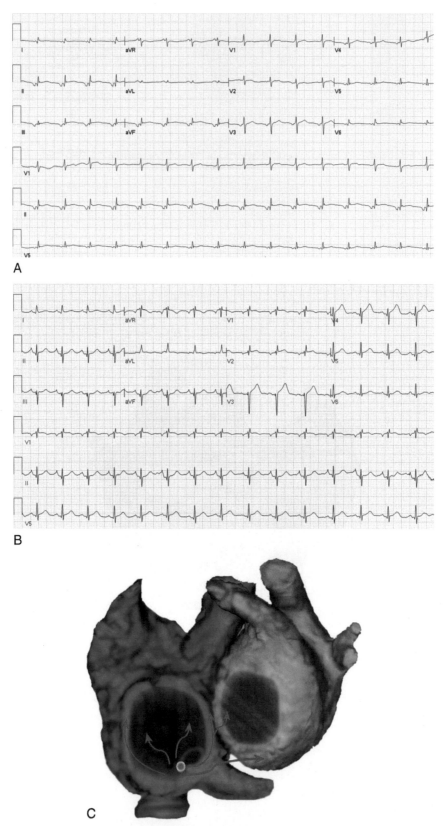

Fig. 7.27 Focal atrial tachycardia (AT) originating from the inferior tricuspid annulus. AT has isoelectric P waves in lead V1 and positive P waves in lead aVR, which suggests a relatively anterior or annular focus of the AT in the right atrium (A). Negative P waves in inferior leads suggest an inferior focus in the right atrium. Negative P waves in leads V3 to V6 (≥3 precordial leads) suggest an annular focus at the low lateral tricuspid annulus. Narrower P waves in AT than P waves in the sinus rhythm (B) suggest the AT focus is close to the septum. Tachycardia originated from the inferior tricuspid annulus close to the septum (C). Anatomic structures as labeled in Fig. 7.25D.

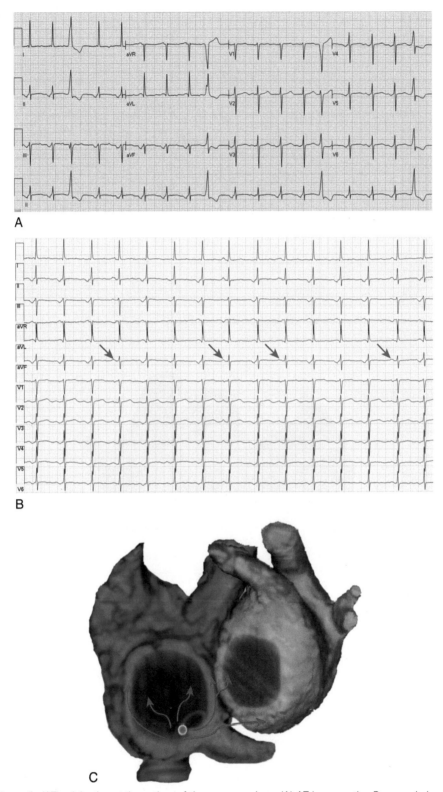

Fig. 7.28 Focal atrial tachycardia (AT) originating at the ostium of the coronary sinus. (A) AT has negative P waves in lead V1 and positive P waves in lead aVR, which suggests a relatively anterior or annular focus of AT in the right atrium. Negative P waves in inferior leads suggest inferior focus in the right atrium. Positive P waves in leads V5 and V6 suggest a septal focus. (B) Patient also had wandering atrial pacemaker with predominant inferior right atrial rhythm with occasional sinus P wave (*arrows*). (C) AT focus was mapped at the low septum at the coronary sinus ostium. Anatomic structures as labeled in Fig. 7.25D.

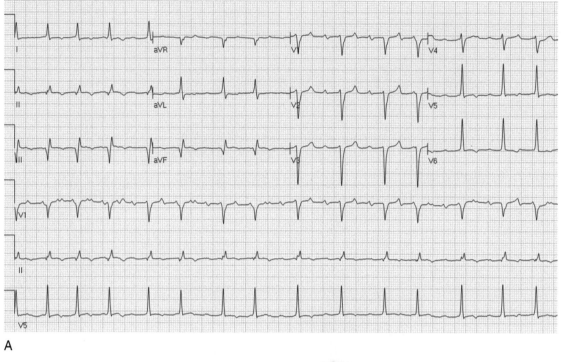

A

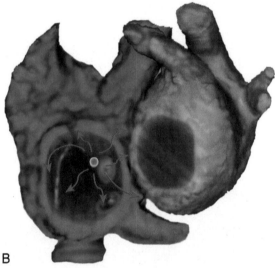

B

Fig. 7.29 Focal atrial tachycardia (AT) originating from the right midseptum. AT shows both low- and high-grade atrioventricular block or atypical Wenckebach. Positive P waves (duration >80 ms) in lead V1 and isoelectric in lead aVL suggest a left atrial origin (A). However, P waves are isoelectric in lead aVR and aVL. AT was mapped at the posterior part of the right interatrial septum and ablated successfully during electrophysiology study (B). Anatomic structures as labeled in Fig. 7.25D.

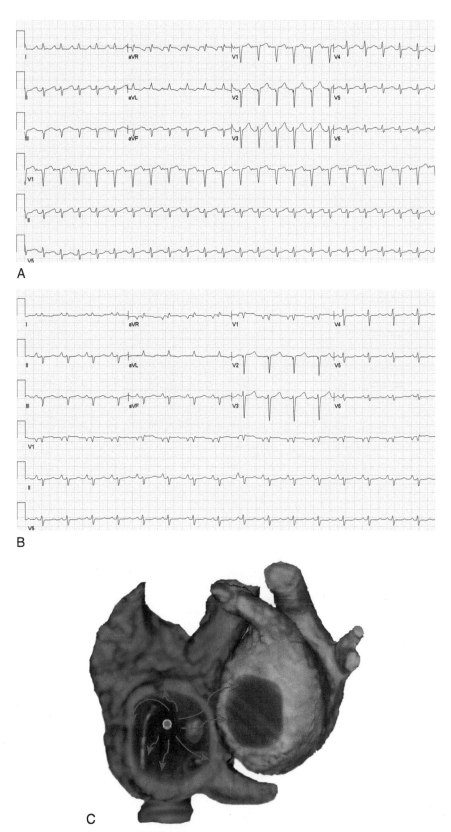

Fig. 7.30 Focal atrial tachycardia (AT) from midposterior right atrium in a 52-year-old woman with nonischemic cardiomyopathy. (A) Electrocardiogram depicts initial negative P waves in leads V1 and aVR along with positive P waves in lead I that suggest a right atrial origin of the AT. Positive P waves in leads V2 to V6 suggest the AT focus is closer to septal location. Electrocardiogram in sinus rhythm (B) shows left atrial enlargement and poor progression of R wave in precordial leads. AT was mapped to the posterior right atrium close to the septum and medial to the crista terminalis (C). Anatomic structures as labeled in Fig. 7.25D.

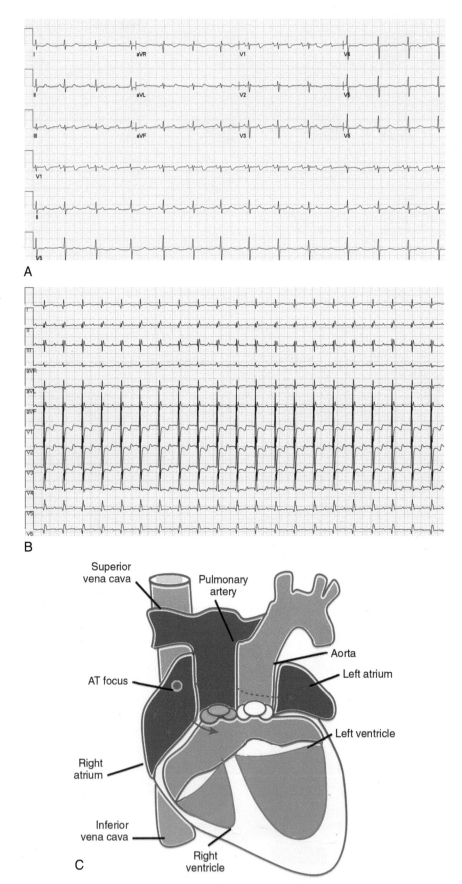

Fig. 7.31 Right atrial tachycardia (AT) near the tricuspid annulus in a 20-year-old patient with mesocardia, double outlet ventricle with hypoplastic right ventricle, and severe pulmonary stenosis. Patient developed ATs of multiple morphologies of both focal and reentrant nature. (A) AT was a focal originating from the anterolateral right atrium. (B) Reentrant AT originating from the same area (C).

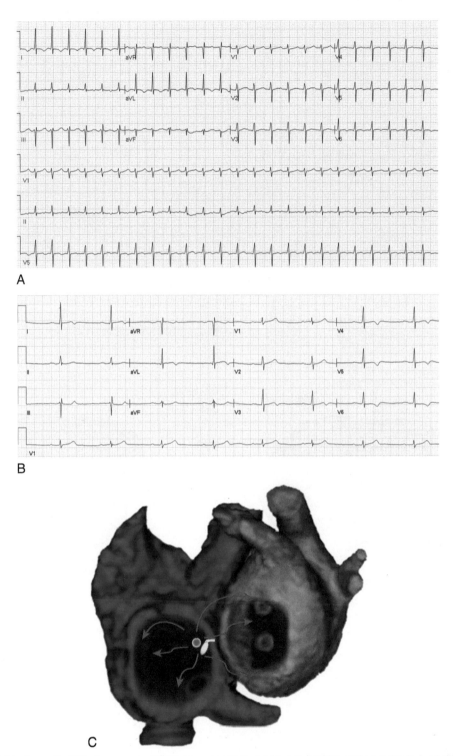

Fig. 7.32 Parahisian atrial tachycardia (AT). P waves in AT (A) are most likely positive in lead V1 and negative in lead aVL, which suggests a left atrial source. However, owing to T wave and P wave fusion, the P wave amplitude and vector cannot be ascertained. Furthermore, the predictive value of P wave morphology for localizing the atrium of origin, a septal AT, is more limited because of variation of activation pattern of both atria. (B) Sinus P waves. (C) Focal AT was mapped to the parahisian area, just anterior and proximal to the His bundle. Anatomic structures as labeled in Fig. 7.25D.

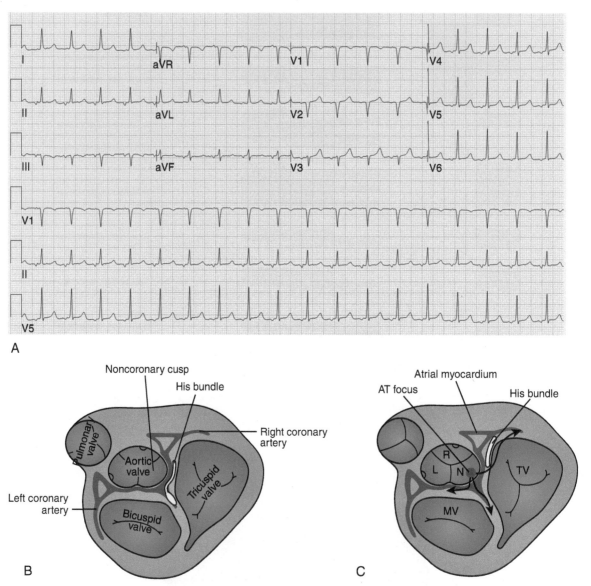

Fig. 7.33 Atrial tachycardia (AT) originating from the noncoronary cusp. (A) P wave morphology is negative-positive in lead V1 and biphasic in inferior leads and lead aVL. (B) AT focus was mapped at the noncoronary cusp of sinus of Valsalva. (C) The activation pattern of atrial impulse during AT from the origin. *L,* Left coronary cusp; *MV,* mitral valve; *N,* noncoronary cusp; *R,* right coronary cusp; *TV,* tricuspid valves.

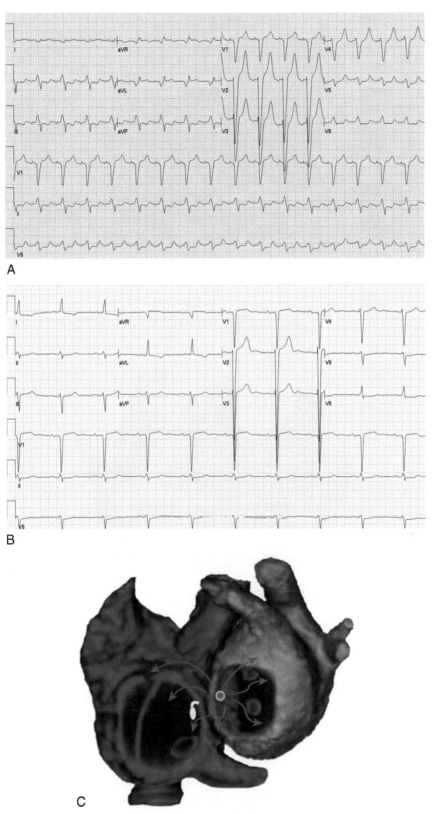

Fig. 7.34 Atrial tachycardia (AT)–induced cardiomyopathy in an 80-year-old patient. P waves during AT (A) are narrow and positive in leads V1, aVR, and aVL, suggesting septal origin. P waves are biphasic in leads II and III, suggesting a lower septal site of origin. However, AT was mapped to the left upper septum (parahisian area). During catheter ablation near the site of the AT focus, transient PR prolongation was noted, suggesting a left septal extension of fast atrioventricular nodal pathway. Tachycardia was ablated successfully just caudal to the site where transient P-R prolongation was observed. Patient also had rate-related left bundle branch block aberrancy with right axis deviation. Electrocardiogram during sinus rhythm (B) shows poor progression of R wave and a left axis deviation. Site of successful catheter ablation is shown in (C). Anatomic structures as labeled in Fig. 7.25D.

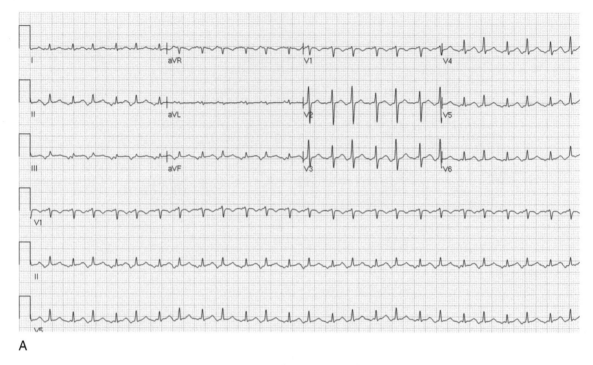

A

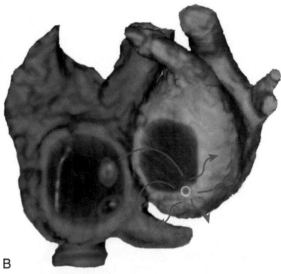

B

Fig. 7.35 Adenosine-sensitive focal atrial tachycardia (AT). P waves are positive-negative in lead V1 and positive in leads I and AVR, suggesting a left atrial focus. (A) P waves are positive in lead aVL and negative in inferior leads, suggesting AT focus in the inferior left atrium. P waves are relatively narrow, suggesting its source is close to the midline. (B) AT focus was mapped at the inferolateral mitral annulus. Anatomic structures as labeled in Fig. 7.25D.

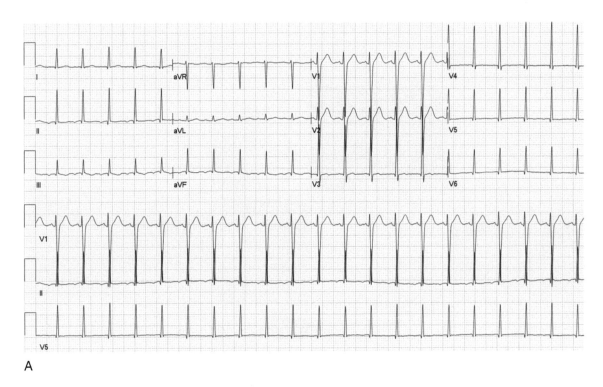

A

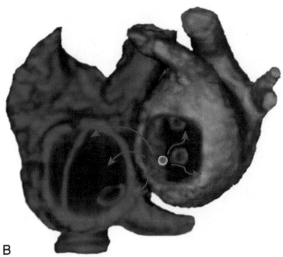

B

Fig. 7.36 Left focal atrial tachycardia (AT) in a 17-year-old male patient. (A) Positive P waves of the AT in lead V1 and isoelectric or mildly positive in aVL suggest a left atrial focus. Negative P waves in inferior leads suggest inferior location in the left atrium. (B) AT focus was mapped at the midinferoseptal region. Anatomic structures as labeled in Fig. 7.25D.

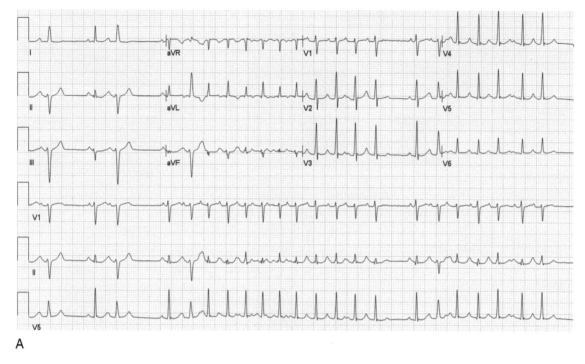

A

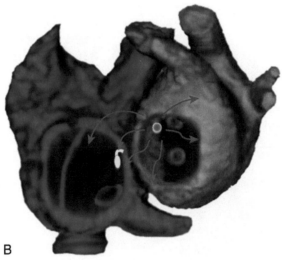

B

Fig. 7.37 Rapid irregular focal atrial tachycardia. P wave is positive in leads V1 and aVL and inferior leads and negative in leads aVR and aVL (A). This focal atrial tachycardia was mapped to the posterosuperior left atrium close to the ostium of the right superior pulmonary vein (B). Anatomic structures as labeled in Fig. 7.25D.

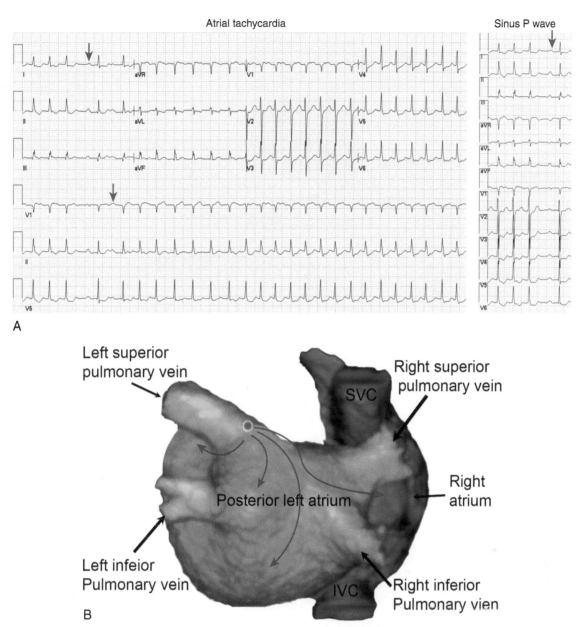

Fig. 7.38 Focal automatic atrial tachycardia (AT). (A) P waves are upright in lead V1 and inferior leads (initiation of the AT is marked by the *red arrow*) and negative in lead aVL. P wave amplitude in lead II is greater than 0.1 mV. The tachycardia later changes to irregular rhythm (atrial flutter/ atrial fibrillation). (B) AT focus was mapped at the superomedial aspect of the left superior pulmonary vein roof. Arrows show the pattern of impulse propagation from the focal source.

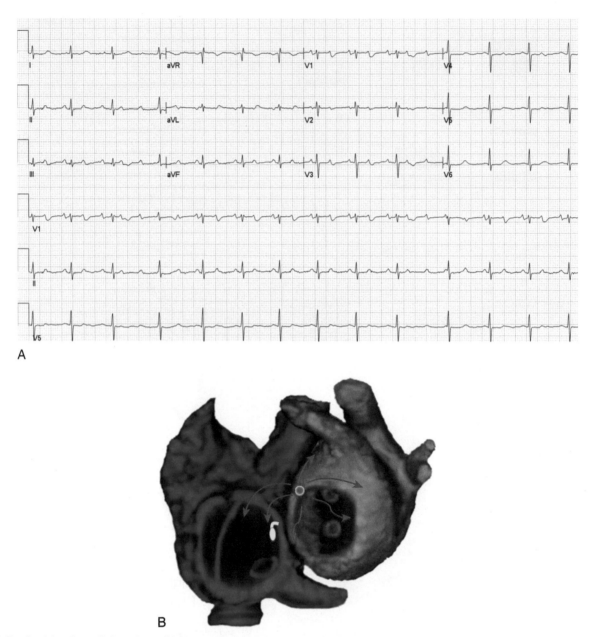

Fig. 7.39 Focal atrial tachycardia in patient with history of mitral valve surgery. (A) P waves are positive-negative in lead V1, isoelectric in lead I, and negative in lead aVL, suggesting a left atrial origin. Positive P waves in the inferior leads suggest an anterior focus in the left atrium. (B) Atrial tachycardia was mapped to the superomedial mitral annulus. Anatomic structures as labeled in Fig. 7.25D.

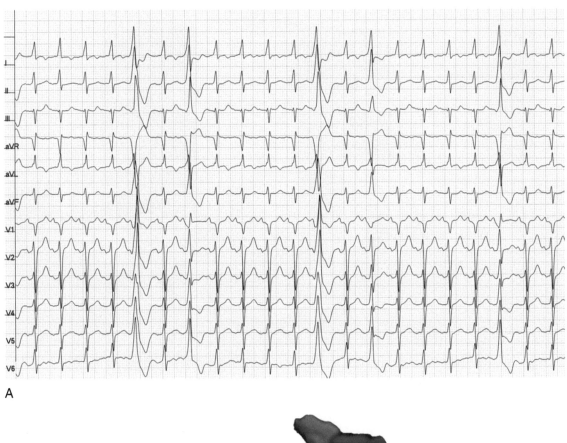

A

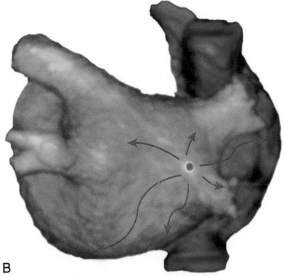

B

Fig. 7.40 Focal atrial tachycardia (AT) in patient with a history of catheter ablation of atrial fibrillation. (A) P waves are better delineated after the monomorphic premature ventricular complex. P waves are positive in lead V1 and isoelectric in lead aVL, suggesting left atrial focus of the AT. P waves are isoelectric in all the limb leads. P wave pattern can vary after a catheter ablation or maze procedure for atrial fibrillation. (B) Focal AT was mapped to the right inferior pulmonary vein. Anatomic structures as labeled in Fig. 7.38B.

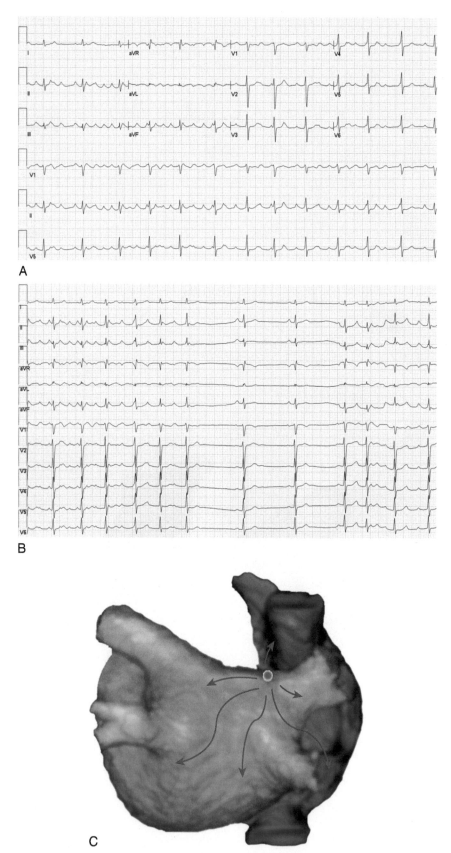

Fig. 7.41 Focal atrial tachycardia and atrial flutter in a patient with a history of catheter ablation of atrial fibrillation. Tachycardia is rapid and irregular with a mild variation in P wave morphology (A and B). P waves are positive in leads V1 and aVL and lead II. Negative P waves in leads aVL and aVR suggest a close to midline focus of the atrial tachycardia. P wave amplitude greater than 50 μV in lead I and greater than 1 mV in lead II suggests a right superior pulmonary vein origin of the tachycardia. (C) Tachycardia was mapped to the superior aspect of the right superior pulmonary vein. Anatomic structures as labeled in Fig. 7.38B.

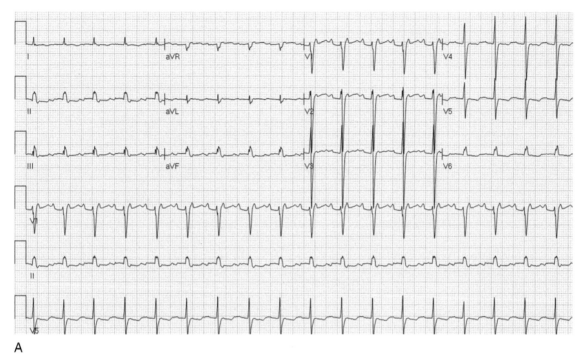

A

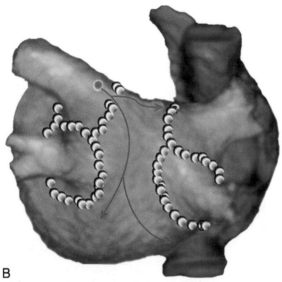

B

Fig. 7.42 Focal atrial tachycardia (AT) in a patient after catheter ablation of atrial fibrillation, which included pulmonary vein isolation. P waves are positive in lead V1 and isoelectric in lead I and aVL, suggesting a left-sided AT (A). P wave amplitude is less than 50 µV, and lead II is greater than 0.1 mV, which is against a left pulmonary vein focus. Focal AT originated from the left superior pulmonary vein (B). Anatomic structures as labeled in Fig. 7.38B. Red arrows show impulse propagation from the focal source. White circles are radiofrequency ablation points.

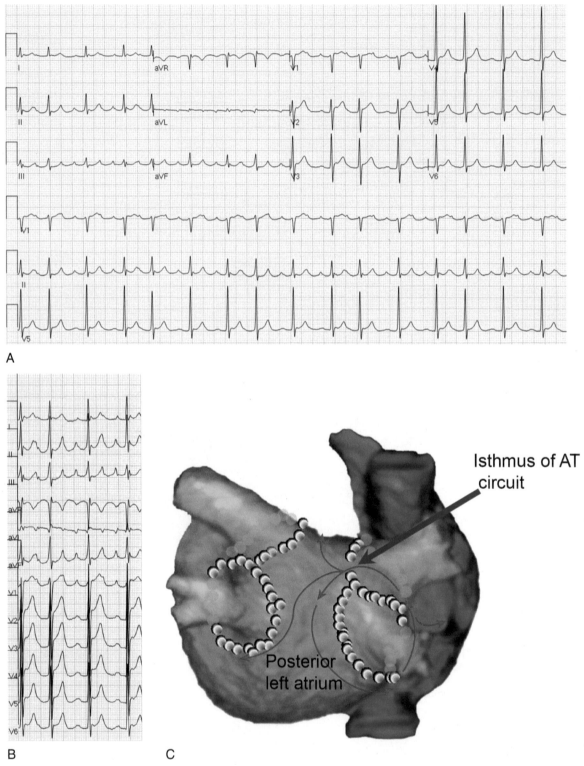

Fig. 7.43 Macroreentrant atrial tachycardia (AT) in a patient after catheter ablation of atrial fibrillation, which included pulmonary vein isolation (A). The 12-lead rhythm (B) strip is gained x2 for better delineation of P waves. P waves are positive in lead V1 and I and negative in aVL, suggesting a left atrial focus close to the interatrial septum. The isthmus of this reentrant AT circuit was mapped between the two right pulmonary veins (*blue arrow*) (C). Anatomic structures as labeled in Fig. 7.38B. White circles denote points of radiofrequency ablation.

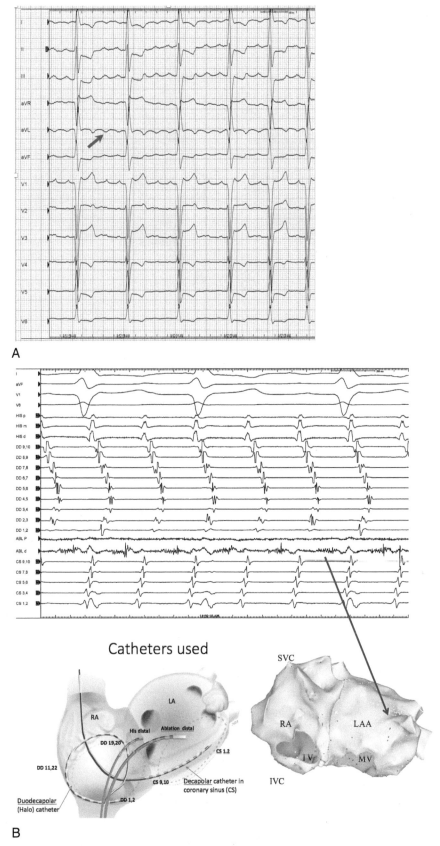

Fig. 7.44 Macroreentrant atrial tachycardia in a patient after catheter ablation of atrial fibrillation, which included pulmonary vein isolation. The 12-lead electrocardiogram rhythm recording, P waves (*arrow*) are positive in lead V1 and inferior leads, and negative in I and negative in aVL, suggesting a left atrial source of the tachycardia (A), atrioventricular block is present. The tachycardia was mapped with electroanatomic mapping system with multipolar catheters placed right (RA) and left atrium (LA). The isthmus of this reentrant atrial tachycardia circuit (*large blue arrow*) was mapped at the base of left atrial appendage (LAA) anteriorly (B), and terminated successfully with catheter ablation at the site of mid-diastolic potential after confirmation with various electrophysiological maneuvers (*smaller blue arrows*, C). *CS,* Coronary sinus; *DD,* multipolar catheter around tricuspid annulus; *IVC,* inferior vena cava; *LIPV,* left inferior pulmonary vein; *LSPV,* left superior pulmonary vein; *MV,* mitral valve; *RIPV,* right inferior pulmonary vein; *RSPV,* right superior pulmonary vein; *SVC,* superior vein; *TV,* tricuspid valves.

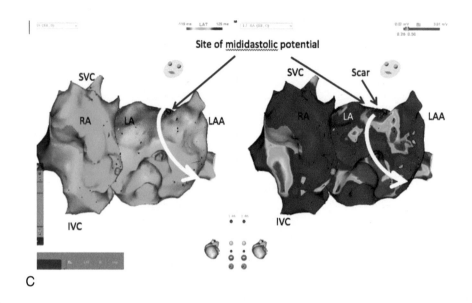

Site of mididastolic potential

C

Fig. 7.44 (Continued).

TABLE 7.2   Right Versus Left Superior Pulmonary Vein Atrial Tachycardias

P Wave	Right Superior PV AT	Left Superior PV AT
Lead V1	Biphasic or positive	Broad P waves
Lead I	Isoelectric	Isoelectric or negative
Lead aVL	Positive or biphasic	Negative
Inferior leads	Positive	Positive
Amplitude in lead III vs. II	Equal	III/II ratio >0.8
Positive notching		Present in ≥ 2 leads

AT, Atrial tachycardia; *PV*, pulmonary vein.

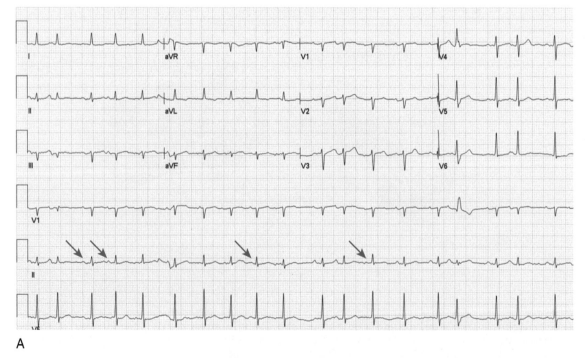

A

Fig. 7.45 Multifocal atrial tachycardia. Note three different morphologies of P waves (*arrows*) in lead V1 in electrocardiograms (ECGs). Atrial rate of 114 bpm is evident in ECG (A), whereas it is 87 bpm in ECG (B), which may be defined as wandering atrial pacemaker.

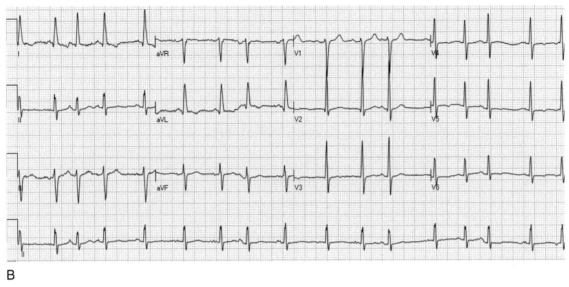

B

Fig. 7.45 (Continued).

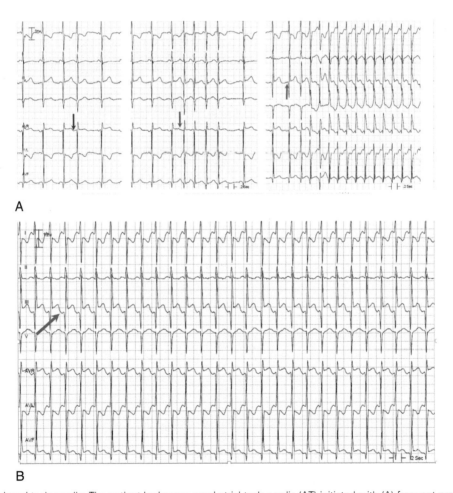

A

B

Fig. 7.46 Tachycardia-induced tachycardia: The patient had paroxysmal atrial tachycardia (AT) initiated with (A) frequent premature atrial complexes (*blue arrow*) and short runs of AT (*red arrow*), which later became sustained (B); and during one of her episodes, the AT induced ventricular tachycardia/ventricular fibrillation (C) and was resuscitated successfully.

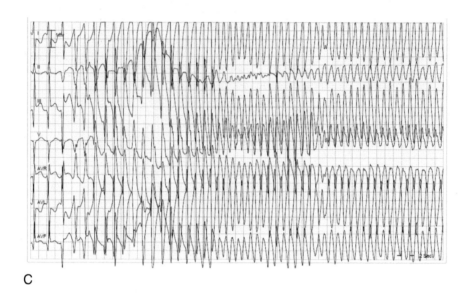

Fig. 7.46 (Continued).

REFERENCES

1. Kistler PM, Roberts-Thomson KC, Haqqani HM, et al. P-wave morphology in focal atrial tachycardia: development of an algorithm to predict the anatomic site of origin. *J Am Coll Cardiol*. 2006;48:1010—1017.
2. Teh AW, Kistler PM, Kalman JM. Using the 12-lead ECG to localize the origin of ventricular and atrial tachycardias. Part 1: focal atrial tachycardia. *J Cardiovasc Electrophysiol*. 2009;20:706—709. quiz 705.
3. Bazan V, Rodriguez-Font E, Vinolas X, et al. Atrial tachycardia originating from the pulmonary vein: clinical, electrocardiographic, and differential electrophysiologic characteristics. *Rev Esp Cardiol*. 2010;63:149—155.
4. Zhou YF, Wang Y, Zeng YJ, et al. Electrophysiologic characteristics and radiofrequency ablation of focal atrial tachycardia arising from non-coronary sinuses of valsalva in the aorta. *J Interv Card Electrophysiol*. 2010;28:147—151.
5. Kistler PM, Fynn SP, Haqqani H, et al. Focal atrial tachycardia from the ostium of the coronary sinus: electrocardiographic and electrophysiological characterization and radiofrequency ablation. *J Am Coll Cardiol*. 2005;45:1488—1493.

8

Atrial Flutter

Atrial flutter (AFL) is an arrhythmia with an electrocardiographic diagnosis based on regular sawtooth-like atrial waves without an underlying isoelectric line between flutter waves, at rates between 240 and 340 bpm. AFLs are considered to be macroreentrant arrhythmias; however, rapid focal firing of impulses in the atrium (mostly from pulmonary veins) can also manifest as fast atrial tachycardia (AT) or atypical AFL with a sawtooth pattern without an isoelectric line between flutter waves on electrocardiogram (ECG).[1] These AFLs are commonly encountered in patients who have had catheter ablation of atrial fibrillation, maze procedure, or prior cardiac surgery with atrial scar. Electrocardiographically, AFL is defined as right atrial cavotricuspid isthmus (CTI)-dependent (typical) and non-CTI-dependent (atypical flutter) (Figs. 8.1 through 8.9).[2]

Typical CTI-dependent AFL: CTI-dependent flutter has a sawtooth pattern of flutter waves at a fixed rate of approximately 300 (+/− 40 bpm) usually with 2:1 atrioventricular (AV) conduction with a ventricular rate of approximately 150 bpm (Figs. 8.4 through 8.15). In fact, any tachycardia presenting with a ventricular rate of 150 bpm should raise the suspicion of AFL. With AV nodal disease or AV nodal drug therapy, 4:1, 6:1, 8:1, or variable AV block is seen during AFL. The majority of AFLs have depolarization counterclockwise around the tricuspid annulus, and only approximately 10% have clockwise wavefronts. The typical counterclockwise AFL waves are negative in the inferior leads, and there are tall positive, small positive, or biphasic flutter waves in lead V1. Flutter pattern in the inferior leads can have prominent negative deflections, negative and then positive deflections that are equal in size, or a small negative and then a larger positive deflection. Leads I and aVL characteristically show low-voltage deflections. Clockwise AFL generally has broad positive deflections in the inferior leads and wide negative deflections in V1. AFL rate can slow with progression of atrial myopathy or with the use of antiarrhythmic drugs, such as amiodarone. Typical sawtooth pattern can also change with the appearance of an isoelectric baseline between flutter waves in these patients and appear as an AT. Additionally, the ECG pattern can be markedly altered in isthmus-dependent typical AFL after catheter ablation of atrial fibrillation owing to the alteration in depolarization pattern in scarred atria.

Rarely, AFL due to double-loop or lower-loop reentry wavefronts always involves CTI. In the lower-loop entry AFL, the activation wavefront traverses the CTI, activates the posterior right atrium, and then skirts the inferior vena cava with breakthrough along the low right atrium. Dual-loop reentry involves CTI with simultaneous two wavefronts or one wavefront involving CTI and other a atriotomy scar. These circuits can occur and may be indistinguishable electrocardiographically from typical AFL. Typical AFL can accelerate during an electrophysiology study after an extrastimulus delivered at the CTI with the same P wave morphology on the 12-lead ECG. The acceleration of the flutter is caused by two successive activation wavefronts circulating in the same direction along the same reentrant circuit (double-wave reentry) (Fig. 8.2). Flutter is usually faster in double-loop reentry, and flutter wave morphology in lower-loop reentry may vary depending on the site of breakthrough in the crista terminalis.

AFL with 1:1 conduction: In the presence of antiarrhythmic drug therapy, the cycle length of AF can prolong and atrial fibrillation can organize to a relatively slower flutter that allows the AV node to conduct 1:1, resulting in a paradoxically faster ventricular response and risk for life-threatening ventricular arrhythmia. A similar scenario can occur in patients with Wolff-Parkinson-White syndrome with rapid 1:1 AV conduction by way of one or more accessory pathways. It can also occur in patients with enhanced AV nodal conduction or during enhanced AV node conduction secondary to high sympathetic tone, such as during exercise.

ATYPICAL ATRIAL FLUTTERS

Atypical AFLs are mostly macroreentrant ATs and occur in diseased atria (Figures 8.16 through 8.47).[3] The circuit of AFL can be mapped during an electrophysiology study. In atypical AFL, the pathway reenters around a scar caused by an atriotomy, suture lines, or scar from a prior catheter ablation or maze procedure. Alternatively, reentry can occur around prosthetic patches and around a scar and anatomic structures, such as venae cavae, tricuspid annulus, mitral annulus, and pulmonary veins. AT and AFL can also result from atrial scarring in patients who have not undergone prior atrial surgery. These AFLs occur around scars in patients with congestive heart disease, valvular heart disease, and primary atrial myopathy.

Right AFLs: ECG pattern depends on the site, complexity, and multiplicity of circuits. Focal ATs and AFLs can also result from rapid focal discharge from pulmonary veins. AFL circuits in adults with repaired congenital heart disease are found in the right atrial lateral wall around the lateral atriotomy scar, atrial septal patch, or intraatrial baffle. However, CTI-dependent typical AFL still remains the most common AT/AFL in this population. Multiple circuits are not common around scars in a dilated right atrium or between the scar and anatomic structures, such as tricuspid annulus and vena cava. Left AFLs are uncommon in patients with congenital heart disease. Right AFL can also occur in patients with a history of pulmonary hypertension, mitral valve surgery, or atrial fibrillation ablation. As mentioned previously, the ECG pattern of typical AFL can change after catheter ablation of AFL or extensive myocardial scarring. Therefore ECG patterns of AFL can range from typical AFL to atypical flutter waves depending on the location and site of exit of the wavefront in the circuits.

Left AFLs: Iatrogenic AFL or AT occurring after catheter ablation of atrial fibrillation and maze procedure is probably the most common atypical form of left AFL or AT encountered in clinical practice. After mitral valve surgery, the most common flutter circuits are around the mitral valve, pulmonary veins, and atriotomy scars.[4]

Perimitral AFL: A counterclockwise perimitral AFL has positive flutter waves in the inferior and precordial leads and negative flutter waves in leads I and aVL. It can mimic AFL/AT arising from left

(Text continues on p. 228)

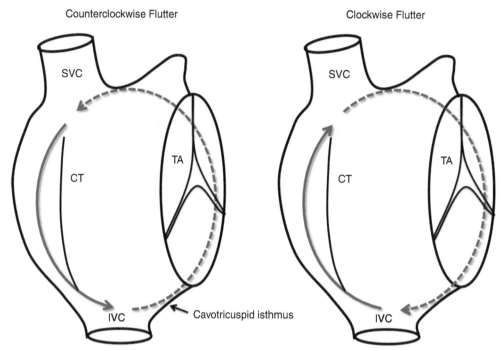

Fig. 8.1 Isthmus-dependent typical atrial flutter. The common variety of typical flutter wavefront travels counterclockwise along the tricuspid annulus and around the superior vena cava and crista terminalis (*red lines*). Clockwise atrial flutter is uncommon (10% of typical flutters). *CT*, Crista terminalis, *IVC*, inferior vena cava; *SVC*, superior vena cava; *TA*, tricuspid annulus.

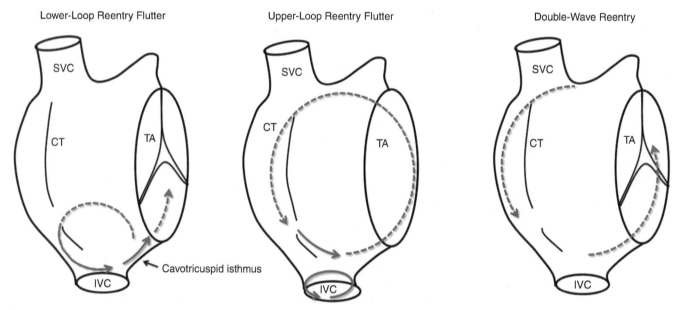

Fig. 8.2 Upper-loop reentry and lower-loop reentry atrial flutters. The upper-loop reentry circuit involves the crista terminalis (CT) with a breakthrough point somewhere in the crista, whereas in lower-loop reentry the circuit involves the cavotricuspid isthmus and turns around with a breakthrough in the physiologic barrier of CT (*red lines*). Presence of two successive activation wavefronts (*blue* and *red curved arrows*) circulating in the same direction along the same reentrant circuit is called *double-wave* or *double-loop reentry*. *IVC*, Inferior vena cava; *PA*, pulmonary artery; *SVC*, superior vena cava; *TA*, tricuspid annulus.

Scar-Related (Reentrant) Right Atrial Flutter/Tachycardia

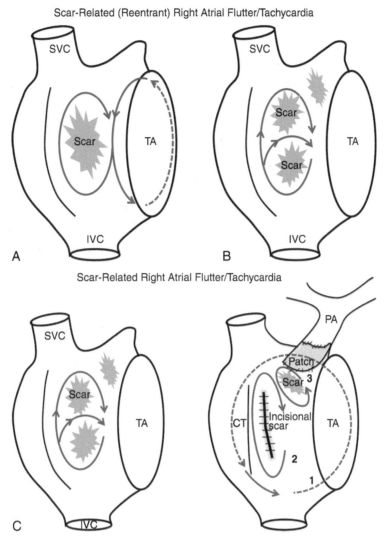

Scar-Related Right Atrial Flutter/Tachycardia

Fig. 8.3 Scar-related right atrial flutter has circuits (*red lines*) around the single (A) or multiple (B) atrial scars, around the incision, or near the anastomosis site (e.g., patch that connects right atrium with the pulmonary artery [Fontan surgery]) (C). *CT*, Crista terminalis; *IVC*, inferior vena cava; *PA*, pulmonary artery; *SVC*, superior vena cava; *TA*, tricuspid annulus.

Scar-Related Left Atrial Flutter/Tachycardia

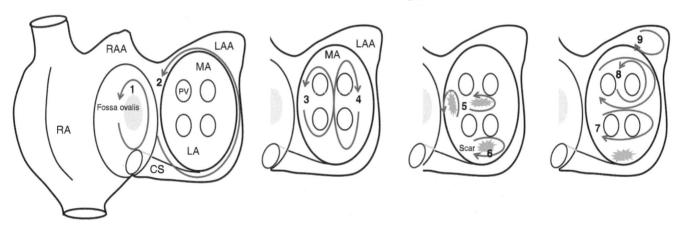

Fig. 8.4 Scar-related left atrial flutter/atrial tachycardia. Single or multiple circuits can exist in patients with a history of mitral valve surgery, catheter ablation of atrial flutter, and maze procedure. Commonly, circuits involve the interatrial septum (1) mitral annulus (mitral isthmus circuit, 2), around one or more pulmonary veins and atrial scars (3–8), at the base of the atrial appendage (9), and in the atrial septum. Red lines indicate direction of impulse propagation. *CS*, Coronary sinus; *LA*, left atrium; *LAA*, left atrial appendage, *MA*, mitral annulus; *PV*, pulmonary vein; *RA*, right atrium; *RAA*, right atrial appendage.

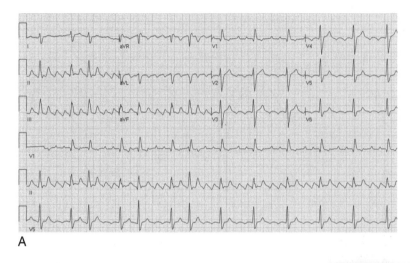

A

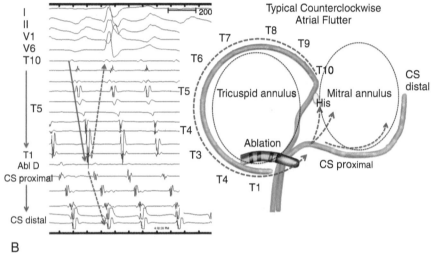

B

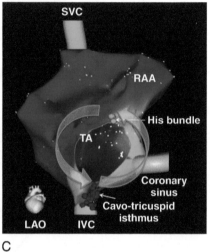

C

Atrial Flutter Termination During Catheter Ablation

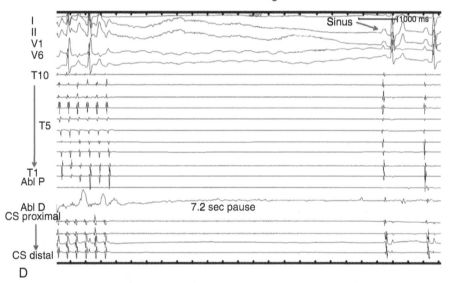

D

Fig. 8.5 Typical counterclockwise atrial flutter (AFL). (A) Electrocardiogram shows typical AFL with 2:1 and 4:1 atrioventricular conduction. (B) Intracardiac electrograms are recorded during an electrophysiology study with a multipolar circular (Halo) catheter (T1–T10) around the tricuspid annulus and another multipolar catheter in the coronary sinus (CS). AFL is terminated by applying radiofrequency energy with an ablation catheter (Abl D) and creating the conduction block along the cavotricuspid isthmus. *Red lines* denote flutter circuit. (C) Electroanatomic activation map shows the counterclockwise reentrant circuit around the tricuspid valve explain colors (D). *Abl P,* Ablation proximal; *IVC,* inferior vena cava; *LAO,* left anterior oblique; *RAA,* right atrial appendage; *SVC,* superior vena cava; *TA,* tricuspid annulus. (E) Flutter terminated during catheter ablation is followed by 7.2 sec sinus pause owing to sinus node dysfunction. *Wavy lines* in E are artifacts. Red and blue lines indicate multipolar catheter recordings from proximal to distal.

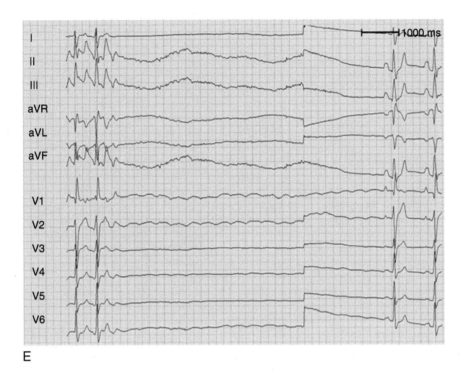

E

Fig. 8.5 (Continued).

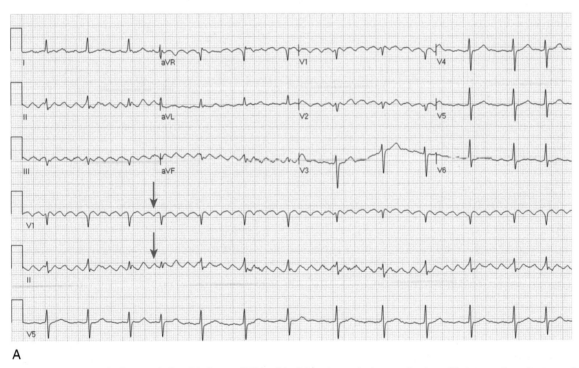

A

Fig. 8.6 (A) Electrocardiogram depicts typical atrial flutter (AFL) with 4:1 atrioventricular conduction. (B) Intracardiac electrocardiograms are recorded during an electrophysiology study with a multipolar circular (Halo) catheter (T1–T10) around the tricuspid annulus and another multipolar catheter in the coronary sinus (CS). They show a clockwise wavefront around the tricuspid annulus (*red lines*). The AFL is terminated by applying radiofrequency energy with an ablation catheter (Abl D) and creating a conduction block along the cavotricuspid isthmus. Arrows show flutter waves. *Abl P*, Ablation proximal.

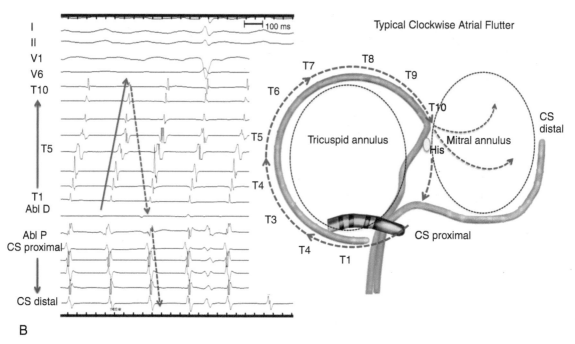

Fig. 8.6 (Continued).

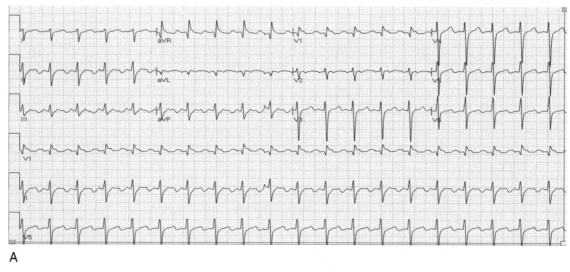

Fig. 8.7 Atrial flutter in a 39-year-old man with nonischemic cardiomyopathy. (A) Electrocardiogram shows positive flutter waves in inferior leads and negative-positive flutter waves in lead V1. The electroanatomic activation map (B) depicts the clockwise reentrant circuit around the tricuspid valve (*arrows*); color code activation from earliest (*red*) to latest (*purple*) timing. *RAA,* Right atrial appendage.

pulmonary veins; however, counterclockwise perimitral AFL is suggested by a more negative component in lead I, initial negative component in lead V2, and lack of any isoelectric interval between flutter waves. A clockwise perimitral AFL has an initial negative component in flutter waves in the lateral precordial leads but positive flutter waves in leads I and aVL.

AFLs with circuits around pulmonary veins and posterior left atrial scars: ECG pattern of these AFLs depend on several factors, including size and anatomy of circuits, amount of atrial scar, atrial anatomy, and

prior catheter ablation or cardiac surgery. Therefore the ECG pattern is most variable.

ATs or AFLs with left septal circuits: Septal circuits manifest as prominent flutter waves in lead V1 or V2 and almost flat waves in most other leads. This pattern is caused by a septal circuit with anterior-posterior forces projecting in lead V1 and the cancellation of caudocranial forces. This pattern is 100% sensitive for a left atrial septal circuit, but the specificity of this pattern for any left atrial AFL is only 64%.

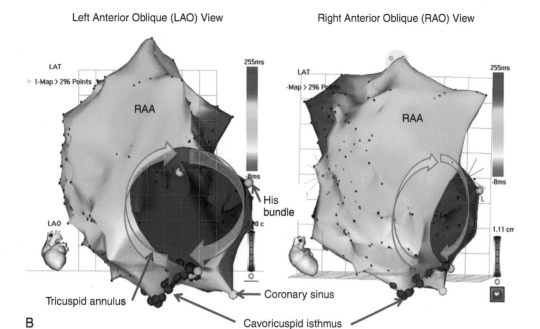

Left Anterior Oblique (LAO) View   Right Anterior Oblique (RAO) View

B

Fig. 8.7 (Continued).

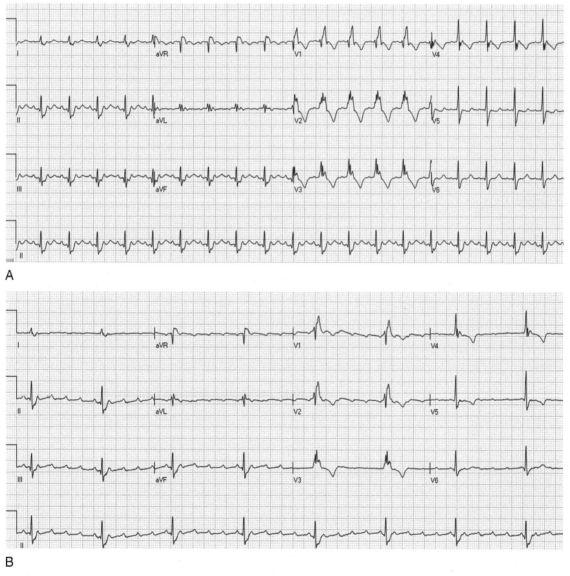

A

B

Fig. 8.8 Clockwise atrial flutter in a 44-year-old woman with chronic obstructive pulmonary disease and right bundle branch block. Electrocardiogram reveals typical clockwise atrial flutter (positive P waves in inferior leads and negative P waves in lead V1) with 2:1 atrioventricular (AV) conduction (A). Therapy with AV nodal–blocking drugs resulted in a decrease in the AV conduction to 5:1 (B).

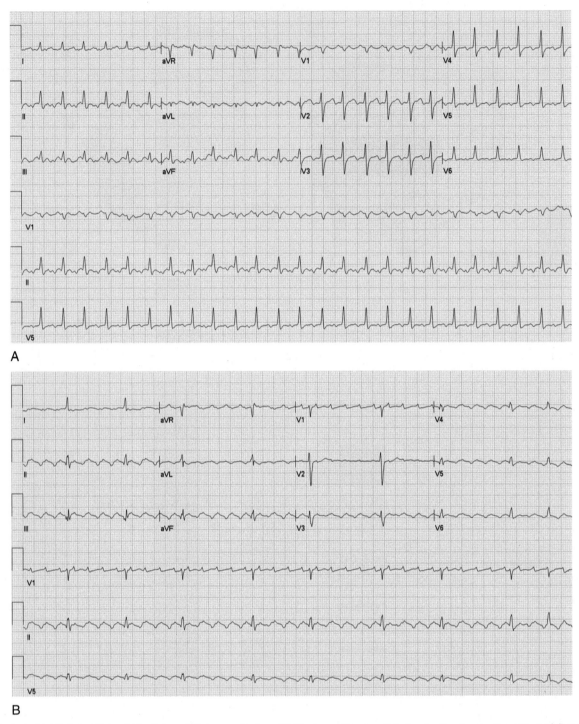

Fig. 8.9 Typical atrial flutter with variable atrioventricular conduction. (A) Electrocardiogram shows negative sawtooth pattern of flutter waves in the inferior leads and positive flutter waves in lead V1 with 2:1 conduction. (B) Typical flutter with 3:1, 4:1, and 5:1 atrioventricular block.

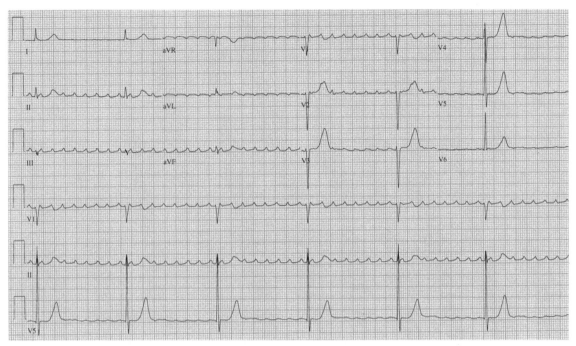

Fig. 8.10 Electrocardiogram depicts typical atrial flutter with an 8:1 atrioventricular block with a ventricular rate of 38 bpm owing to advanced atrioventricular nodal disease.

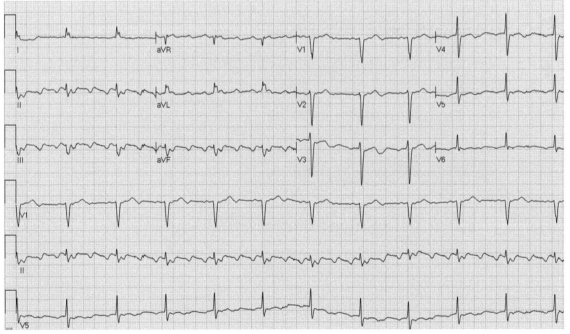

Fig. 8.11 Atrial flutter (AFL) with 3:1 atrioventricular (AV) conduction. AFL is commonly associated with 2:1 or 4:1 AV block; 3:1 or 5:1 AV block is very uncommon in a typical AFL.

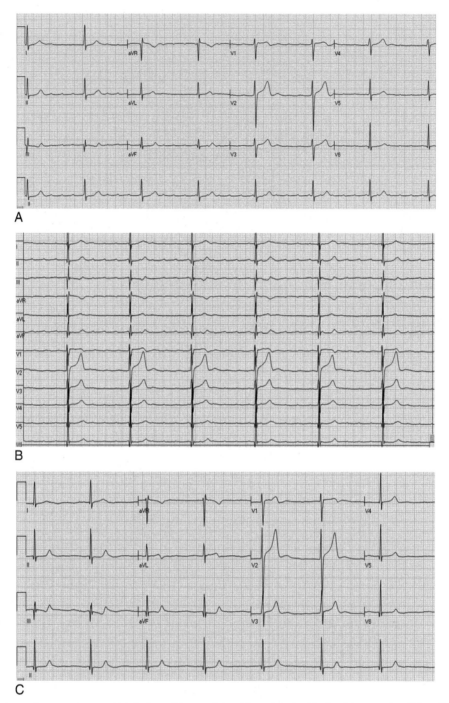

Fig. 8.12 (A and B) Electrocardiogram shows atrial flutter with complete atrioventricular block with a varying flutter-R interval and a fixed R-R interval. (C) Termination of atrial flutter resulted in sinus arrest with a junctional rhythm (with narrow QRS).

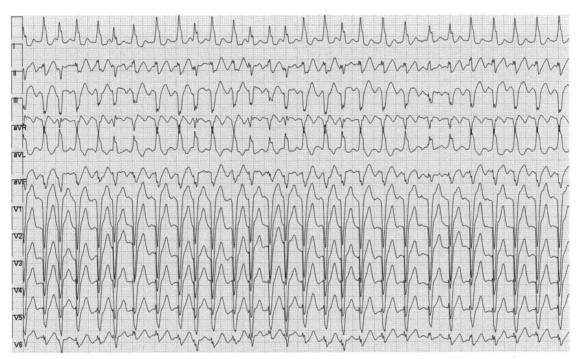

Fig. 8.13 Atrial flutter with variable atrioventricular conduction and a rapid ventricular response mimicking atrial fibrillation.

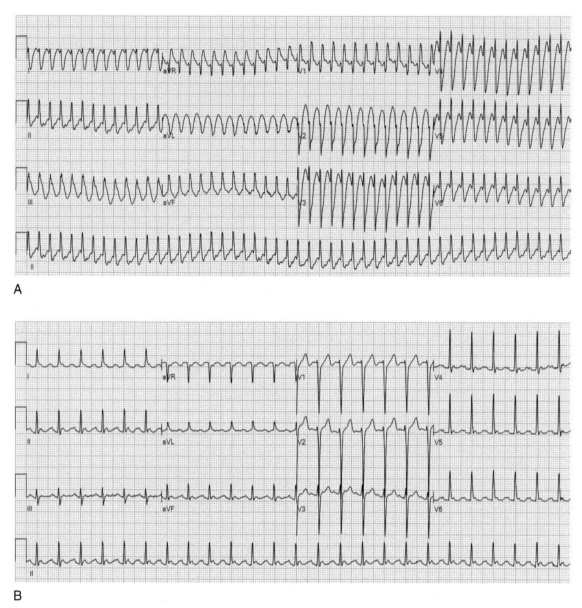

A

B

Fig. 8.14 A 43-year-old man presented with paroxysmal wide complex tachycardia (A). After giving atrioventricular (AV) nodal blocking drugs, the tachycardia was recognized to be atrial flutter with 2:1 AV nodal conduction and narrow QRS complexes (B). During electrophysiology (EP) study, the typical clockwise atrial flutter was mapped and ablated successfully at the cavotricuspid isthmus (C). During EP study, atrial pacing at the atrial flutter rate demonstrated right bundle branch block aberrancy similar to the presenting wide complex tachycardia rhythm, proving that the AV node is capable of 1:1 AV conduction with right bundle branch block aberrancy at the fast atrial rate during atrial flutter (S: stimulus artifact, A: atrial electrogram, V: ventricular electrogram). (D) 12-lead electrocardiograms are not in perfect position during EP study due to large Carto patches on the chest and spuriously depict a tall R wave.

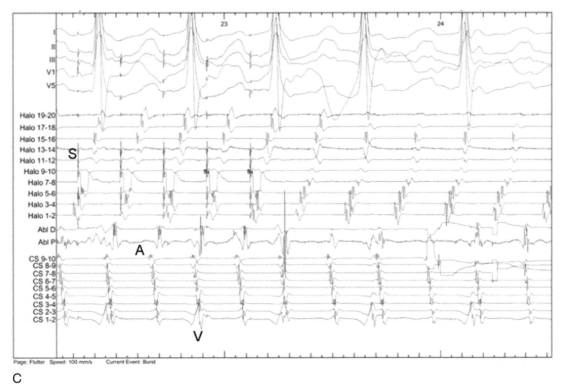

C

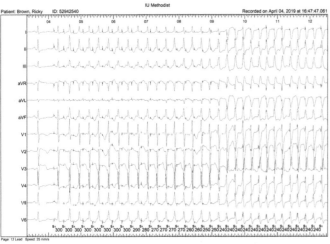

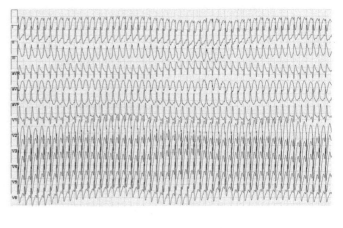

D

Fig. 8.14 (Continued).

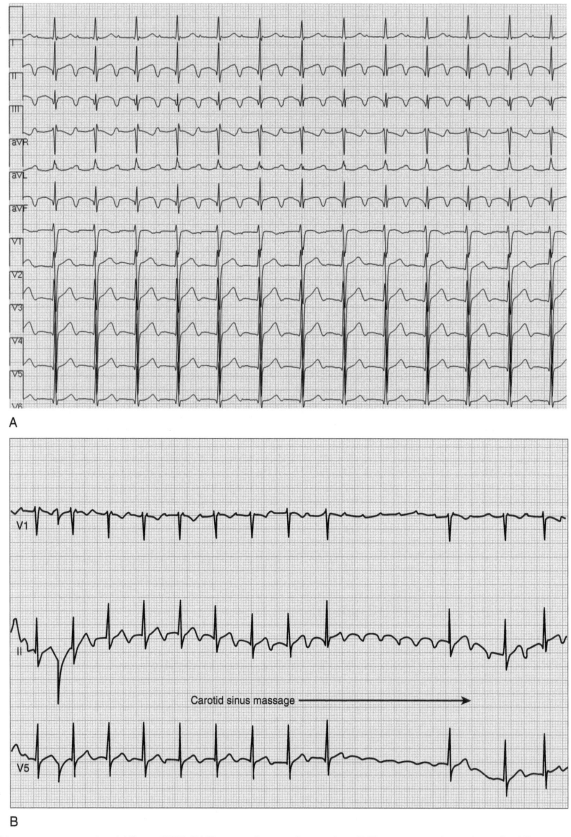

Fig. 8.15 Maneuvers to unmask atrial flutter (AFL). (A) Electrocardiogram shows a long R-P' narrow complex tachycardia. AFL waves are not well distinguished from T waves. (B) Carotid sinus massage results in advanced atrioventricular block and unmasking of AFL waves. AFL waves are also unmasked after a spontaneous premature ventricular complex (*red arrows*) (C) and after administration of intravenous diltiazem (D).

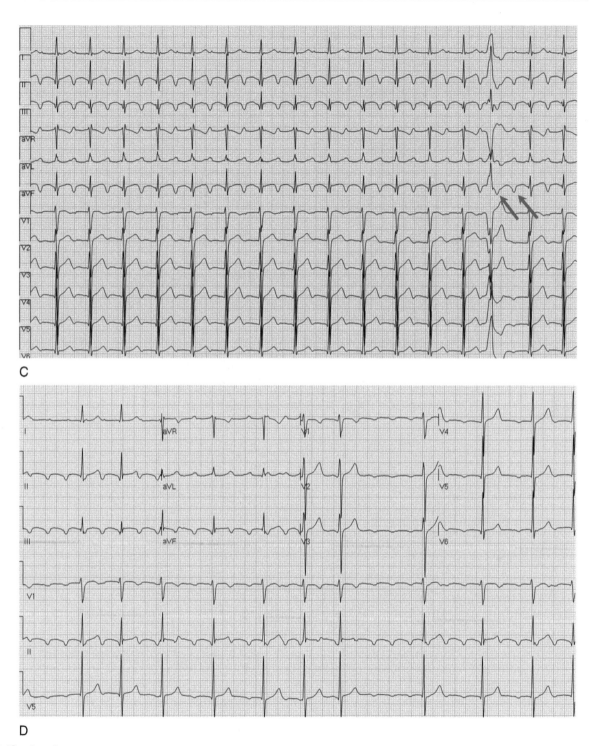

C

D

Fig. 8.15 (Continued).

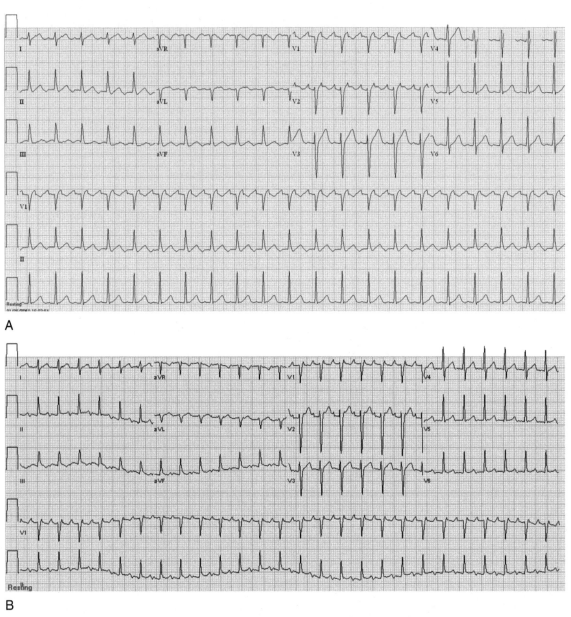

A

B

Fig. 8.16 Two types of left atrial flutter with positive flutter waves in lead V1, after catheter ablation of atrial fibrillation (A and B). These were mapped in the left atrial posterior wall close to the right pulmonary veins. Of note, even the cavotricuspid isthmus–dependent atrial flutter may appear atypical flutter in patient with history of atrial fibrillation due to extensive left and right atrial scar.

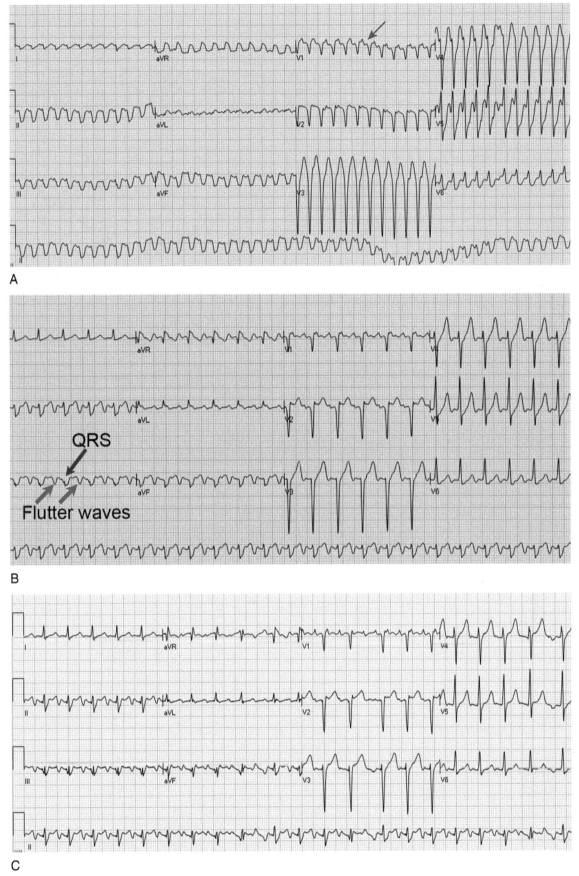

Fig. 8.17 Atrial flutter (AFL; *arrow*) presenting as a wide complex tachycardia owing to 1:1 atrioventricular (AV) conduction. (A) Patient presented with a hemodynamically unstable wide complex tachycardia with positive P waves in lead V1. Flutter waves are not well recognized. (B) Administration of intravenous calcium blocker induced 2:1 AV block, and AFL waves are unmasked (*red arrows*). The R-R interval during 1:1 AV conduction is half the R-R interval after 2:1 AV block. (C and D) Typical AFL waves are better recognized after further AV block. (E) Patient later developed atrial fibrillation.

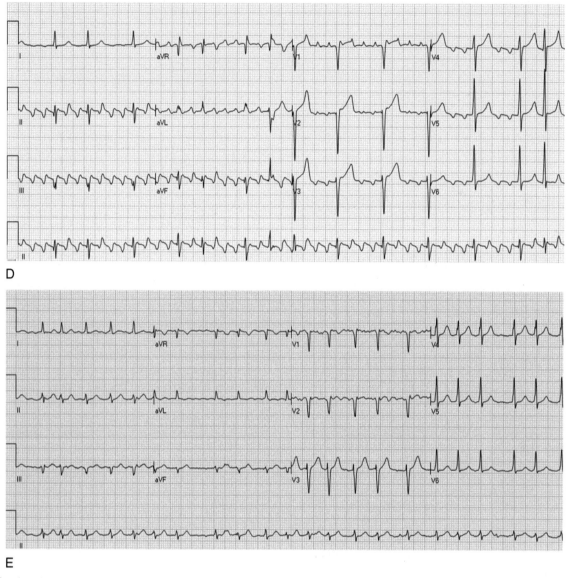

D

E

Fig. 8.17 (Continued).

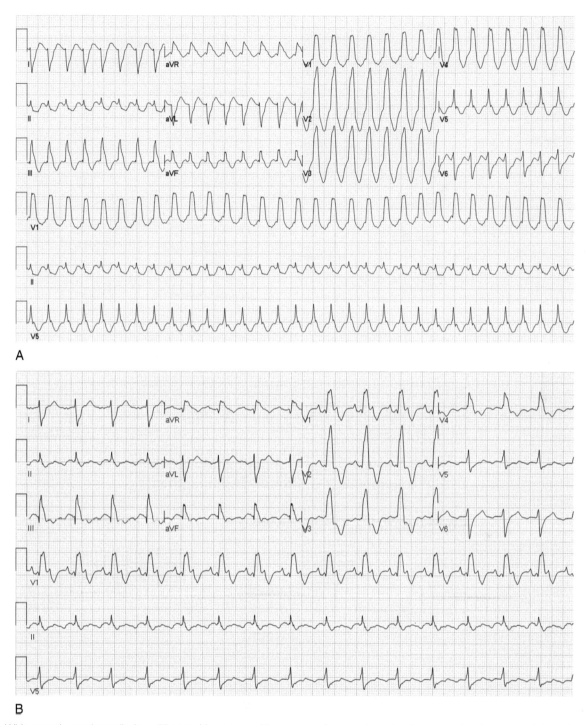

Fig. 8.18 Wide complex tachycardia in a 35-year-old woman with severe pulmonary hypertension secondary to recurrent thromboemboli. (A) Electrocardiogram shows wide complex tachycardia with right bundle branch block and right axis deviation. Electrocardiogram features are consistent with a supraventricular tachycardia with aberrancy. This is a typical counterclockwise atrial flutter (AFL) with 1:1 atrioventricular conduction. (B) Typical AFL with 2:1 atrioventricular conduction. AFL cycle length is 320 ms because of a significantly enlarged right atrium with slow atrial myocardial conduction of AFL waves.

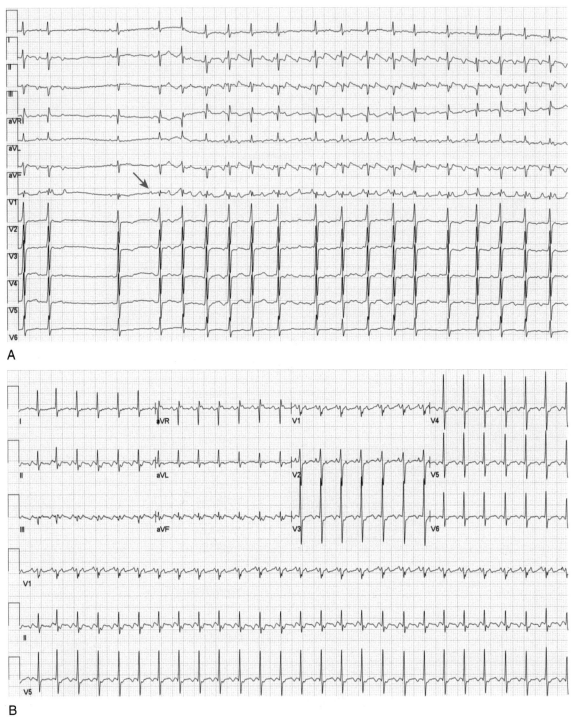

Fig. 8.19 Initiation of atrial flutter (*arrow*) with an premature atrial complex (A). Typical atrial flutter is a reentrant arrhythmia and is typically initiated by a premature atrial complex. Atrial flutter later shows 2:1 AV response (B).

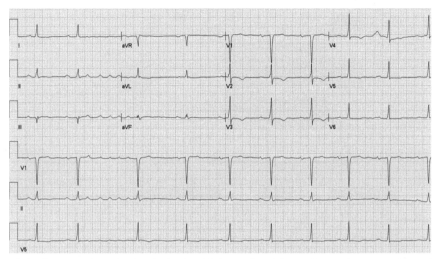

Fig. 8.20 Focal atrial flutter. Atrial flutter can be a focal arrhythmia, which usually originates from pulmonary veins and can be a precursor of atrial fibrillation. Focal atrial flutters are usually paroxysmal, and its origin can be mapped during electrophysiology study.

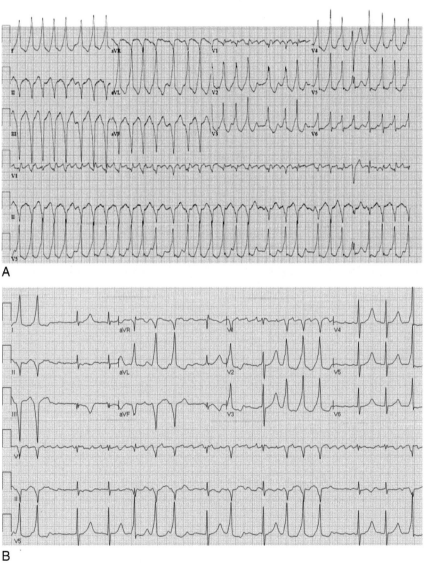

Fig. 8.21 Atrial flutter with Wolff-Parkinson-White syndrome. (A) Patient presented with atrial flutter with rapid ventricular response with a short R-R interval of 210 ms. Short R-R interval can result in rapid ventricular tachycardia, ventricular fibrillation, and sudden cardiac death. (B) Patient later developed atrial fibrillation with intermittent preexcitation.

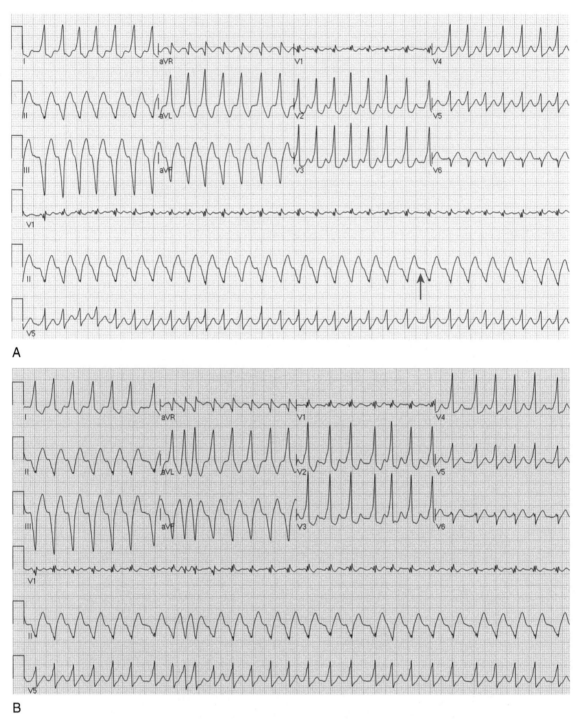

A

B

Fig. 8.22 Wide complex tachycardia in a 58-year-old man with hypotension. (A) Electrocardiogram (ECG) reveals a wide complex tachycardia with slurred upstroke in R waves in V2-V5 and in slurred QS pattern in inferior leads (*arrow*). The tachycardia appears to be regular; however, close observation reveals atrial flutter/fibrillation with Wolff-Parkinson-White syndrome. The arrow shows slower RR interval. (B) ECG shows atrial fibrillation with an irregular ventricular rhythm. (C) After direct current cardioversion, the ECG shows right bundle branch block morphology with positive delta waves in lead V1 and negative delta waves in inferior leads (*arrows*) suggestive of a left posteroseptal accessory pathway. (D) ECG after catheter ablation shows normal sinus rhythm and normal P-R interval without any delta waves. Atrial arrhythmia did not recur during a 2-year follow-up.

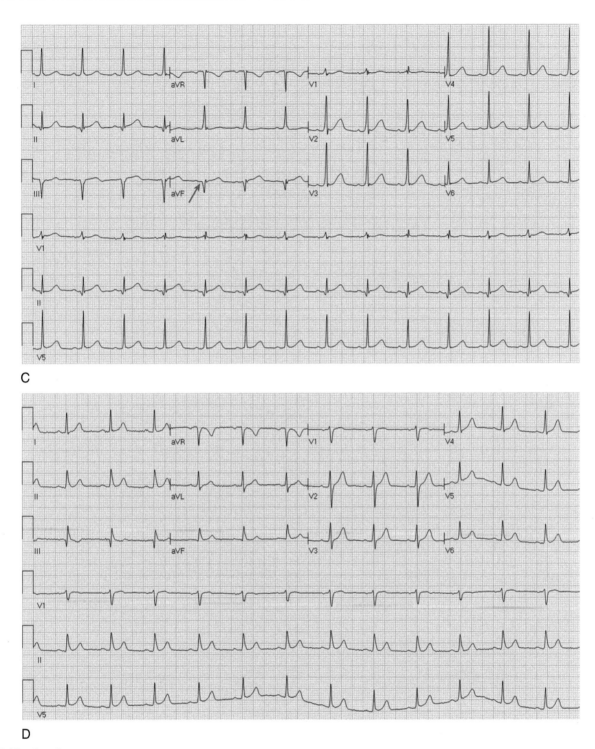

C

D

Fig. 8.22 (Continued).

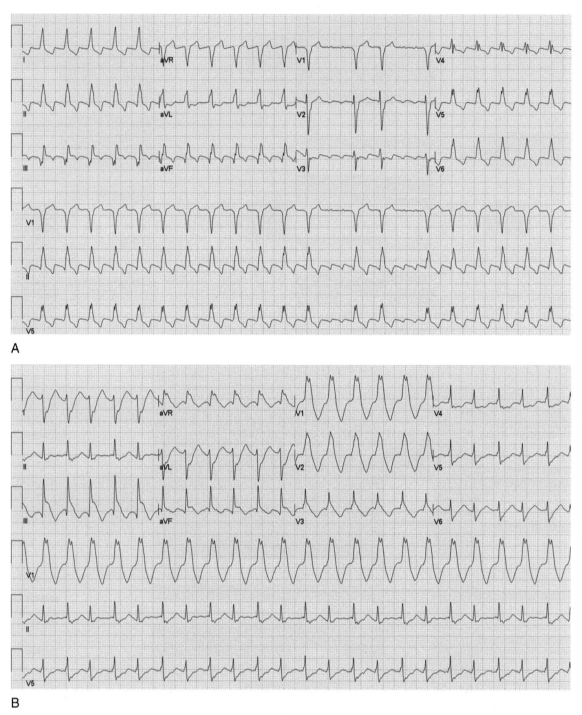

A

B

Fig. 8.23 Atrial flutter with ventricular aberrancy. (A) Electrocardiogram shows atrial flutter with left bundle branch block. (B) Electrocardiogram shows right bundle branch block aberrancy owing to rapid ventricular rates.

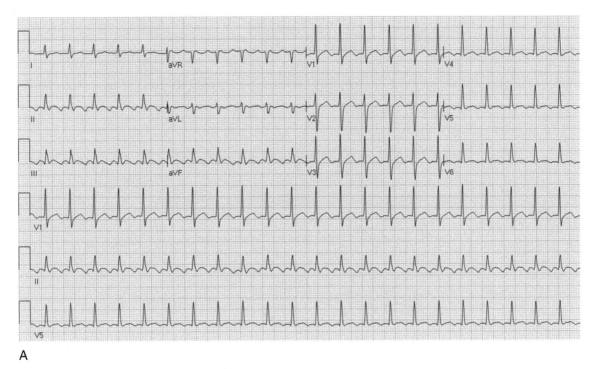

A

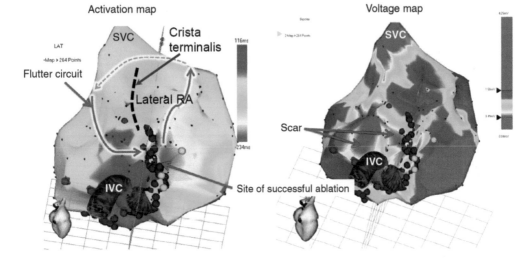

B

Fig. 8.24 Right atrial flutter (AFL) with upper-loop reentry. (A) Electrocardiogram reveals AFL with flutter wave vector similar to a typical counterclockwise AFL. However, during the electrophysiologic study the arrhythmia was found to have upper-loop reentry (see also Fig. 8.2). The electroanatomic (right anterior oblique view) shows that, unlike a typical AFL circuit, the wavefronts break through the inferior part of the crista terminalis (B). *IVC*, Inferior vena cava; *SVC*, superior vena cava.

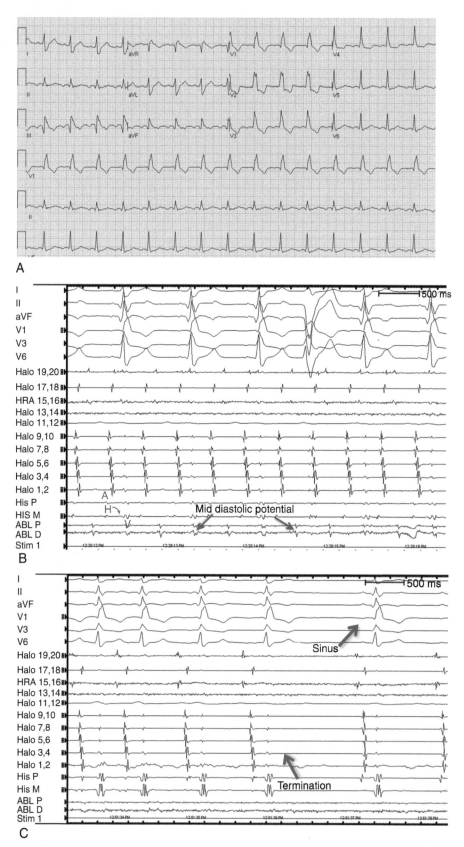

Fig. 8.25 Scar-related right atrial flutter (AFL). (A) Electrocardiogram shows AFL with 2:1 atrioventricular conduction in a patient with no significant risk factor for AFL. Isthmus of AFL circuit is localized at the lower crista terminalis region. (B) Intracardiac electrocardiogram shows a mid-diastolic potential at the isthmus of the reentrant circuit. (C) Tachycardia terminated (*upright arrow*) at that site with progressive prolongation of the tachycardia cycle length before termination. Electroanatomic map shows a localized area of reentry (D) with earliest activation (*red zone*) followed by later activation zones as *yellow*, *green*, and *purple areas*. There is extensive right atrial scarring with interatrial septal scarring (*red zone*) and scarring in the posterior wall of left atrium (E) suggestive of atrial myopathy. Other areas are relative healthy (*purple areas*), green (mild scar), yellow (scar boarder zone). *A,* Atrial electrogram, *Abl,* ablation; *CS,* coronary sinus; *H,* His bundle electrogram; *His M,* middle His; *His P,* proximal His; *HRA,* high right atrium; *IVC,* inferior vena cava; *LIPV,* left inferior pulmonary vein; *LSPV,* left superior pulmonary vein; *SVC,* superior vena cava; *V,* ventricular electrogram.

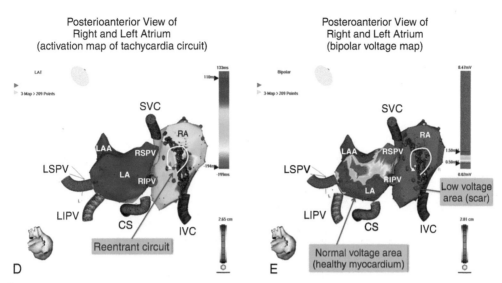

Posterioanterior View of
Right and Left Atrium
(activation map of tachycardia circuit)

Posteroanterior View of
Right and Left Atrium
(bipolar voltage map)

D

E

Fig. 8.25 (Continued).

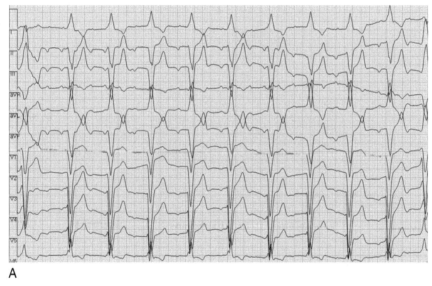

A

Fig. 8.26 Right atrial tachycardia/atrial flutter with 3:1 atrioventricular conduction. (A) Tachycardia shows negative P waves in lead V1 and inferior leads and positive P waves in lead aVR. (B) Isthmus of tachycardia circuit was mapped to the inferoposterolateral right atrium (RA). Reentrant mechanism was confirmed by entrainment mapping. The atrial tachycardia circuit is shown anatomically on the computerized tomography (CT) scan of the heart, and different colors are used to show different parts of the heart. *AO,* Aorta; *IVC,* inferior vena cava; *LA,* left atrium; *PA,* pulmonary artery; *PV,* pulmonary vein; *RV,* right ventricle.

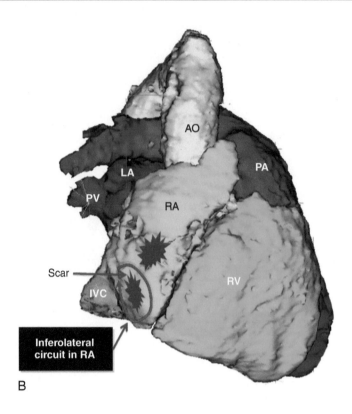

B

Fig. 8.26 (Continued).

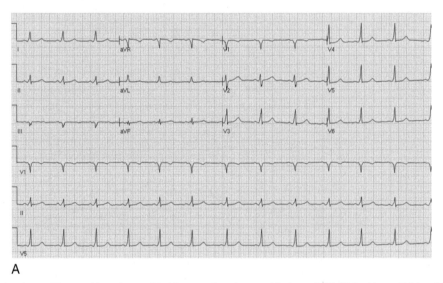

A

Fig. 8.27 Atrial arrhythmias in a 58-year-old patient with history of catheter ablation of Wolff-Parkinson-White (WPW) syndrome and an anterolateral right atrial circuit. (A) Electrocardiogram (ECG) shows sinus rhythm with short P-R interval and delta wave (*arrow*) of right inferolateral accessory pathway, which recurred after an attempted surgical correction. (B) Patient later underwent a successful catheter ablation of the accessory pathway with abolition of delta waves. However, she developed several episodes of atrial flutter (AFL). (C) The ECG shows inverted flutter wave in leads V1, aVR, and inferior leads. The AFL circuit was mapped at the inferolateral RA. (D) The ECG shows similar inverted flutter wave in leads V1, aVR, and inferior leads. The AFL circuit was mapped at the anterolateral RA. (E) The ECG shows inverted flutter wave in leads V1, aVR, and inferior leads. The AFL circuit was mapped at the inferolateral RA. (F) Diagram showing the location of anterolateral and inferolateral RA scar and reentrant circuit for AFL shown in D and E, respectively. The atrial tachycardia circuit is shown anatomically on the CT scan of the heart, and different colors are used to depict different parts of the heart. *AO,* Aorta; *IVC,* inferior vena cava; *LA,* left atrium; *PA,* pulmonary artery; *PV,* pulmonary vein; *RA,* right atrium; *RV,* right ventricle.

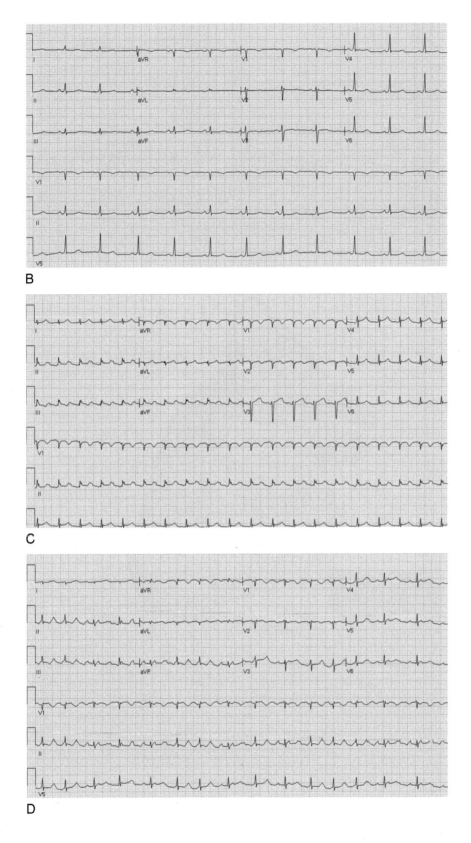

B

C

D

Fig. 8.27 (Continued).

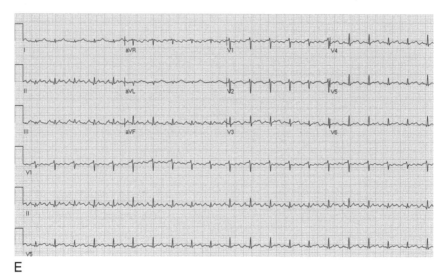

E

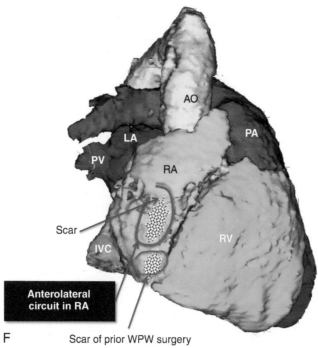

F

Scar

IVC

Anterolateral circuit in RA

Scar of prior WPW surgery

AO

LA

PV

RA

PA

RV

Fig. 8.27 (Continued).

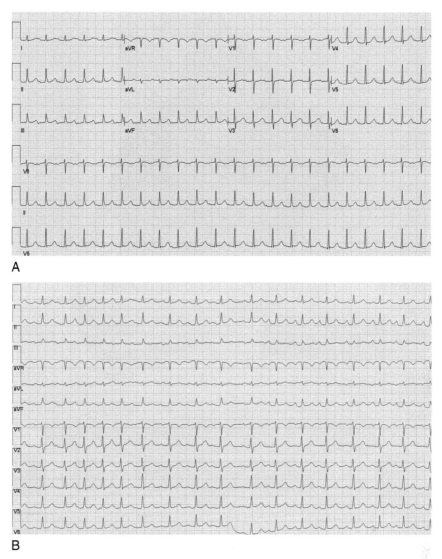

Fig. 8.28 Atrial flutter/atrial tachycardia with 1:1 atrioventricular (AV) conduction in a 60-year-old woman with pulmonary hypertension. The flutter wave morphology cannot be ascertained in many leads because of 1:1 AV conduction (A). However, the 12-lead electrocardiogram during AV nodal drug therapy (B) clearly shows biphasic flutter waves in lead V1 and positive flutter waves in leads I, aVL, and inferior leads. The isthmus of reentrant circuit was mapped arising from the anterosuperior RA (C). The atrial tachycardia circuit is shown anatomically on the CT scan of the heart, and different colors are used to depict different parts of the heart. *AO*, Aorta; *IVC*, inferior vena cava; *LA*, left atrium; *PA*, pulmonary artery; *PV*, pulmonary vein; *RA*, right atrium; *RV*, right ventricle.

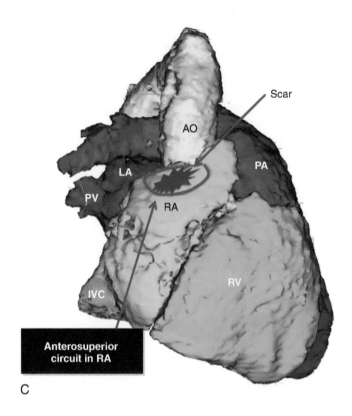

Fig. 8.28 (Continued).

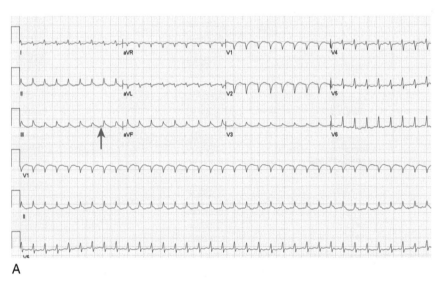

Fig. 8.29 Macroreentrant atrial flutter in a 48-year-old woman with atrial myopathy. (A) Electrocardiogram (ECG) shows negative flutter waves in lead V1 and inferior leads (*arrow*) and positive flutter waves in leads I, aVL, and aVR. (B) ECG depicts negative flutter waves in lead V1 and aVR and positive flutter waves in lead I and inferior leads. The isthmus of tachycardia circuit of ECGs A and B were mapped at the lateral and mid inferolateral right atrium. (C) Diagram of the lateral RA circuit around scar. The atrial tachycardia circuit is shown anatomically on the CT scan of the heart, and different colors are used to depict different parts of the heart. *A* and the inferolateral circuit around scar *B. AO*, Aorta; *IVC*, inferior vena cava; *LA*, left atrium; *PA*, pulmonary artery; *PV*, pulmonary vein; *RA*, right atrium; *RV*, right ventricle.

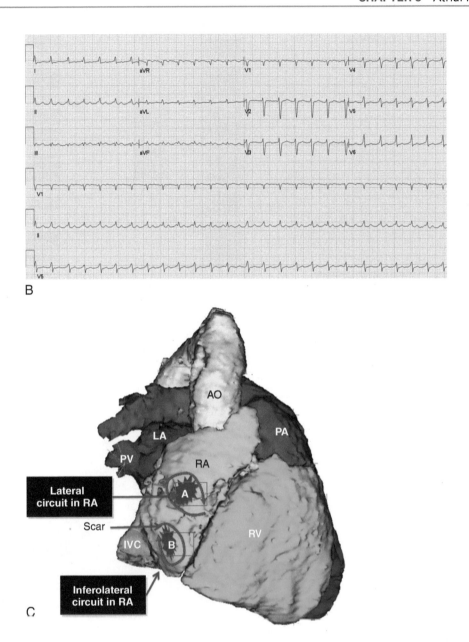

Fig. 8.29 (Continued).

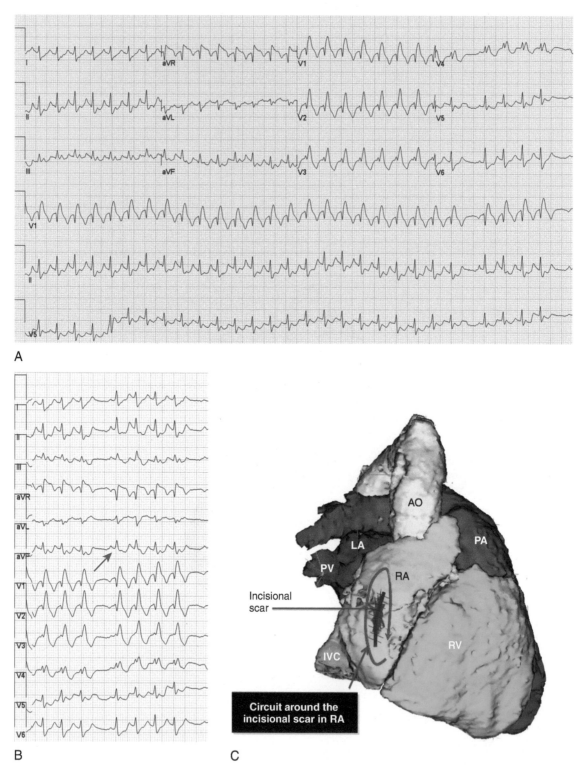

Fig. 8.30 Macroreentrant atrial tachycardia/atrial flutter around the lateral atriotomy scar in a 53-year-old man with history of cardiac surgery for the treatment of atrioventricular nodal reentrant tachycardia. The electrocardiogram (A) and its 12-lead rhythm strip (B) show negative flutter waves in lead V1 and inferior leads (*arrow*) and positive flutter waves in leads I, aVL, and aVR. Tachycardia circuit was mapped around the incisional scar in the lateral right atrium (C). *AO,* Aorta; *IVC,* inferior vena cava; *LA,* left atrium; *PA,* pulmonary artery; *PV,* pulmonary vein; *RA,* right atrium; *RV,* right ventricle.

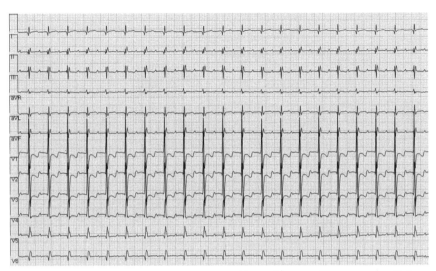

Fig. 8.31 Scar-related atrial tachycardia/flutter in a 20-year-old man with congenital heart disease and Fontan surgery. He has mesocardia with double outlet ventricle, hypoplastic right ventricle, juxtaposition of atrium, and severe pulmonary stenosis. Electrocardiogram reveals positive flutter waves in lead V1 and inferior leads and isoelectric flutter waves in leads I, aVL, and aVR. Tachycardia circuit was mapped at the junction of the right atrium and pulmonary artery.

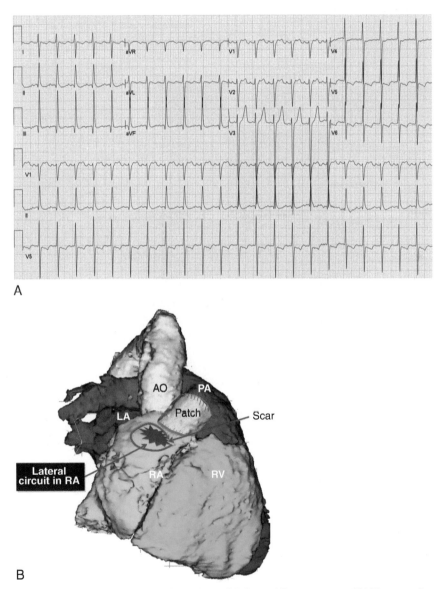

Fig. 8.32 Scar-related atrial flutter/tachycardia in a patient with tetralogy of Fallot and Fontan surgery. (A) Electrocardiogram depicts negative flutter waves in lead V1 and inferior leads and positive flutter waves in leads I, aVL, and aVR. Atrial tachycardia/flutter circuit was mapped during the electrophysiology study around the junction of the right atrial appendage and pulmonary artery anastomosis (classic Fontan shunt) (B) and was ablated successfully. The atrial tachycardia circuit is shown anatomically on the CT scan of the heart, and different colors are used to depict different parts of the heart. *AO,* Aorta; *LA,* left atrium; *PA,* pulmonary artery; *RA,* right atrium; *RV,* right ventricle.

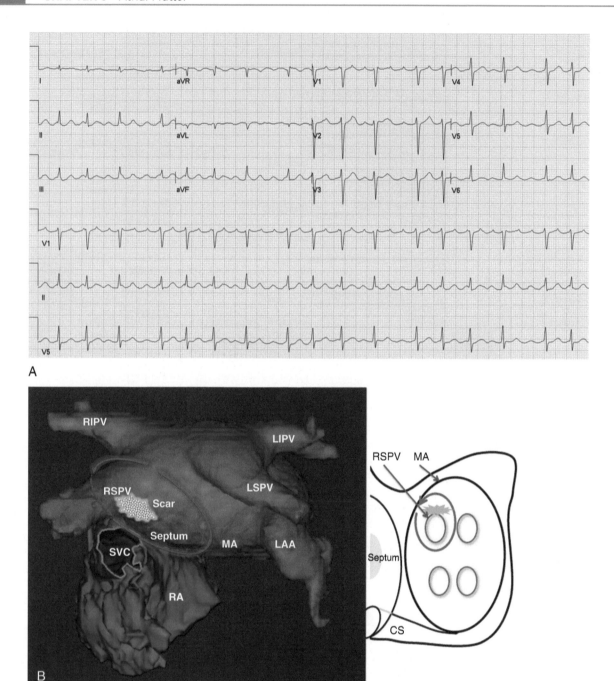

Fig. 8.33 Macroreentrant atrial flutter in a patient after catheter ablation of atrial fibrillation. (A) Electrocardiogram reveals positive flutter waves in lead V1 and inferior leads and negative flutter waves in leads I, aVL, and aVR. (B) Isthmus of reentrant circuit was mapped between the right superior pulmonary vein (RSPV) and the anterior mitral annulus (MA). The picture shows superior view of the CT scan of the heart with right atrium (*purple*) and left atrium (*brown*). *CS,* Coronary sinus; *LAA,* left atrial appendage; *LIPV,* left inferior pulmonary vein; *LSPV,* left superior pulmonary vein; *RA,* right atrium; *RIPV,* right inferior pulmonary vein; *SVC,* superior vena cava.

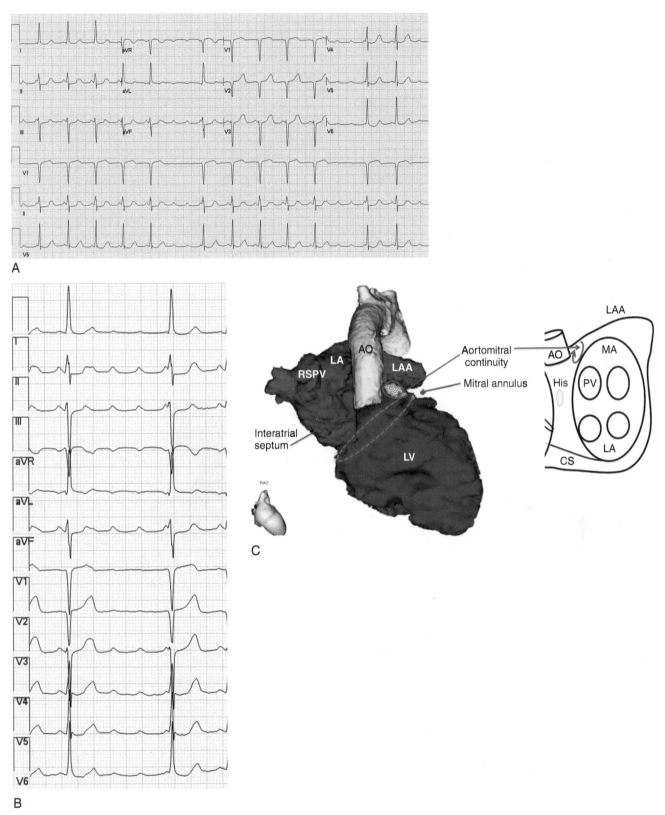

Fig. 8.34 Microreentrant atrial flutter in a patient after catheter ablation of atrial fibrillation. Electrocardiogram (A) and rhythm strip of the same electrocardiogram (B) show isoelectric flutter waves in lead V1 and I; mildly negative in lead aVL; positive flutter waves in inferior leads (*arrow*); and positive flutter waves in leads I, aVL, and aVR. The atrial flutter circuit was mapped near the aortomitral continuity (C). The picture shows the right anterior oblique view of the CT scan of the heart showing the left atrium (LA), left ventricle (LV), and the aorta (AO), and the image shows the site of the circuit in a simplified way. *CS,* coronary sinus; *LAA,* left atrial appendage; *MA,* mitral annulus; *PV,* pulmonary vein; *RSPV,* right superior pulmonary vein.

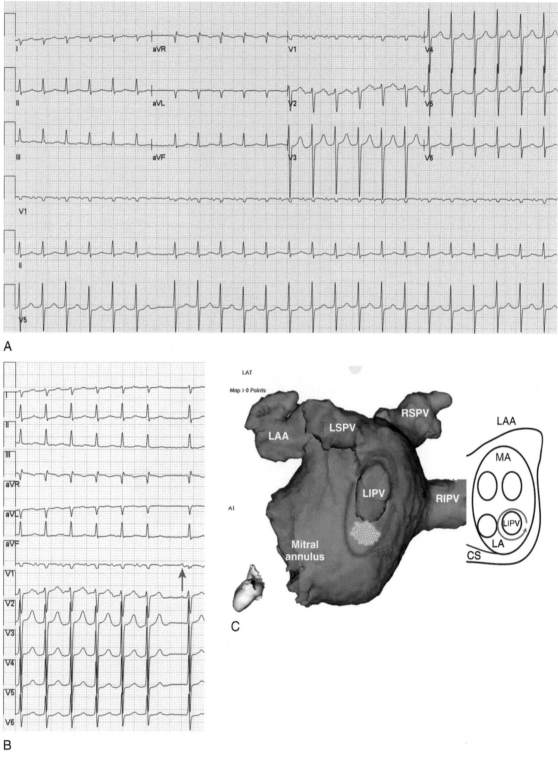

Fig. 8.35 Macroreentrant atrial tachycardia/flutter occurred after catheter ablation of atrial fibrillation (pulmonary vein isolation). Electrocardiogram (A) and rhythm strip of the same electrocardiogram (B) show isoelectric flutter waves in lead V1 and isoelectric low-voltage flutter waves. During an electrophysiology study, the tachycardia isthmus was at the lateral mitral annulus (MA) (C) and was terminated successfully by creating a line of block between the lateral MA and left inferior pulmonary vein (LIPV). The picture shows the CT scan of the lateral view of the left atrium (LA) and the cartoon shows the site of the circuit in a simplified way. The two oval circuits around the pulmonary veins represent line of circumferential ablation around right and left pulmonary veins for the treatment of atrial fibrillation. *CS,* Coronary sinus; *LAA,* left atrial appendage; *LSPV,* left superior pulmonary vein; *RIPV,* right inferior pulmonary vein; *RSPV,* right superior pulmonary vein.

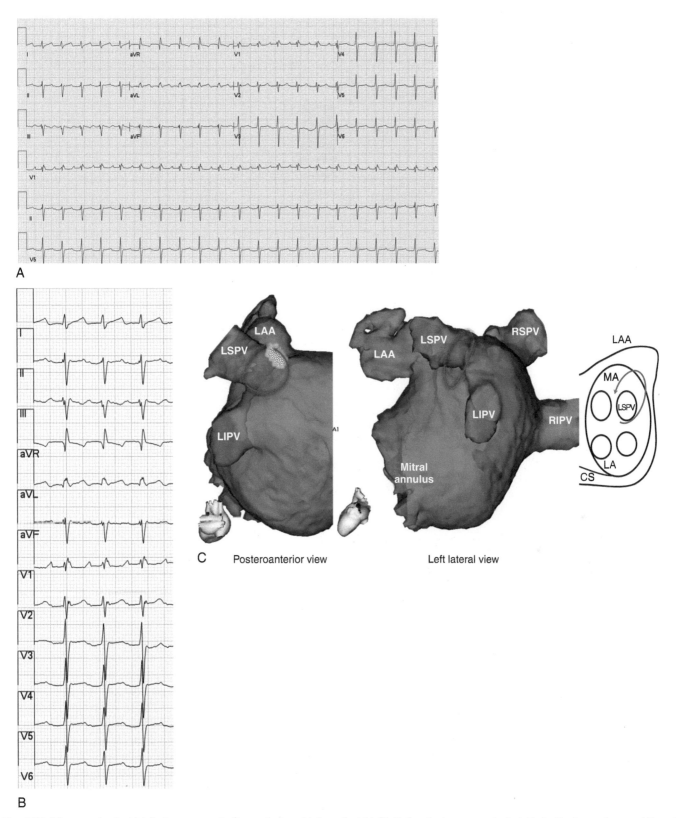

Fig. 8.36 Microreentrant atrial flutter occurred after catheter ablation of atrial fibrillation (pulmonary vein isolation). Electrocardiogram (A) and rhythm strip of the same electrocardiogram (B) show isoelectric flutter waves in lead V1, mildly negative in lead aVL, and positive flutter waves in inferior leads. During an electrophysiology study, the tachycardia circuit (C) was mapped at the anterior ridge of the left superior pulmonary vein (LSPV). After its reentrant mechanism was determined with entrainment, the tachycardia was terminated successfully during catheter ablation. The picture shows the CT scan of the anteroposterior and lateral view of the left atrium (LA) and the cartoon shows the site of the circuit in a simplified way. The two oval circuits around the pulmonary veins represent line of circumferential ablation around right and left pulmonary veins for the treatment of atrial fibrillation. *CS,* Coronary sinus; *LA,* left atrium; *LAA,* left atrial appendage; *LIPV,* left inferior pulmonary vein; *MA,* mitral annulus; *RIPV,* right inferior pulmonary vein; *RSPV,* right superior pulmonary vein.

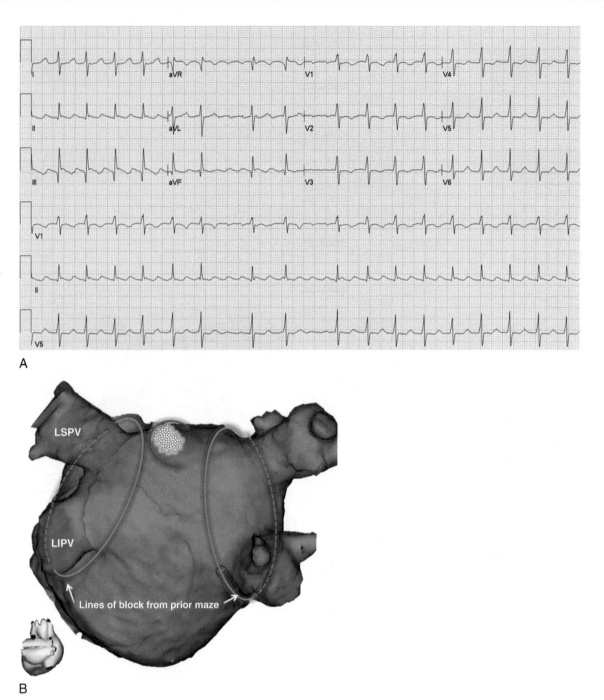

Fig. 8.37 Atrial flutter after mitral valve repair and maze procedure. (A) Electrocardiogram depicts negative flutter waves in lead V1, aVR, and lead I; mildly negative in lead aVL; positive flutter waves in inferior leads; and positive flutter waves in lead I. The flutter circuit was mapped at the left atrial roof close to the left superior pulmonary vein (LSPV) origin (B). The picture shows the posteroanterior view of the CT scan of the heart showing the left atrium, and shows the site of the circuit in a simplified way. The two oval circuits around the pulmonary veins represent line of circumferential ablation around right and left pulmonary veins for the treatment of atrial fibrillation. The arrhythmia was terminated by ablation at the roof of the left atrium. *LIPV*, Left inferior pulmonary vein.

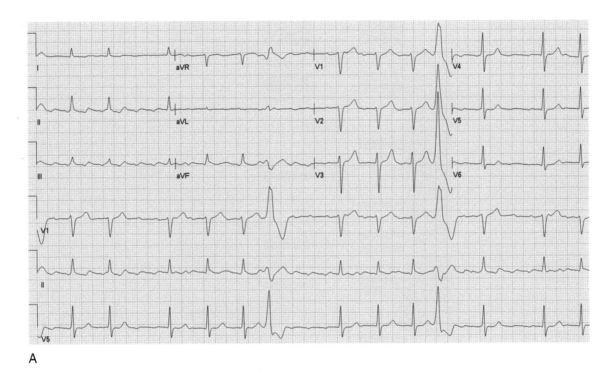

A

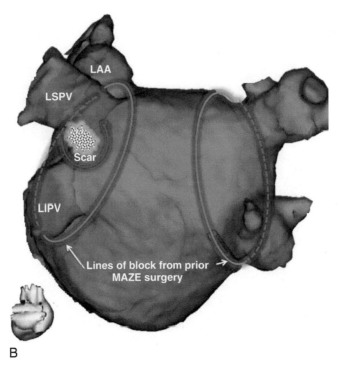

B

Fig. 8.38 Post–maze procedure macroreentrant atrial flutter. (A) Electrocardiogram shows positive flutter waves in lead V1 and negative-positive waves in inferior leads and isoelectric flutter waves in lead aVL and I. (B) The isthmus of the circuit was mapped at the carina of left pulmonary veins. The picture shows the posteroanterior view of the CT scan of the heart showing the left atrium, and the image shows the site of the circuit in a simplified away and at the roof of the left atrium, where the arrhythmia was terminated with ablation. *LAA,* Left atrial appendage; *LIPV,* left inferior pulmonary vein; *LSPV,* left superior pulmonary vein.

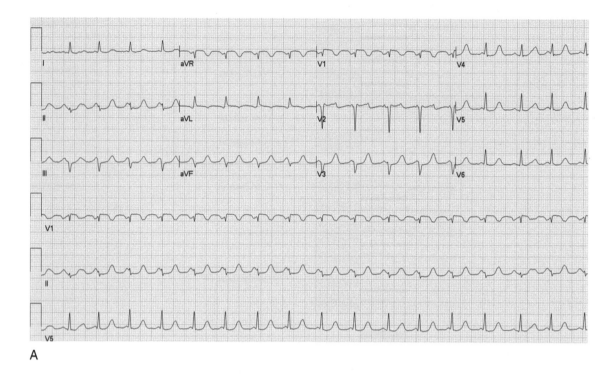

A

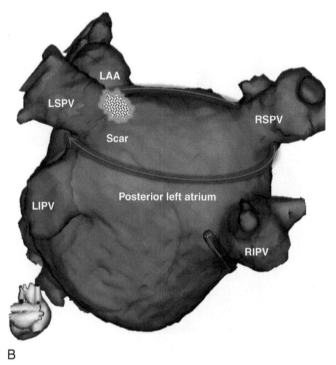

B

Fig. 8.39 Macroreentrant atrial flutter after catheter ablation of atrial fibrillation. (A) Electrocardiogram shows isoelectric flutter waves in lead I; mildly negative in lead aVL; and positive in inferior leads. Flutter waves are negative in leads aVL and aVR. (B) The circuit was mapped around right and left superior pulmonary veins. *LAA,* Left atrial appendage; *LIPV,* left inferior pulmonary vein; *LSPV,* left superior pulmonary vein; *RIPV,* right inferior pulmonary vein; *RSPV,* right superior pulmonary vein.

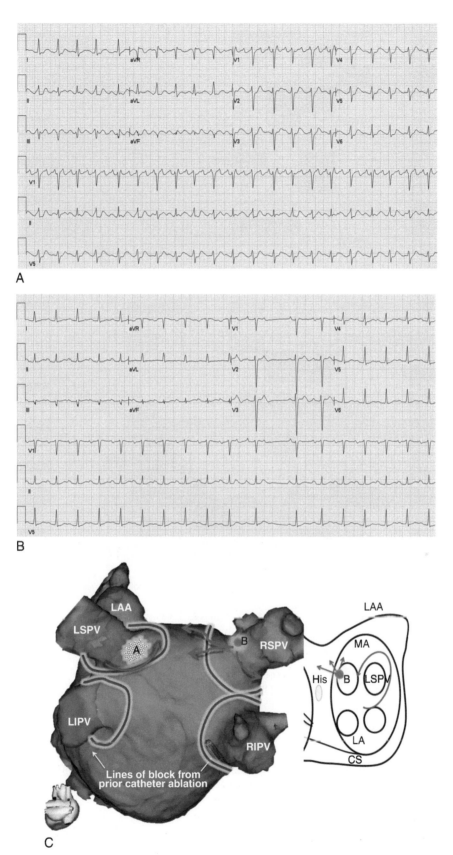

Fig. 8.40 Macroreentrant and focal atrial flutter after catheter ablation of atrial fibrillation. (A) Electrocardiogram reveals positive flutter waves in lead V1 and inferior lead and negative flutter waves in leads I, aVL, and in inferior leads. The circuit was mapped to be around the left superior pulmonary veins (LSPV). (B) The slow atrial flutter/atrial tachycardia also occurred during flecainide therapy. Electrocardiogram shows biphasic flutter waves in lead V1 and positive flutter waves in the inferior and precordial leads. The tachycardia most likely is originating from the right superior pulmonary vein (RSPV) (C). Red arrows show the direction of impulse propagation. *CS*, Coronary sinus; *LA*, left atrium; *LAA*, left atrial appendage; *LIPV*, left inferior pulmonary vein; *MA*, mitral annulus; *RIPV*, right inferior pulmonary vein.

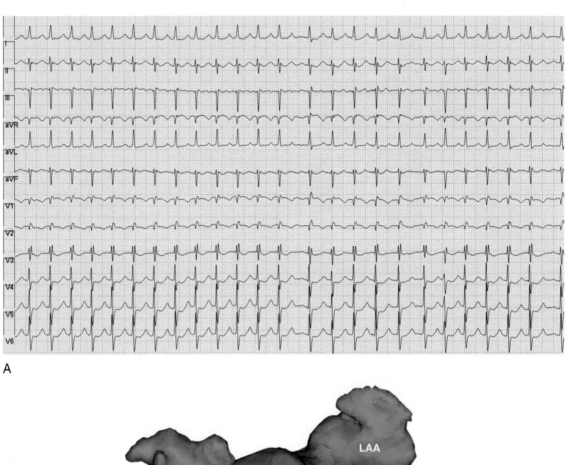

A

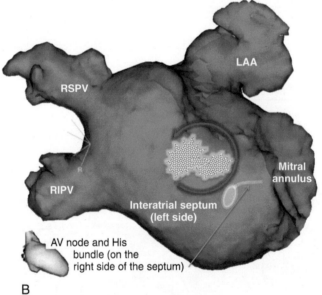

B

Fig. 8.41 Macroreentrant atrial tachycardia/flutter in a patient after catheter ablation of atrial fibrillation. (A) Electrocardiogram is the 12-lead rhythm strip showing negative flutter waves in lead V1 and aVR; positive in lead I and aVL; and positive flutter waves in inferior leads. Flutter waves are also positive in precordial leads. (B) The tachycardia circuit was mapped to the left anteroseptal (parahisian) area. *AV*, Atrioventricular; *LAA*, left atrial appendage; *RIPV*, right inferior pulmonary vein; *RSPV*, right superior pulmonary vein.

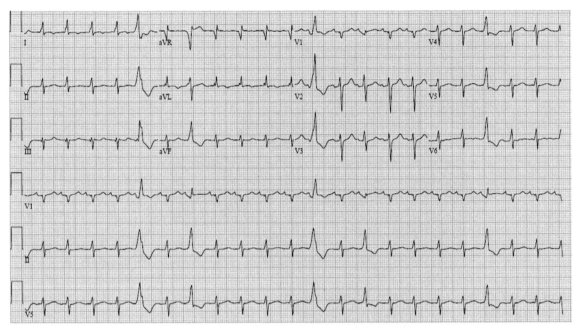

Fig. 8.42 Atrial flutter in a patient with prior mitral valve surgery. Electrocardiogram depicts positive P waves in leads V1 to V3 and isoelectric P waves in all other leads, suggestive of an atrial flutter/tachycardia with a left septal circuit in an area similar to that shown in Fig. 8.41.

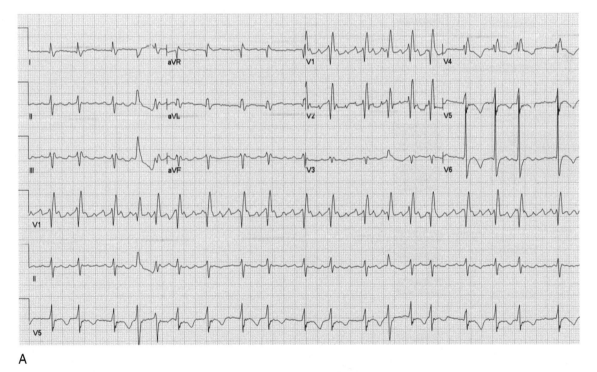

A

Fig. 8.43 Macroreentrant atrial tachycardia/atrial flutter after mitral valve repair. (A) The electrocardiogram shows positive flutter waves in lead V1 and inferior leads. The flutter waves are negative in lead aVL. (B) A figure-eight circuit was mapped around the scars between the two left pulmonary veins. *CS*, Coronary sinus; *LA*, left atrium; *LAA*, left atrial appendage; *LIPV*, left inferior pulmonary vein; *LSPV*, left superior pulmonary vein; *MA*, mitral annulus; *RIPV*, right inferior pulmonary vein; *RSPV*, right superior pulmonary vein.

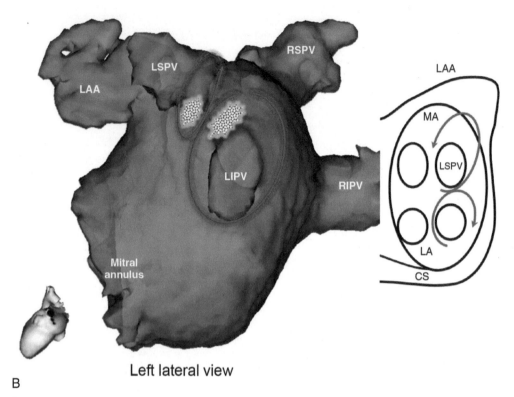

B

Fig. 8.43 (Continued).

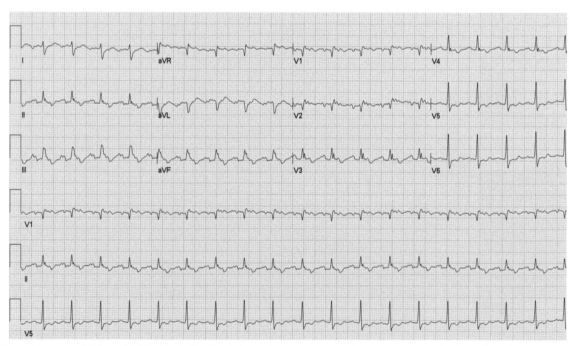

Fig. 8.44 Macroreentrant atrial flutter/atrial tachycardia after heart transplant. Flutter waves are negative in lead V1 and aVL and positive in inferior leads and leads V2 to V4. During an electrophysiology study the reentrant mechanism of atrial flutter was demonstrated, originating from the anterolateral left superior pulmonary vein at the site of reconnection from the native and donor left atrium.

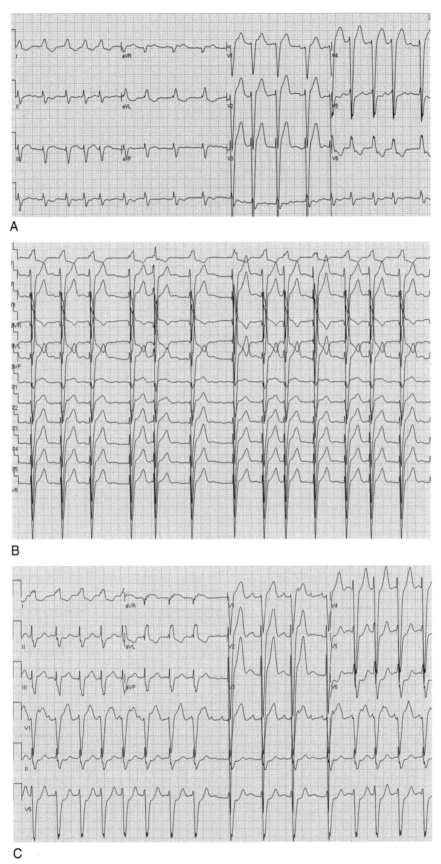

Fig. 8.45 Atrial flutter. (A) Electrocardiogram shows atrial fibrillation in a patient with coronary artery disease and left ventricular hypertrophy. Patient was inappropriately treated with quinidine without prior administration of an atrioventricular blocking drug. The rhythm organized to atrial flutter/tachycardia on quinidine therapy (B and C). Quinidine and other class IA and class IC drugs can enhance atrioventricular nodal conduction by slowing the atrial rate, and atrial flutter/atrial tachycardia can conduct 1:1 to the ventricle (D), which can result in a rapid ventricular tachycardia or ventricular fibrillation.

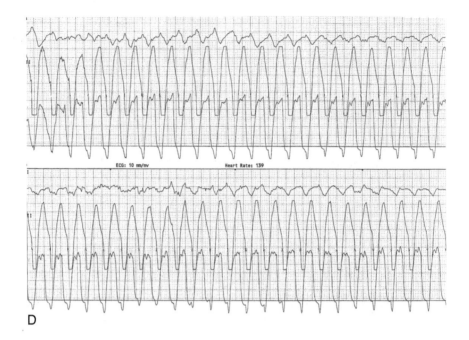

ECG: 10 mm/mv   Heart Rate: 139

D

Fig. 8.45 (Continued).

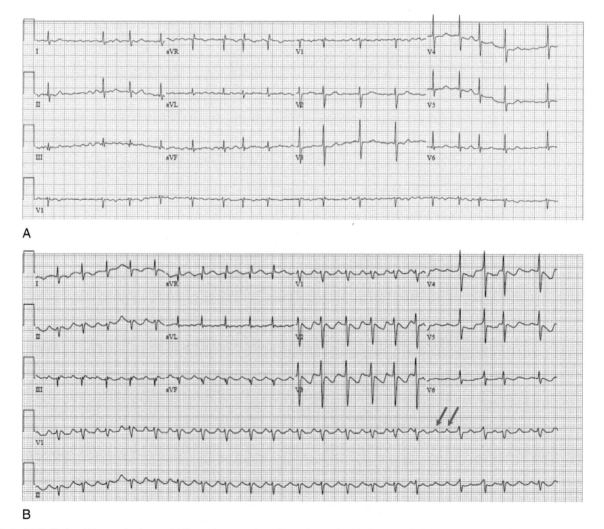

A

B

Fig. 8.46 Atrial fibrillation (A) organized to atrial flutter (*arrows* show flutter waves) with the use of dofetilide therapy (B).

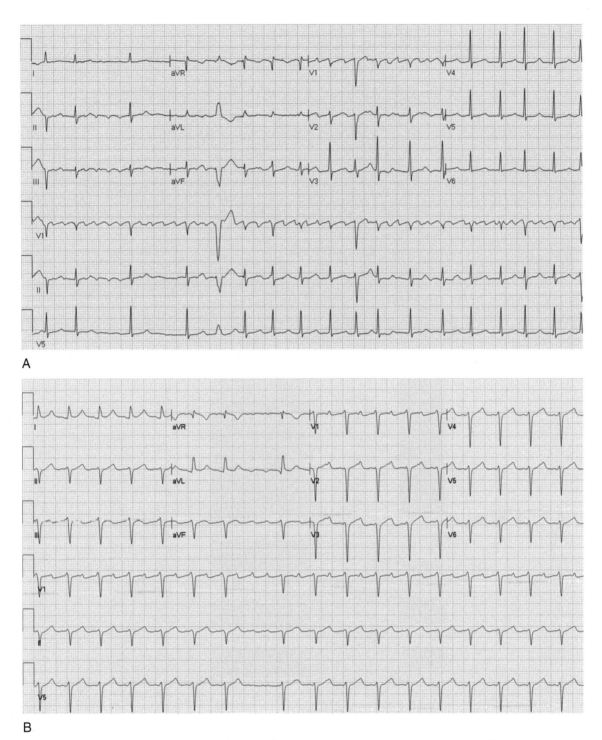

Fig. 8.47 Atrial fibrillation organized to atrial flutter with the use of dofetilide therapy (A) and amiodarone therapy (B).

REFERENCES

1. Markowitz SM, Thomas G, Liu CF, Cheung JW, Ip JE, Lerman BB. Atrial tachycardias and atypical atrial flutters: mechanisms and approaches to ablation. *Arrhythm Electrophysiol Rev.* 2019;8:131−137.
2. Uhm JS, Shim J, Wi J, et al. An electrocardiography algorithm combined with clinical features could localize the origins of focal atrial tachycardias in adjacent structures. *Europace.* 2014;16:1061−1068.
3. Cosio FG. Atrial flutter, typical and atypical: a review. *Arrhythm Electrophysiol Rev.* 2017;6:55−62.
4. Orczykowski M, Derejko P, Urbanek P, et al. Ablation of macro-re-entrant atrial arrhythmia late after surgical aortic valve replacement. *J Heart Valve Dis.* 2016;25:574−579.

9

Atrial Fibrillation

Atrial fibrillation (AF), the most common cardiac tachyarrhythmia, is classified as paroxysmal, persistent, and long-standing or permanent. Paroxysmal AF can evolve into persistent or long-standing AF. AF is characterized by rapid (300–600 bpm) and irregular atrial fibrillatory waves (f waves) with an undulating baseline. Initially, f waves can be coarse, but as the disease progresses, they can become fine or appear as a nearly flat line. These waves are generally best seen in lead V1 and in the inferior leads. Sometimes AF can organize and appear like atrial flutter in the same electrocardiogram (ECG) recording and is often designated as fibrillation/flutter. The ventricular rate is typically irregular (usually ≤ 200 bpm). The ventricular rate in AF can become rapid (> 200 bpm) in young patients, during peak exercise, with excessive catecholamine administration, during parasympathetic withdrawal, thyrotoxicosis, or in patients with the Wolff-Parkinson-White (WPW) syndrome (see Chapter 6). Ventricular rate below 60 bpm during AF occurs in patients with atrioventricular (AV) nodal disease and patients receiving AV nodal–blocking drug therapy (Figs. 9.1 through 9.3). Patients with AF are at greater risk for dementia, strokes, heart failure, death, and sudden death.[1,2]

REGULAR VENTRICULAR RATE DURING ATRIAL FIBRILLATION

Regular ventricular rate in AF suggests complete AV nodal block or AV dissociation with a junctional, subjunctional, or ventricular rhythm (Figs. 9.4 through 9.7). This commonly occurs in the presence of severe AV nodal disease, AV nodal drug therapy, or drug (e.g., digoxin) overdose. Rarely, the R-R interval can be regularly irregular and show group beating with the combination of complete heart block and a lower nodal pacemaker with a Wenckebach type of exit block (see Chapter 3). A very rapid ventricular rate can appear to be regular but on careful measurement actually exhibits slight cycle length variations.

PAROXYSMAL ATRIAL FIBRILLATION

Most episodes of paroxysmal AF are initiated from a focal source, usually in one of the pulmonary veins.[3,4] This phenomenon can be recorded during Holter monitoring. Sometimes, it can be recorded on a routine 12-lead ECG as a short burst of irregular atrial tachycardia or AF initiated by a single premature atrial complex (Figs. 9.8 through 9.10). The morphology of the initiating premature atrial complex (by applying the P wave algorithm for atrial tachycardia, see Chapter 7) can help determine the site of origin of the AF or atrial tachycardia.

QRS MORPHOLOGY DURING ATRIAL FIBRILLATION

The QRS complexes during AF are usually narrow (i.e., normal, not prolonged duration). Wide QRS complexes occur in the presence of functional or fixed bundle branch block (BBB) or WPW syndrome with conduction via the accessory pathway or during a premature ventricular

complex or ventricular tachycardia. Rate-related BBB aberrancy (see Chapter 10) is caused by the physiologic refractoriness of the conduction system that is directly related to heart rate. Therefore aberrant conduction can result from a long R-R interval followed by a short R-R interval. The QRS complex ending the long pause conducts normally, but the bundle branches now have a longer refractory period. The right bundle branch has a longer refractory period than the left bundle branch at slower heart rates. Therefore if the next supraventricular impulse initiates a QRS complex that occurs after a short R-R interval, it can be conducted aberrantly because one of the bundle branches (usually the right bundle branch) is still refractory as a result of the lengthened refractory period (Ashman phenomenon) (Figs. 9.11 through 9.22). The left anterior fascicle is also frequently involved, often in combination with right BBB. In contrast, functional aberration is uncommon in the His bundle or the left posterior fascicle. The correct diagnosis of ventricular aberrancy, as opposed to a premature ventricular complex, can at times be challenging on a single 12-lead ECG recording; however, in most cases it can be accomplished by careful analysis of the ECG and rhythm strip.

ATRIAL FIBRILLATION WITH WOLFF-PARKINSON-WHITE SYNDROME

In patients with WPW syndrome, AF can conduct to the ventricles at rapid rates by way of rapidly conducting single or multiple accessory pathways, which can result in ventricular fibrillation and sudden cardiac death (Figs. 9.23 and 9.24).

TACHYCARDIA-INDUCED TACHYCARDIA

AF can lead to monomorphic ventricular tachycardia, polymorphic ventricular tachycardia, or ventricular fibrillation. Patients with severe underlying heart disease can develop the combination of AF and ventricular tachycardia, leading to a rapid, regular, wide QRS complex tachycardia (Figs. 9.25 and 9.26).

AUTONOMIC-MEDIATED ATRIAL FIBRILLATION

There are two distinct varieties of AF: adrenergically mediated, which occurs during exercise or emotional stress (Fig. 9.27); and vagally mediated, which can be initiated during bradycardia (e.g., during sleep). Vagally mediated paroxysmal AF occurs more commonly in men than in women. The age of onset is usually between 30 and 50 years. It hardly ever occurs in a structurally diseased heart, probably because any cardiac disease tends to shift the vagosympathetic balance toward a sympathetic predominance. Ganglionated plexi in the left atrium, which concentrate more in the left atrial posterior wall around the pulmonary vein ostium, may play a role in initiation of vagal AF. During catheter ablation of AF, stimulation of these areas of the left atrium can result in bradycardia and significant pauses (Fig. 9.28 and Table 9.1).

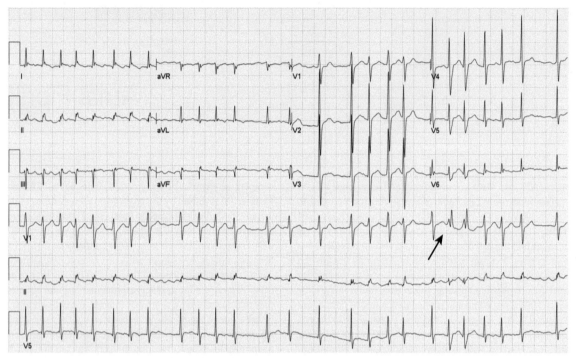

Fig. 9.1 Atrial fibrillation (AF) with a rapid ventricular rate. The most common presentation of AF is a rapid, irregular, ventricular rate. Electrocardiogram shows AF with an average rate of 170 bpm. The tachycardia is also associated with two consecutive ventricular complexes with right bundle branch block aberrancy (*arrow*).

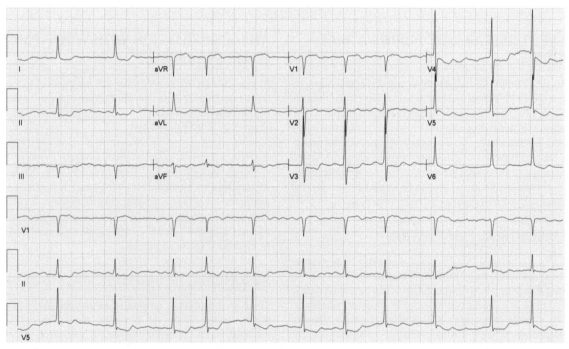

Fig. 9.2 Atrial fibrillation with a controlled ventricular rate of 68 bpm.

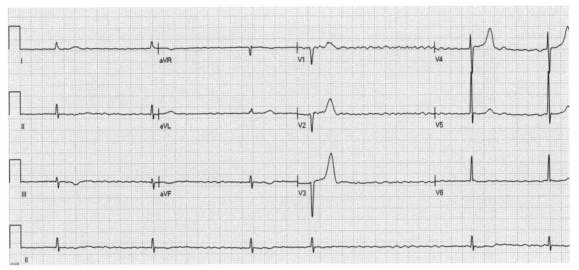

Fig. 9.3 Atrial fibrillation (AF) with slow ventricular rate. Electrocardiogram shows AF with a ventricular rate of 34 bpm. This is the second most common presentation of AF and results from atrioventricular nodal disease or atrioventricular nodal–blocking drug therapy.

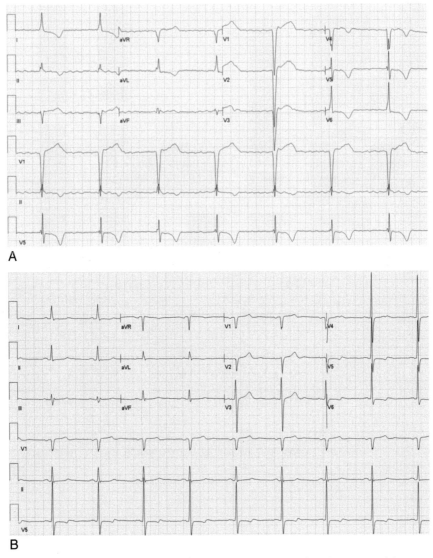

A

B

Fig. 9.4 (A) Electrocardiogram depicts atrial fibrillation with a regular ventricular rate of 42 bpm caused by complete atrioventricular block. (B) Baseline electrocardiogram is sinus with narrow QRS complexes. The QRS complexes during atrial fibrillation in this same patient are wide (duration 130 ms) and represent a ventricular escape rhythm.

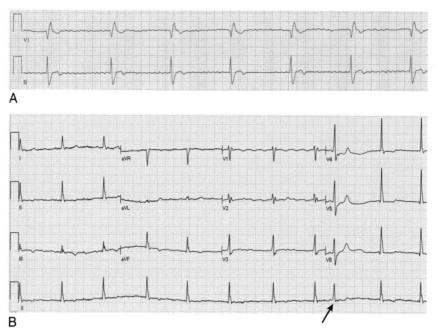

Fig. 9.5 Electrocardiograms reveal atrial fibrillation with a regular slow ventricular rate caused by complete atrioventricular block (A). The *arrow* identifies a premature ventricular complex in the presence of complete atrioventricular block (B).

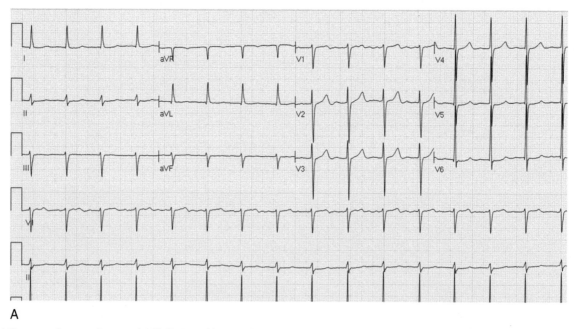

Fig. 9.6 (A) Electrocardiogram shows atrial fibrillation with a regular ventricular rhythm of 95 bpm. This rhythm was recorded during a high digoxin level and is called *nonparoxysmal junctional tachycardia*, likely caused by digoxin toxicity. (B) Electrocardiogram depicts atrial fibrillation with junctional tachycardia at 80 bpm in a different patient.

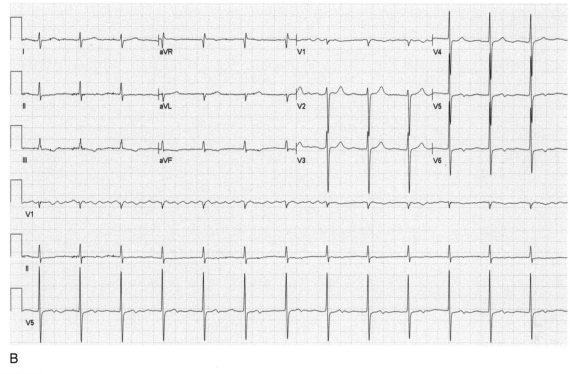

B

Fig. 9.6 (Continued)

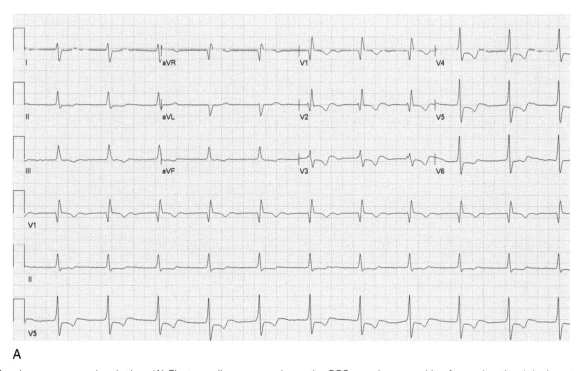

A

Fig. 9.7 Regular narrow complex rhythm. (A) Electrocardiogram reveals regular QRS complexes resulting from a junctional rhythm at an average rate of 70 bpm with some degree of atrioventricular block caused by digitalis toxicity. (B) This electrocardiogram shows similar QRS complexes, but the rhythm is irregular, consistent with atrial fibrillation now conducting with variable atrioventricular block as the digitalis effects have worn off.

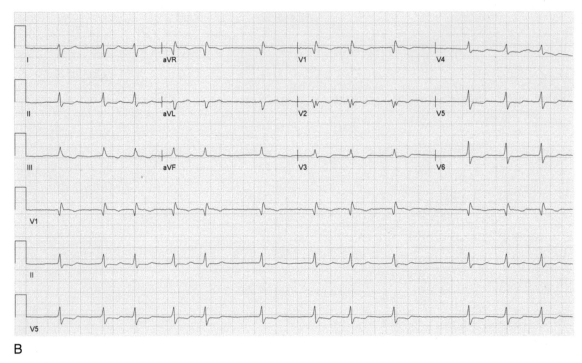

B

Fig. 9.7 (Continued)

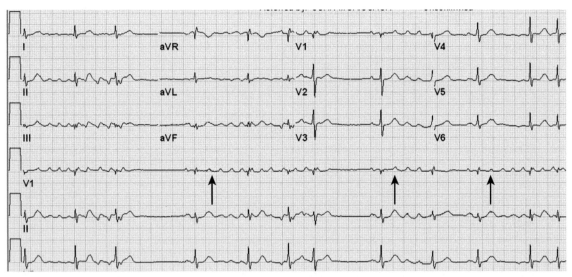

Fig. 9.8 Electrocardiogram depicts atrial fibrillation/flutter with a rapid ventricular response initiated by single premature atrial complex originating from the right superior pulmonary vein (*arrows*).

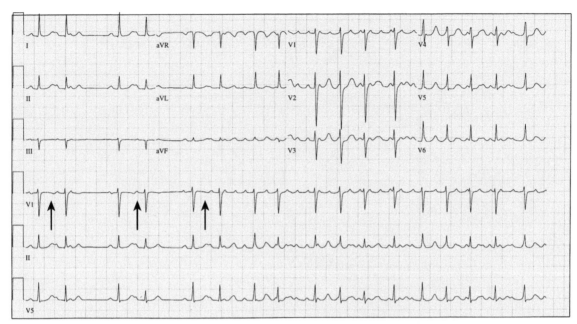

Fig. 9.9 Paroxysmal atrial fibrillation. Electrocardiogram shows sinus rhythm with frequent premature atrial complexes (*arrows*). A single premature atrial complex originating from the right superior pulmonary vein initiates atrial fibrillation/flutter with a rapid ventricular response.

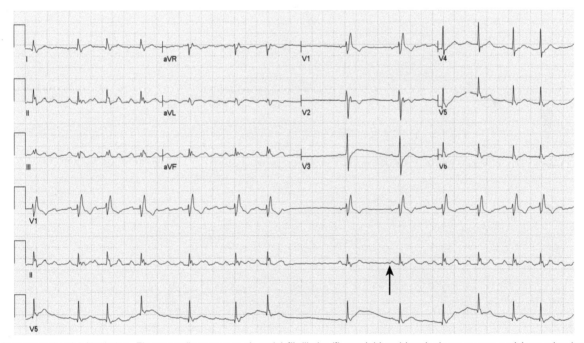

Fig. 9.10 Paroxysmal atrial fibrillation. Electrocardiogram reveals atrial fibrillation/flutter initiated by single premature atrial complex (*arrow*), most likely from the right superior pulmonary vein.

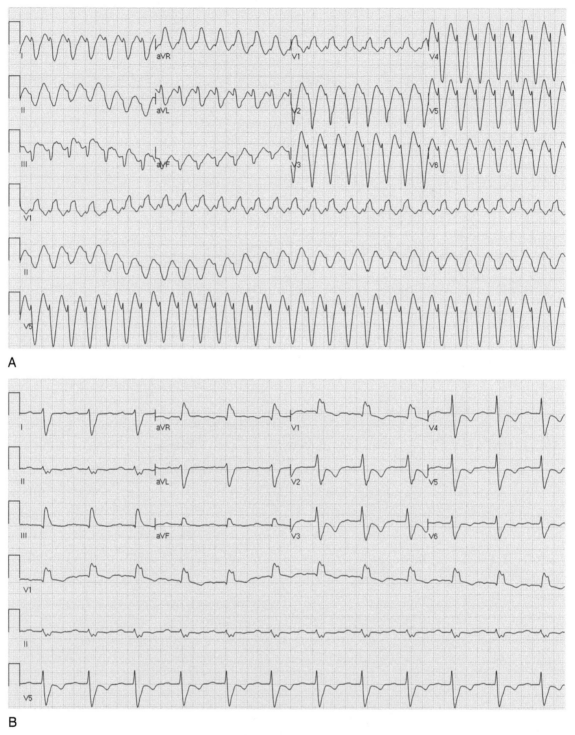

Fig. 9.11 Wide complex tachycardia (WCT). (A) Electrocardiogram (ECG) shows a fairly regular WCT at a rate of 166 bpm, which later became irregular (B). Baseline ECG reveals sinus rhythm with right bundle branch block and a superior axis, similar to the QRS complexes in the WCT. Therefore ECG (A) is most likely atrial flutter with 2:1 conduction.

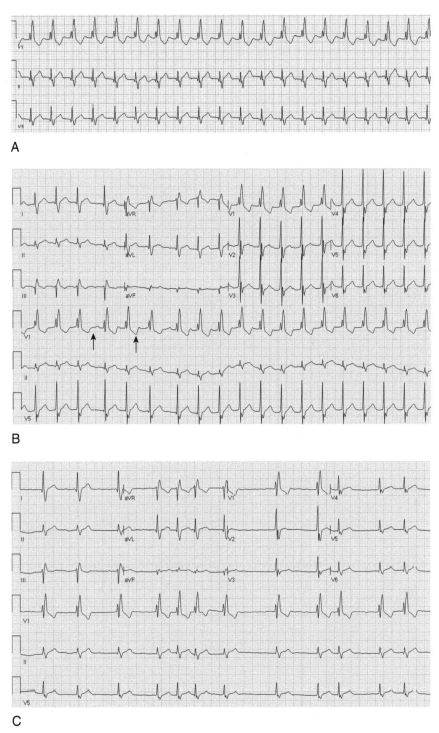

Fig. 9.12 Atrial fibrillation with a rapid ventricular response. (A and B) Electrocardiogram shows a regular wide complex tachycardia with a subtle variation in cycle length (*arrows*). The atrioventricular nodal block later increased with the use of intravenous diltiazem and confirmed the underlying rhythm as atrial fibrillation (C) and atrial flutter (D). (E) Electrocardiogram shows sinus rhythm of the same patient.

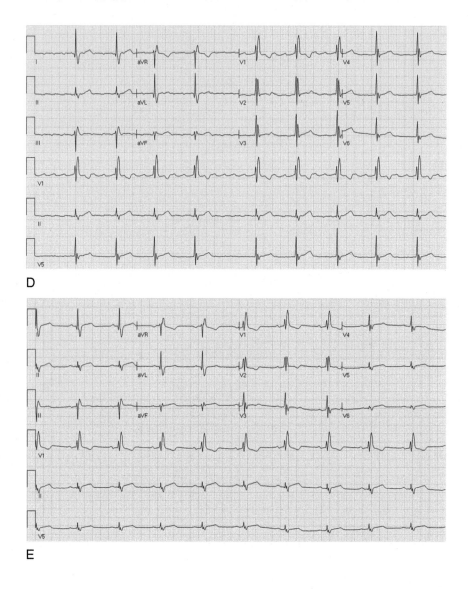

D

E

Fig. 9.12 (Continued)

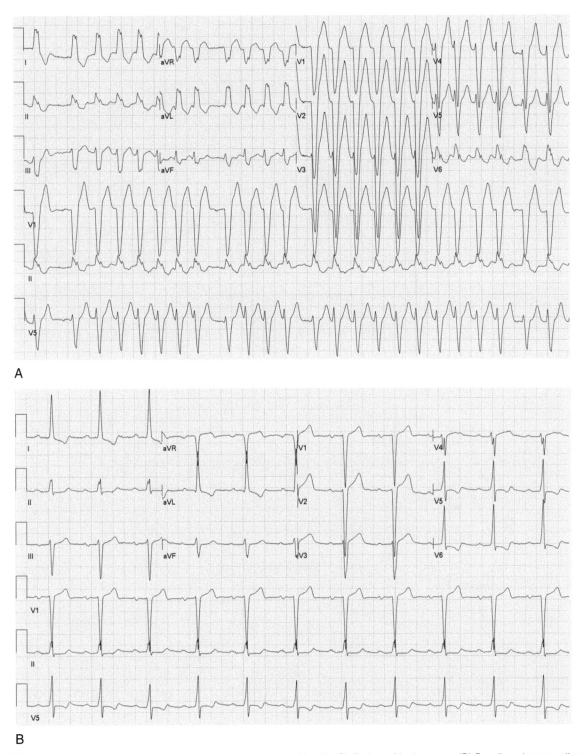

A

B

Fig. 9.13 (A) The irregular wide complex tachycardia is most consistent with atrial fibrillation with aberrancy. (B) Baseline electrocardiogram of the same patient shows sinus rhythm, first-degree atrioventricular block, and narrower QRS duration (118 ms). QRS complexes similar in appearance to the wide complex tachycardia.

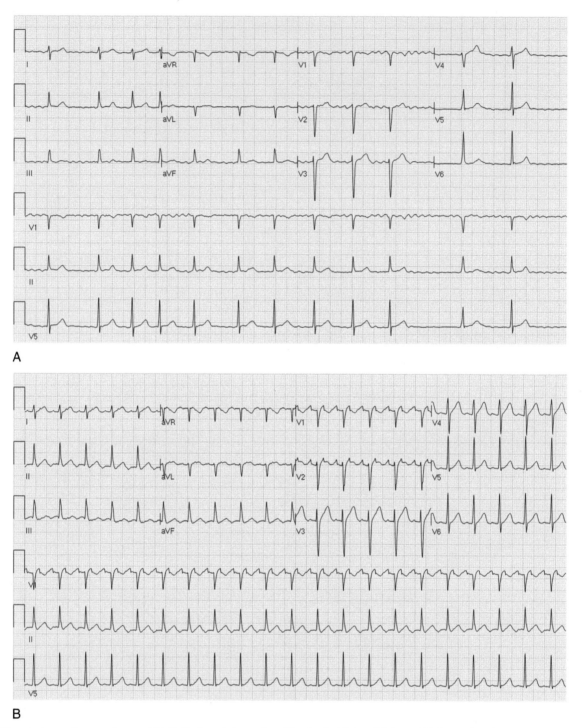

Fig. 9.14 The electrocardiogram shows atrial fibrillation of the patient (A) who had left atrial flutter (B) 3 months after catheter ablation. It was mapped to have circuit around right pulmonary veins.

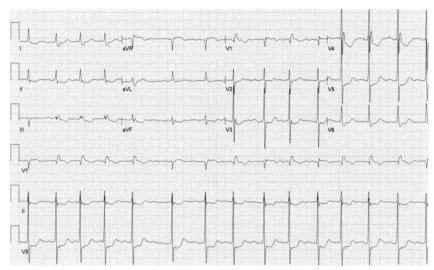

Fig. 9.15 Atrial fibrillation with intermittent right bundle branch block aberrancy at a rate below 100 bpm. This may denote underlying right bundle branch block disease.

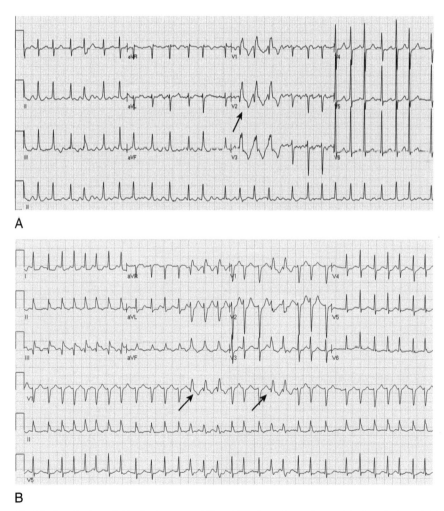

Fig. 9.16 Atrial fibrillation with right bundle branch block aberrancy. (A) and (B) show intermittent right bundle branch block aberrancy during short R-R cycles (see *arrows* in V1). However, sometimes the aberrancy does not occur during the same or shorter R-R intervals as those producing ventricular aberrancy, possibly owing to subtle changes in the preceding R-R cycle length that alter refractoriness.

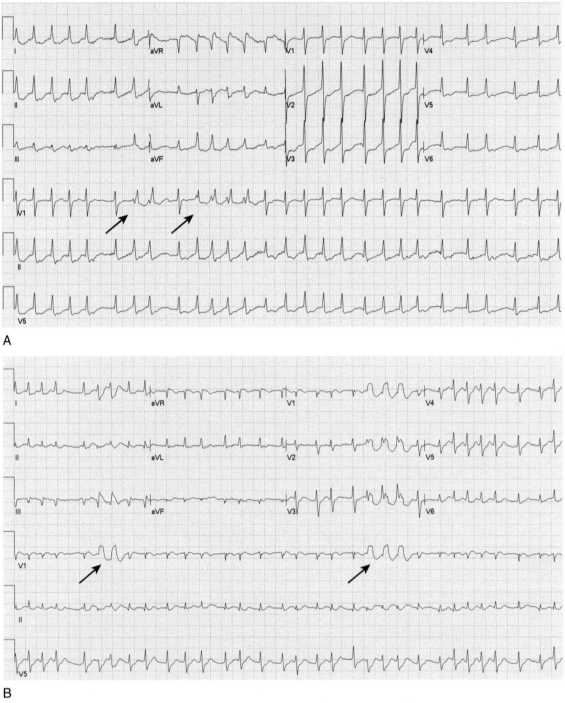

A

B

Fig. 9.17 Atrial fibrillation with Ashman phenomenon in two different patients (*arrows*). The right bundle branch block aberrancy during atrial fibrillation is initiated by a short-long-short R-R sequence (Ashman phenomenon) in (A) and (B).

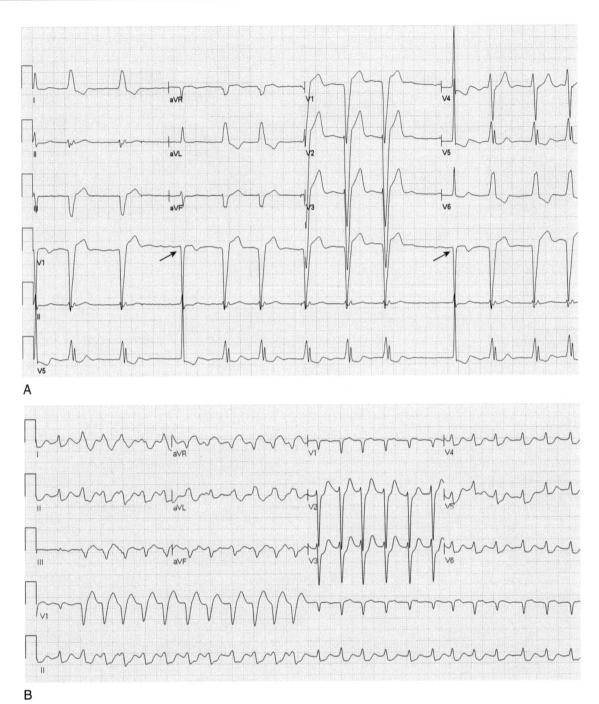

Fig. 9.18 Atrial fibrillation (AF) with left bundle branch block aberrancy. (A) Electrocardiogram shows AF with an average heart rate of 75 bpm. The aberrancy disappears when the R-R cycle length is greater than 1100 ms (*arrows*). (B) Electrocardiogram from a different patient reveals AF with an average heart rate of 150 bpm and left bundle branch block aberrancy.

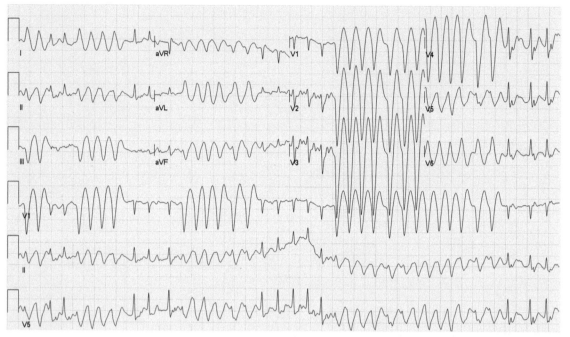

Fig. 9.19 Atrial fibrillation with wide complex tachycardia. Electrocardiogram depicts atrial fibrillation with left bundle branch block aberrancy with a shortest R-R cycle length of 200 ms. The salvos of wide complex tachycardia can also be frequent nonsustained ventricular tachycardia.

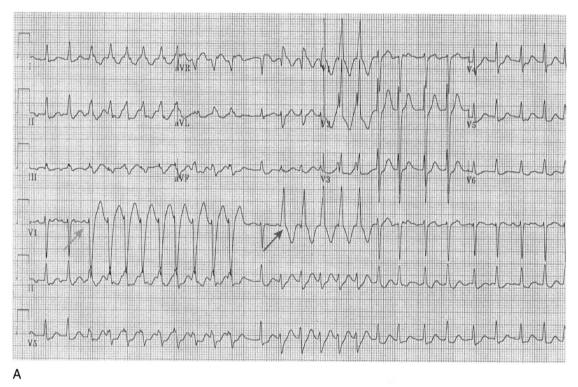

A

Fig. 9.20 Atrial fibrillation with intermittent left bundle branch block (*blue arrows*) and right bundle branch block (*red arrows*) aberrancy in two different patients (A and B). Right bundle branch aberrancy is more common because refractory period of right bundle is longer than the left bundle branch at slower heart rates.

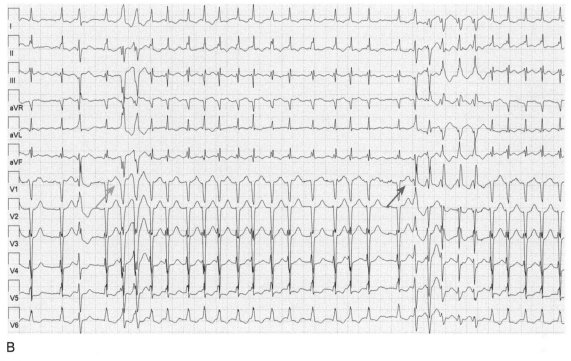

B

Fig. 9.20 (Continued)

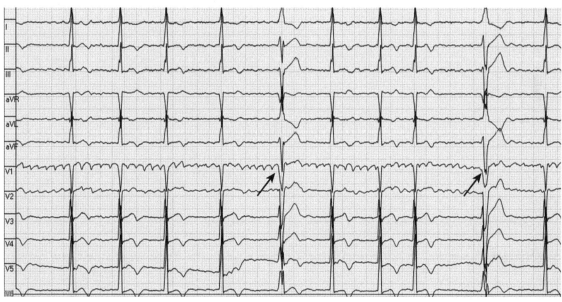

Fig. 9.21 Deceleration-dependent aberrancy. Electrocardiogram shows atrial fibrillation with left bundle branch block aberrancy during long R-R cycles (*arrows*).

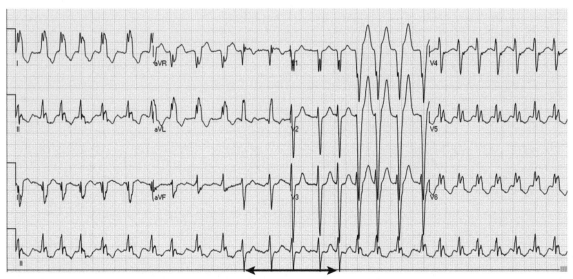

Fig. 9.22 Atrial fibrillation with normalization of the QRS, perhaps owing to supernormal conduction via the left bundle branch (LBB). Electrocardiogram depicts LBB aberrancy with a five-beat run of narrow QRS complexes (*horizontal arrow*). These complexes may represent supernormal conduction via the LBB, resulting in narrow QRS complexes. Alternatively, equal delay in both bundle branches can result in narrow QRS complexes but PR interval is usually longer by 20 to 30 ms owing to delay in conduction in both bundles.

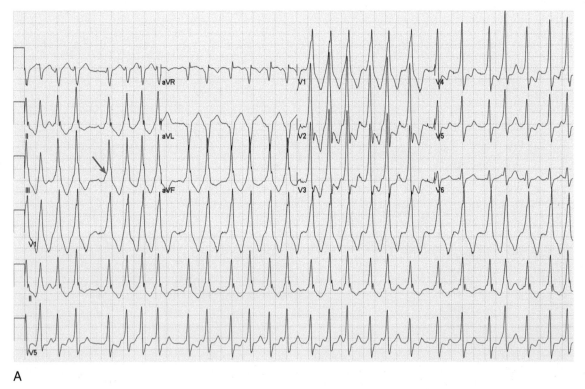

A

Fig. 9.23 Irregular wide complex tachycardia. (A) Electrocardiogram shows irregular wide complex tachycardia with slurred upstrokes in inferior and precordial leads suggestive of Wolff-Parkinson-White syndrome. (B) Another electrocardiogram of the same patient reveals sinus rhythm with positive delta waves (*arrows*) in precordial and inferior leads confirming Wolff-Parkinson-White syndrome. The location of the accessory pathway is most likely parahisian.

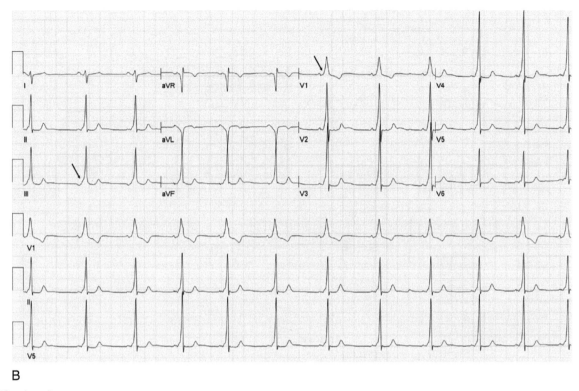

B

Fig. 9.23 (Continued)

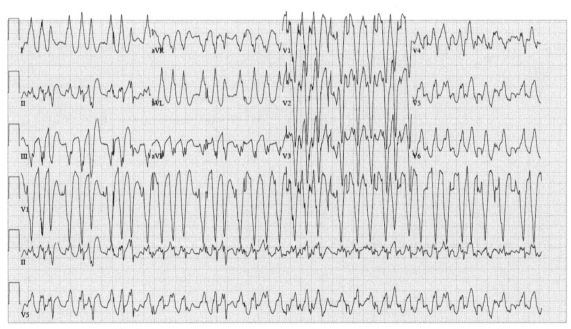

Fig. 9.24 Atrial fibrillation with a rapid irregular wide complex tachycardia requiring prompt direct current cardioversion. Tachycardia is the result of anterodromic conduction via a right accessory pathway. Patient presented with loss of consciousness and was resuscitated with direct current shock and later underwent a successful catheter ablation.

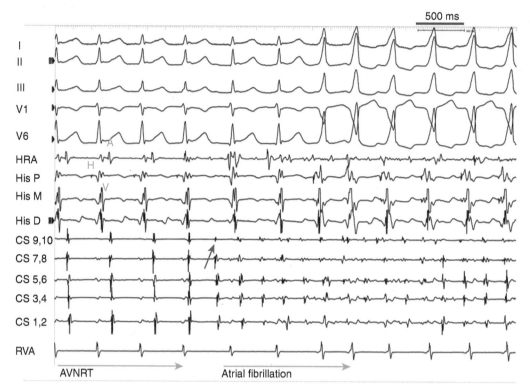

Fig. 9.25 Tachycardia-induced tachycardia. Electrocardiogram and intracardiac recordings show a short R-P′ tachycardia, which was an atrioventricular nodal reentrant tachycardia (AVNRT) that initiated atrial fibrillation (*red arrow*). Coronary sinus (CS) electrograms show rapid irregular tachycardia consistent with atrial fibrillation. QRS complexes became aberrant when the rate increased during the atrial fibrillation. *A*, Atrial electrogram; *AVNRT*, atrioventricular nodal reentrant tachycardia; *CS 1,2*, distal coronary sinus; *CS 9,10*, proximal coronary sinus; *H*, His bundle; *His D*, distal His bundle; *His M*, middle His bundle; *His P*, proximal His bundle; *HRA*, high right atrium; *V*, right ventricular electrogram.

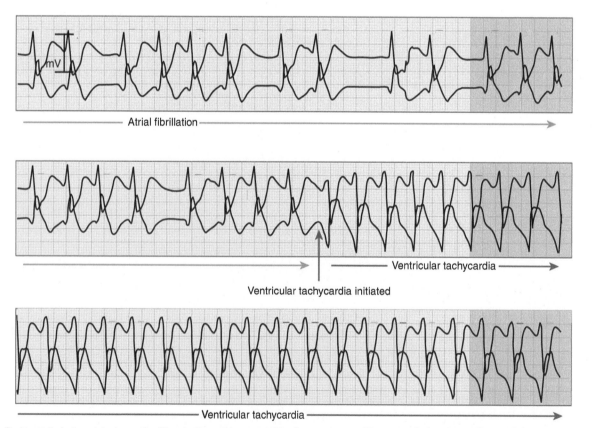

Fig. 9.26 Tachycardia-induced tachycardia. The rhythm strip was taken from a man with severe ischemic cardiomyopathy and advanced heart failure who developed atrial fibrillation. The premature ventricular complex on the T wave during atrial fibrillation (*vertical red arrow*) initiated ventricular tachycardia that required direct current shock to convert to sinus rhythm.

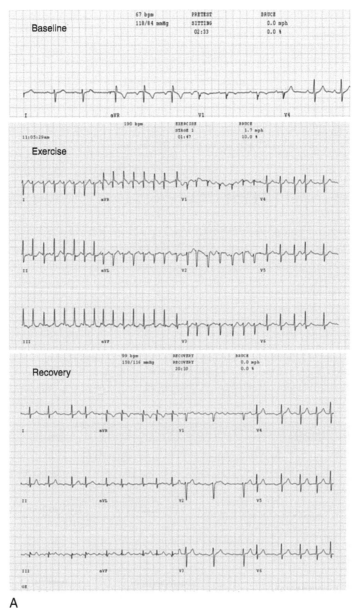

A

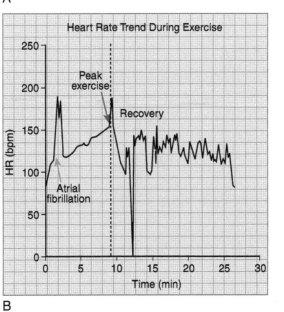

B

Fig. 9.27 (A) Electrocardiogram recordings at baseline, during exercise, and during recovery period. Patient developed atrial fibrillation (AF) during exercise, which resolved spontaneously during the latter part of the stress test, and the patient remained in AF during recovery period. (B) Graph depicts the heart rate trend during the stress test. AF was triggered by exercise, and the rhythm converted to sinus spontaneously.

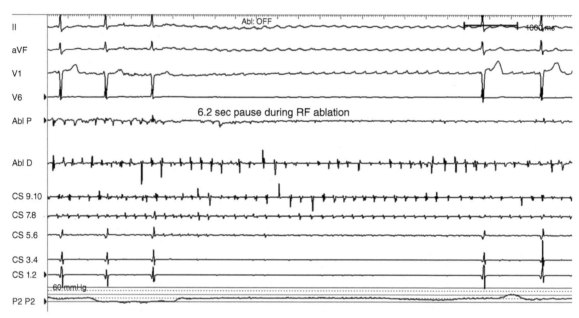

Fig. 9.28 Electrocardiogram demonstrates 6.2-second pause during catheter ablation of atrial fibrillation. Pause resulted from stimulation of vagal ganglionated plexi at the posterosuperior aspect of the left atrium close to the left superior pulmonary vein ostium. *Abl D*, Ablation distal; *Abl P*, ablation proximal; *CS 1,2*, distal coronary sinus; *CS 9,10*, proximal coronary sinus; *P2P2*, systemic arterial pressure; *RF*, radiofrequency.

TABLE 9.1	Atrial Fibrillation With Aberrancy Versus Premature Ventricular Contractions	
Electrocardiogram Characteristics	**AF With Aberrancy**	**AF with PVC**
Long-short cycle	+	Usually followed by a longer R-R cycle owing to a compensatory pause, secondary to retrograde conduction into the AV node and anterograde block of the impulse originating in the atrium.
Random wide complex	Appears like a BBB (mostly right BBB)	Wide QRS, unlike BBB.
Fixed coupling interval between a narrow supraventricular QRS and wide complex	–	+

AF, Atrial fibrillation; *AV*, atrioventricular; *BBB*, bundle branch block; *PVC*, premature ventricular contraction.

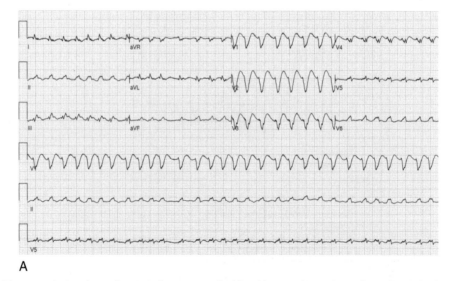

A

Fig. 9.29 The patient with severe ischemic cardiomyopathy presented with wide complex tachycardia and was inadvertently initially treated for ventricular tachycardia in the emergency room with intravenous diltiazem, and after cardioversion the electrocardiogram in sinus rhythm (*arrow* depict sinus P wave) showed similar left bundle branch block QRS complexes.

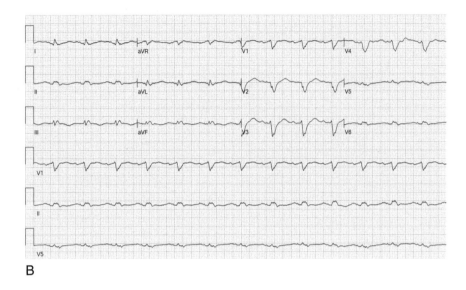

Fig. 9.29 (Continued)

REFERENCES

1. Bisbal F, Baranchuk A, Braunwald E, Bayes de Luna A, Bayes-Genis A. Atrial failure as a clinical entity: JACC review topic of the week. *J Am Coll Cardiol.* 2020;75:222—232.
2. Calkins H, Hindricks G, Cappato R, et al. 2017 HRS/EHRA/ECAS/APHRS/ SOLAECE expert consensus statement on catheter and surgical ablation of atrial fibrillation: executive summary. *J Arrhythm.* 2017;33:369—409.
3. Lau DH, Linz D, Sanders P. New findings in atrial fibrillation mechanisms. *Card Electrophysiol Clin.* 2019;11:563—571.
4. Issa ZF, Miller JM, Zipes DP. Atrial fibrillation. In: Issa ZF, Miller JM, Zipes DP, eds. *Arrhythmology and Electrophysiology.* 3rd ed. Philadelphia, PA: Elsevier; 2009:421—548.

10

Wide Complex Tachycardia

A wide complex tachycardia (WCT) is defined by a QRS duration greater than 120 ms and rate greater than 100 bpm. The majority (80%) of WCTs are ventricular tachycardias (VTs), especially in the setting of structural heart disease. Supraventricular tachycardia (SVT) with pre-existing or rate-related aberrancy accounts for 15% to 20% of WCTs. Less commonly, WCT results from Wolff-Parkinson-White syndrome with antidromic atrioventricular reentrant tachycardia (see Chapter 6) or an atrial tachyarrhythmia (atrial fibrillation, atrial flutter, and atrial tachycardia; see Chapters 7–9) with bystander preexcitation (1%–6%). SVT or sinus tachycardia with intraventricular conduction delays and QRS prolongation caused by antiarrhythmic drug therapy or hyperkalemia, as well as ventricular paced rhythm (especially when pacing spikes are not obvious) can also mimic a WCT.[1] A thorough history, physical examination, knowledge of drug therapy, and careful inspection of rhythm strips or prior electrocardiograms (ECGs) (if available) may help in determining the arrhythmia. Vagal maneuvers or drugs may also be useful. However, it can sometimes be difficult to distinguish VT from SVT with aberrancy by ECG alone, because most of the associations between the QRS morphology and type of tachycardia are based on statistical correlations, which have a substantial overlap (Table 10.1 and Fig. 10.1). Symptoms of tachycardia (palpitations, lightheadedness) or heart rate ranges do not help in differentiating a VT from an SVT. Atrioventricular dissociation, fusion beat, capture beat, QRS concordance in precordial leads (positive QRS concordance: all precordial leads are positive; negative QRS concordance: all precordial leads are negative), and QRS morphology, unlike typical bundle branch, support VT[2] (Figs. 10.2 and 10.3). QRS alternans, defined as alternate-beat variation in the amplitude of complexes greater than 0.1 mV, is commonly found in narrow complex SVT. QRS alternans is also present in as many as 25% of WCTs with an equal frequency in SVT and VT. An algorithm measuring V_i/V_t ratio published by Vereckei and associates[3,4] has a diagnostic accuracy of 83.5% compared with the Brugada algorithm's predictive accuracy for SVT of 65.2% ($P < 0.05$) (Fig. 10.4). The V_i is the voltage excursion in the initial 40 ms, and V_t is the voltage excursion in the last 40 ms of a QRS complex. Because in an SVT with aberrancy, only one portion of the His-Purkinje system is blocked while another portion mediates initial ventricular activation, the first part of the QRS should have relatively rapid voltage changes compared with the terminal part of the QRS. In VT, slower muscle-to-muscle spread of activation at the onset of the QRS yields slower voltage changes. Therefore V_i/V_t ratio is greater than 1 in SVT with aberrancy. More recently, a simplified algorithm using the lead aVR has been shown to be valuable in differentiating a VT from an SVT with aberrancy (Fig. 10.4).

REFERENCES

1. Tordini A, Leonelli FM, De Ponti R, et al. Challenging cases of wide complex tachycardias: use and limits of algorithms. *Card Electrophysiol Clin.* 2019;11:301–314.
2. Hanna EB, Johnson CJ, Glcy DL. Wide-QRS complex tachycardia. *Am J Cardiol.* 2018;121:275–276.
3. Vereckei A, Duray G, Szenasi G, Altemose GT, Miller JM. Application of a new algorithm in the differential diagnosis of wide QRS complex tachycardia. *Eur Heart J.* 2007;28:589–600.
4. Vereckei A, Duray G, Szenasi G, Altemose GT, Miller JM. New algorithm using only lead aVR for differential diagnosis of wide QRS complex tachycardia. *Heart Rhythm.* 2008;5:89–98.

TABLE 10.1 Differentiating Ventricular Tachycardia From Supraventricular Tachycardia

		VT	SVT with Aberrancy
Clinical	Structural heart disease	CAD, MI, DCM	Normal heart
	Long history	Only with idiopathic VT.	>3 years
	Syncope	Common	Not common
	Termination with Valsalva maneuvers, adenosine, beta blocker, or calcium blocker	Idiopathic VT	Likely
	Calcium blocker (not beta blocker)	Idiopathic left fascicular VT.	Likely
Electrocardiogram	Baseline QRS	Infarct, aberrancy, IVCD.	Normal, aberrancy
	QRS duration	RBBB >140 ms[a] LBBB >160 ms[b]	
	QRS duration (WCT vs. baseline)	The QRS during tachycardia is narrower than baseline wide QRS complexes (such as BBB pattern), contralateral BBB pattern than the baseline BBB pattern in a WCT.	
	>1 QRS configurations during WCT	Present in 50% VTs.	Only in 8% of SVTs
	QRS axis	−180 to −90 (northwest). Change of >40° from baseline. RBBB + LAD (−30° or more) LBBB + RAD (+ 90° or more).	RBBB with normal QRS axis.[f]
	AV relationship	AV ratio <1.	AV ratio ≥ 1
		AV dissociation (sensitivity 100%, specificity 20%−50%).	
		1:1 VA relation (30%), 2:1 or Wenckebach (15%−20%).	1:1 VA relation in AVNRT or AVRT with aberrancy, antidromic AVRT.
		Fusion beat (diagnostic of VT).[c]	
		Capture beat (diagnostic of VT).[c]	
	Concordance	Positive or negative concordance (sensitivity >90%, specificity 20%).	Rarely positive concordance in antidromic SVT with left posteroseptal pathway.
	RBBB-like pattern	Monophasic R, biphasic qR, or broad R (> 40 ms) in lead V1.[d] Double-peaked R in lead V1 with the amplitude of first peak greater than the second peak (likelihood ratio >50:1). rS complex in lead V6.	RSR′, rSr′, rR′, or rSR′ complex in lead V1 Rs complex in lead V6 (likelihood ratio >50:1).
	LBBB-like pattern (negative QRS polarity in lead V1)[e]	R wave ≥ 40 ms in lead V1 or V2 favors VT. Slow descent to the nadir of the S wave (an RS interval >70 ms) in lead V1 or V2. Notching in the downstroke of the S waveQ or QS wave in lead V6 favors VT (likelihood ratio ≥ 50:1).	Absence of an initial R wave (or a small initial R wave <40 ms) in lead V1 or V2. No Q wave in lead V6.
	Lead aVR	R wave; q or R >40 ms.	
	V_i/V_t of QRS complexes	≤ 1	>1

AV, Atrioventricular; AVNRT, atrioventricular nodal reentrant tachycardia; AVRT, atrioventricular reentrant tachycardia; BBB, bundle branch block; CAD, coronary artery disease; DCM, dilated cardiomyopathy, IVCD, intraventricular conduction delays; LAD, left axis deviation; LBBB, left bundle branch block; MI, myocardial infarction; RAD, right axis deviation; RBBB, right bundle branch block; SVT, supraventricular tachycardia; VA, ventriculoatrial; V_i, voltage excursion in the initial 40 ms of QRS; V_t, voltage excursion in the last 40 ms of QRS; VT, ventricular tachycardia; WCT, wide complex tachycardia. V_i/V_t ratio ≤ 1 indicates VT, and V_i/V_t ratio >1 signifies SVT with aberrancy, with positive predictive accuracy for SVT with aberrancy of 83.5%.

[a]Fascicular VT or septal VT can be <140 ms.

[b]There is a greater than 95% chance for VT except in patients with preexisting BBB or preexcitation.

[c]Usually seen in a slower VT.

[d]Capital letter (R) indicates large-wave amplitude and/or duration, and the lower case letter (r) indicates small-wave amplitude and/or duration.

[e]Presence of either slow descent to the nadir of the S wave or notching in the downstroke of the S wave or an RS interval (from the onset of the QRS complex to the nadir of the S wave) of ≥ 70 ms in lead V1 or V2 favors VT, with a likelihood >50:1.

[f]Only 3% of VTs have RBBB with normal QRS axis.

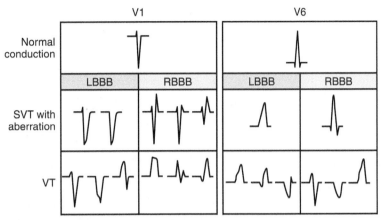

Fig. 10.1 Common QRS morphologies encountered in ventricular tachycardia (VT) and supraventricular tachycardia (SVT), with aberration in leads V1 and V6 for both left bundle branch block (LBBB) and right bundle branch block (RBBB) QRS patterns. Note the initial portions of the QRS complex in normal and aberrant QRS complexes, contrasted with the initial QRS forces in VT complexes. The QRS configurations can be designated as an RBBB or an LBBB type (grouped with LBBB-type morphologies). (From Miller JM, Das MK, Arora R, Alberte-Lista C. Differential diagnosis of wide QRS complex tachycardia. In: Zipes DP, Jalife J, eds. *Cardiac Electrophysiology: From Cell to Bedside*. 4th ed. Philadelphia, PA: Saunders; 2004:747-757.)

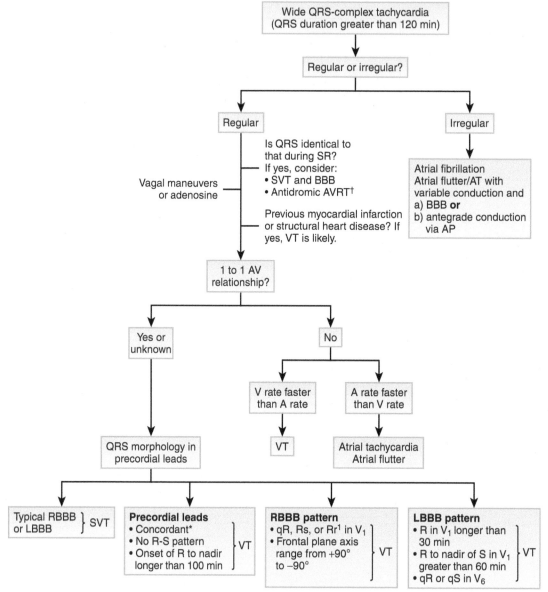

Fig. 10.2 A QRS conduction delay during sinus rhythm, when available for comparison, reduces the value of QRS morphology analysis. Adenosine should be used with caution when the diagnosis is unclear because it can produce ventricular fibrillation (VF) in patients with coronary artery disease and in patients with Wolff-Parkinson-White syndrome during atrial fibrillation with a rapid ventricular rate in preexcited tachycardia. *A*, Atrial; *AP*, accessory pathway; *AT*, atrial tachycardia; *AV*, atrioventricular; *AVRT*, atrioventricular reciprocating tachycardia; *BBB*, bundle branch block; *LBBB*, left bundle branch block; *QRS*, ventricular activation on electrocardiogram; *RBBB*, right bundle branch block; *SR*, sinus rhythm; *SVT*, supraventricular tachycardias; *V*, ventricular; *VT*, ventricular tachycardia. *Concordant* indicates that all precordial leads show either positive or negative deflections. Fusion complexes are diagnostic of VT. [†]In preexcited tachycardia, the QRS is generally wider (i.e., more preexcited) compared with SR. (Reprinted with permission. *Circulation.* 2003;108:1871–1909. © 2003 American Heart Association, Inc.)

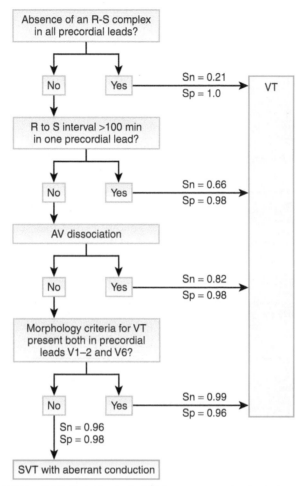

Fig. 10.3 Brugada algorithm for distinguishing ventricular tachycardia (VT) from supraventricular tachycardia (SVT). The R-S interval is the interval between the onset of the R wave and the nadir of the S wave. *AV,* Atrioventricular; *Sn,* sensitivity; *Sp,* specificity. (From Brugada P, Brugada J, Mont L, et al. A new approach to the differential diagnosis of a regular tachycardia with a wide QRS complex. *Circulation.* 1991;83:1649.)

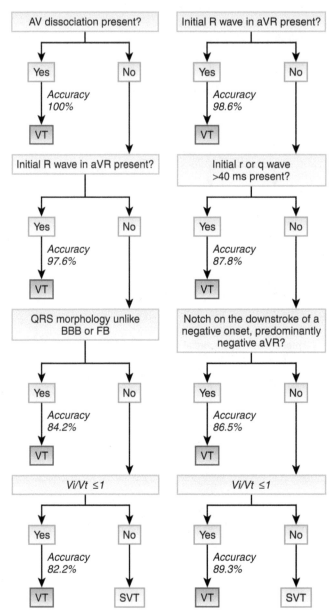

Fig. 10.4 Algorithms by Vereckei and associates use V_i/V_t in differentiating VT from SVT. *AV,* Atrioventricular; *BBB,* bundle branch block; *FB,* fascicular block; *SVT,* supraventricular tachycardia; *VT,* ventricular tachycardia.[3-4]

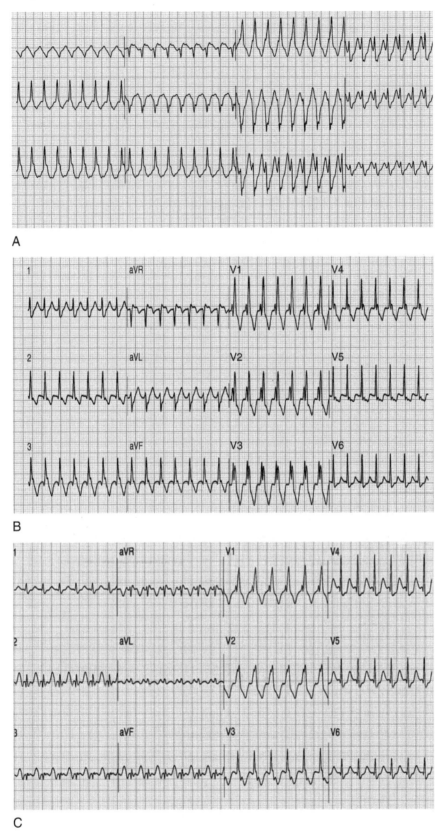

Fig. 10.5 Wide complex tachycardia resulting from right bundle branch block aberrancy in three different patients. There is no initial R wave in lead aVR in electrocardiograms (ECGs) (A) and (B), which favors supraventricular tachycardia with aberrancy, but an R wave is present in lead aVR in (C), incorrectly favoring ventricular tachycardia. Lead V1 shows typical right bundle branch block aberrancy, and lead V6 has r-S pattern with wide S waves in these ECGs. No atrioventricular dissociation is present. The V_i/V_t is greater than 1 in all three ECGs. These findings are suggestive of a supraventricular tachycardia, which was confirmed by electrophysiology studies.

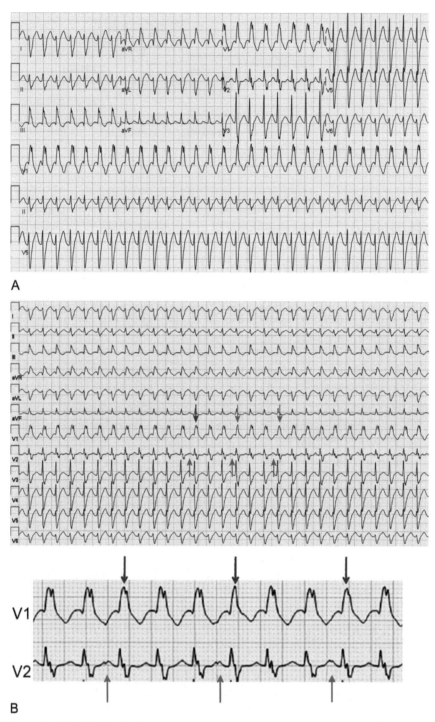

Fig. 10.6 Wide complex tachycardia with right bundle branch block morphology in a 27-year-old man with no structural heart disease. The QRS duration during the wide complex tachycardia is 125 ms with a nearly typical right bundle branch block pattern suggestive of a supraventricular tachycardia. However, the 12-lead rhythm strip (B) of the same patient shows discernible P waves (*red arrows*) with fusion beats (*blue arrows*), which confirm ventricular tachycardia. This is a fascicular ventricular tachycardia.

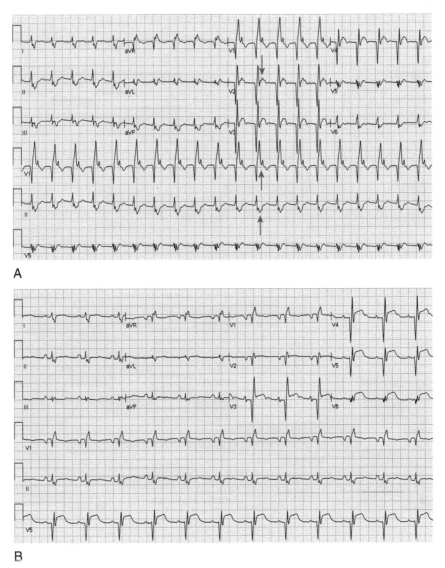

Fig. 10.7 Wide complex tachycardia (WCT) with right bundle branch block and right axis deviation morphology in a 58-year-old woman with a history of anterolateral myocardial infarction. (A) Electrocardiogram (ECG) shows a short R-P′ tachycardia. The QRS morphology has an initial Q-S pattern and S-T elevation in the precordial leads V3-V6 (suggestive of a left ventricular aneurysm) with QRS duration of 160 ms and does not represent a typical right bundle branch block pattern. There is 1:1 ventriculoatrial relation with P waves (*arrows*) having a superior axis (negative in lead II) suggestive of ventricular tachycardia (VT) with retrograde atrial capture. However, the V_i/V_t is greater than 1, and no R wave in aVR, which are suggestive of a supraventricular tachycardia. (B) The baseline ECG of the same patient shows a QRS duration of 150 ms with similar QRS morphology and axis when compared, which suggests that tachycardia in (A) was a supraventricular tachycardia with a short R-P′ interval. The arrhythmia in ECG (A) responded to adenosine. (C) ECG shows junctional rhythm after adenosine therapy. However, the patient later developed another WCT (D) with QRS duration of 180 ms and a different QRS morphology suggestive of a VT. This VT was successfully cardioverted with a direct current shock. (E) ECG of the same patient later showed a WCT with a very short P-R interval. P waves almost extend into the QRS, and the QRS morphology is similar to the QRS morphology during sinus rhythm (B and F). This rhythm (E) cannot be an atrioventricular nodal reentry or atrioventricular reentry tachycardia because P waves are upright in inferior leads (*blue arrows*). It also cannot be an atrial tachycardia (AT) because the P-R interval is too short (shorter than the P-R interval during sinus rhythm) to conduct. The P wave during the AT conducts to the next QRS (*red arrows*). (F) The same sinus rhythm ECG after termination of the AT.

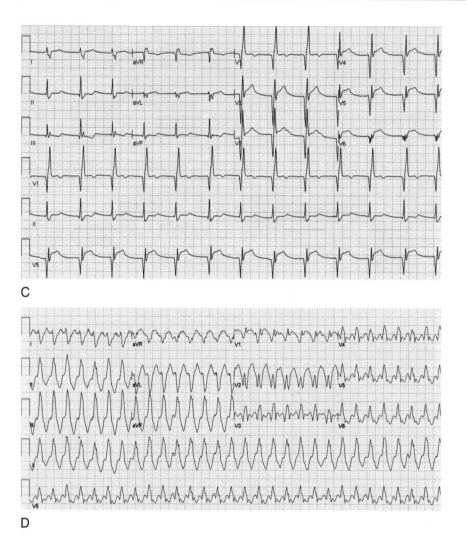

C

D

Fig. 10.7 (Continued).

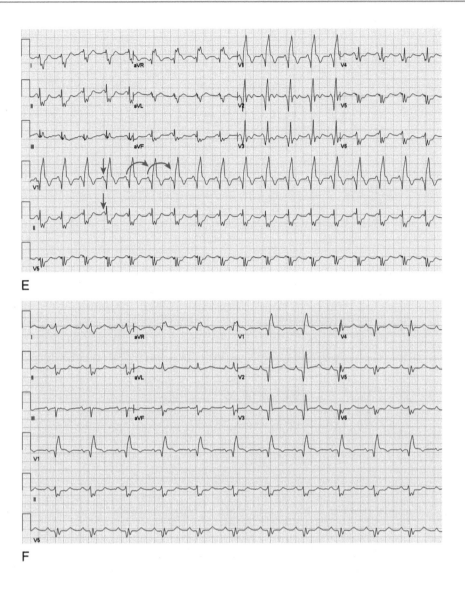

E

F

Fig. 10.7 (Continued).

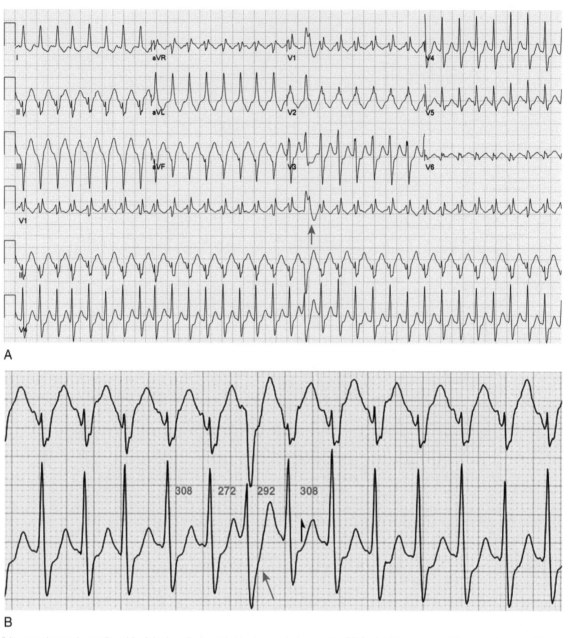

Fig. 10.8 Wide complex tachycardia with right bundle branch block morphology with QRS of 140 ms in an 84-year-old man with coronary artery disease (A). QRS morphology during the wide complex tachycardia has a slurred initial upstroke, unlike a typical right bundle branch block, and suggests ventricular tachycardia (VT). (B) The enlarged view of a part of the same electrocardiogram (leads II, V4) shows that the tachycardia cycle length is 308 ms. The *arrow* shows a PVC. A spontaneous premature ventricular complex (*arrow*) during the VT advances the timing of the next QRS wave by 16 ms and suggests a reentrant mechanism of the VT because the ventricular impulse during the premature ventricular complex enters the VT circuit earlier. The R-R intervals shown on the electrocardiogram are in ms.

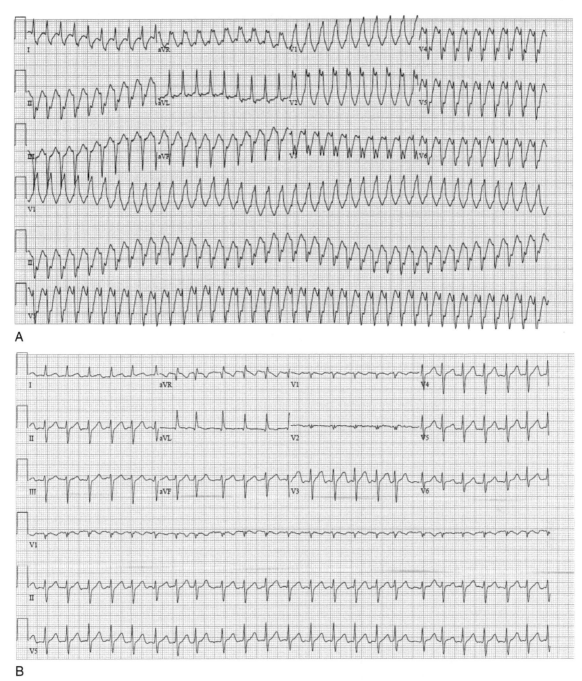

A

B

Fig. 10.9 Wide complex tachycardia with right bundle branch block pattern. (A) Electrocardiogram of a 60-year-old man with wide complex tachycardia shows a QRS duration of 124 ms with a rapid upstroke, rSR pattern in lead V1, V_i/V_t QRS complex in lead aVR more than 1, and Rs pattern in lead V6. This suggests supraventricular tachycardia with aberrancy. (B) The electrocardiogram after the infusion of diltiazem on the same patient shows atrial flutter with 2:1 atrioventricular block with narrow QRS.

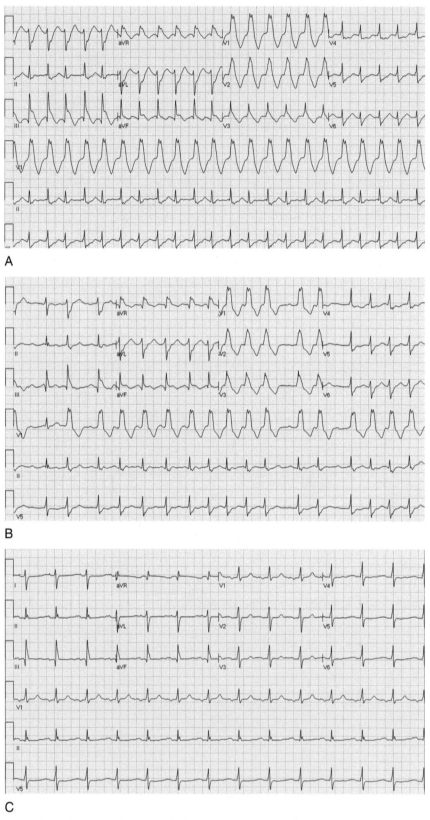

Fig. 10.10 (A) Electrocardiogram of a patient with history of mitral valve replacement and maze procedure who presented with a wide complex tachycardia depicts a right bundle branch block pattern with RsR′ pattern in lead V1 and an Rs pattern in lead V6. (B) With the use of AV nodal–blocking drug, electrocardiogram shows atrial tachycardia with variable atrioventricular block and right bundle branch block aberrancy (*arrow* points toward P waves). (C) Tachycardia was eliminated by catheter ablation in the left atrium, and the sinus rhythm shows baseline narrow QRS complexes.

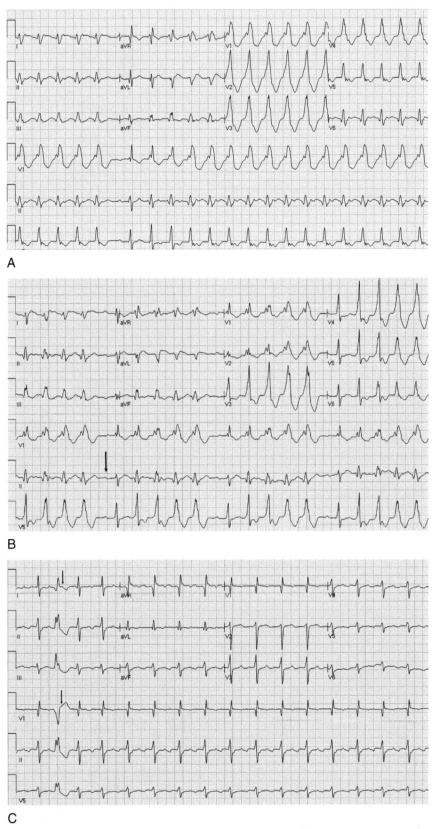

Fig. 10.11 (A) Electrocardiogram (ECG) of a 32-year-old man with nonischemic dilated cardiomyopathy after the maze procedure who presented with a wide complex tachycardia with right bundle branch block pattern. Lead V1 shows RsR′ pattern with qRs pattern in lead V6. (B) ECG in the same patient reveals atrial tachycardia with salvos of 5- to 6-beat run of wide complex tachycardia preceded by a P wave (*arrow*). This is an acceleration-dependent right bundle branch block along with acceleration-dependent left posterior fascicular block, as demonstrated by the axis shift in the lead II rhythm strip. R-R shortening is a result of Wenckebach periodicity. (C) ECG shows a premature ventricular complex with retrograde (*arrow*) concealed conduction during sinus rhythm.

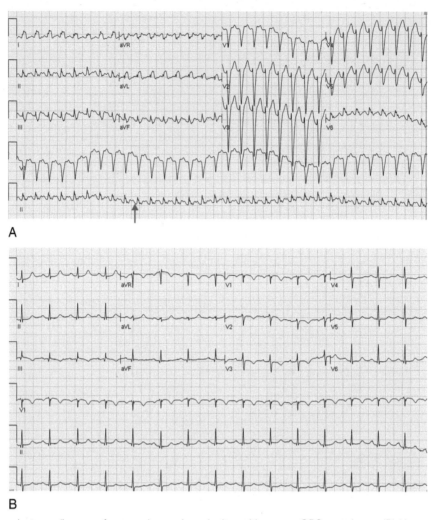

A

B

Fig. 10.12 (A) The baseline electrocardiogram of a man shows sinus rhythm with narrow QRS complexes. (B) He presented with wide complex tachycardia that depicts left bundle branch block pattern with no R wave in lead V1, narrow R wave in lead V2 (<40 ms), and no Q wave in lead V6, suggestive of a supraventricular tachycardia with aberrancy. There is 1:1 ventriculoatrial conduction with inverted P waves (*arrow*) in inferior leads in A. This is an atrial tachycardia, which was mapped to the low right atrial lateral wall.

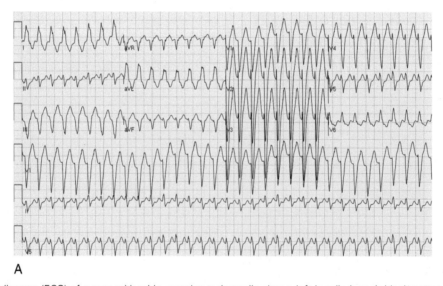

A

Fig. 10.13 (A) Electrocardiogram (ECG) of a man with wide complex tachycardia shows left bundle branch block pattern with narrow R waves in lead V1-V2 (<40 ms) and no Q wave in lead V6, suggestive of a supraventricular tachycardia with aberrancy. (B) ECG depicts the same tachycardia with narrow complexes. The tachycardia in ECG (C) is initiated by a premature atrial complex (*arrow*), which is conducted with a narrow QRS complex. The arrow is present in B. This is an atrial tachycardia (slightly irregular). QRS complexes become narrow when the R-R cycle lengthens (C and D). Atrial tachycardia was mapped at the right atrial lateral wall.

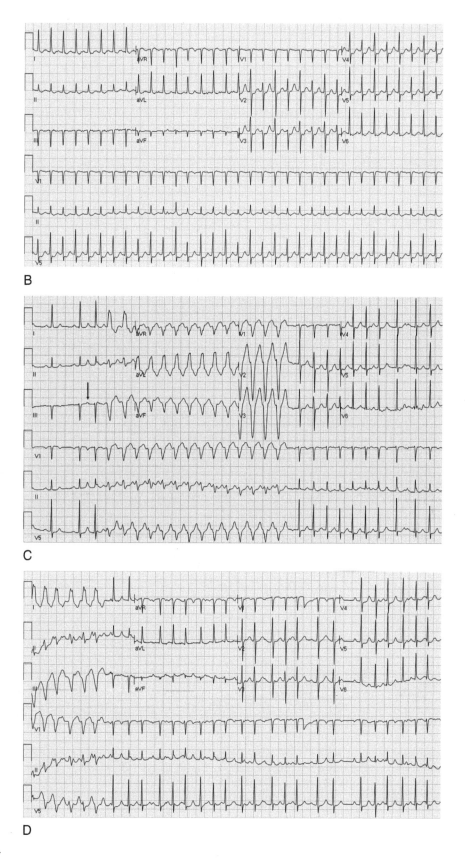

B

C

D

Fig. 10.13 (Continued).

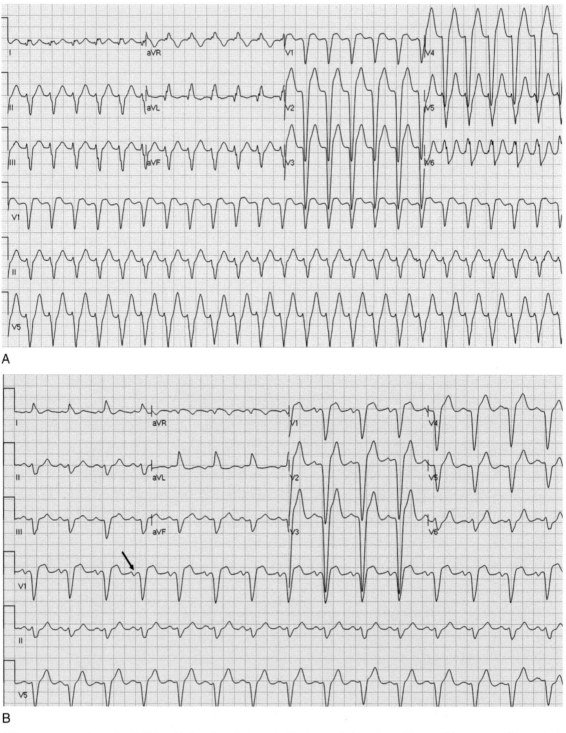

Fig. 10.14 Wide complex tachycardia (WCT) with left bundle branch block morphology in a 76-year-old woman with nonischemic dilated cardiomyopathy. (A) Electrocardiogram (ECG) reveals a WCT with a positive R wave in lead aVR, almost northwest axis, and V_i/V_t less than 1. These ECG signs suggest a ventricular tachycardia. However, the baseline ECG (B) in sinus rhythm (*arrow*) shows similar QRS morphology with a poor progression of R waves in precordial leads and atypical left bundle branch block or intraventricular conduction delay caused by severe cardiomyopathy. Therefore the WCT is most likely a sinus tachycardia recorded during the exacerbation of heart failure.

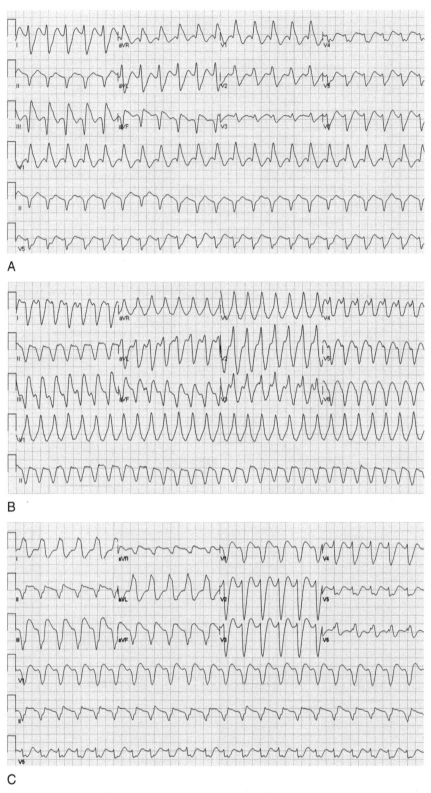

Fig. 10.15 Wide complex tachycardia of three different morphologies in a patient with history of myocardial infarction. (A) QRS morphology shows right bundle branch block with a QRS duration of 180 ms, a monophasic R wave in lead V1, rS in lead V6, and QRS axis that is 230° (northwest) and suggests ventricular tachycardia (VT). (B) QRS morphology shows right bundle branch block with a QRS duration of 188 ms, a monophasic R wave in lead V1, and QRS axis that is 260° (northwest) and suggests VT. (C) QRS morphology shows left bundle branch block pattern with a QRS duration of 184 ms, R wave that is wide (>40 ms) in lead V2, and slow descent to the nadir of the S wave (an R-S interval >70 ms) in lead V1 and suggestive of VT.

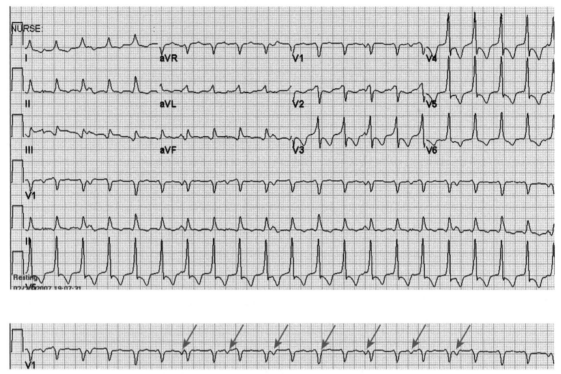

Fig. 10.16 Wide complex tachycardia with relatively narrow QRS complexes. QRS duration is 136 ms, and there is atrioventricular dissociation (*arrows*) with upright P waves in lead II that confirms ventricular tachycardia. This was mapped to be a septal ventricular tachycardia after acute myocardial infarction.

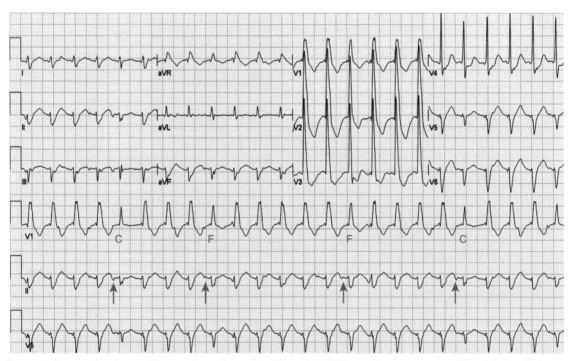

Fig. 10.17 Electrocardiogram showing a wide complex tachycardia with marked QRS complexes as capture (*C*) and fusion (*F*) beats. The *arrows* show the P waves.

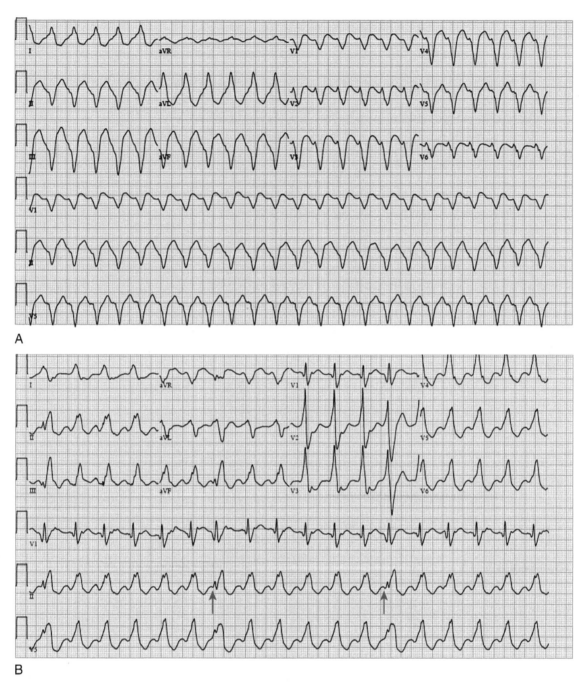

A

B

Fig. 10.18 Wide complex tachycardia (WCT) with positive (predominant direction of QRS complexes are positive in all precordial leads) and negative (predominant direction of QRS complexes are negative in all precordial leads) concordances. (A) WCT has left bundle branch block–like pattern (negative QRS polarity in lead V1) with QRS duration of 200 ms, R wave greater than 40 ms in lead V2, rS pattern in lead V6, and a negative concordance of QRS in precordial leads, suggesting ventricular tachycardia (VT). (B) WCT of a different patient has right bundle branch block–like pattern (positive QRS polarity in lead V1) with QRS duration of 180 ms, the R wave greater than 40 ms in lead V2, rS pattern in lead V6, and a positive concordance of QRS in precordial leads, suggesting VT. The *arrows* show probable fusion beats, confirming VT diagnosis.

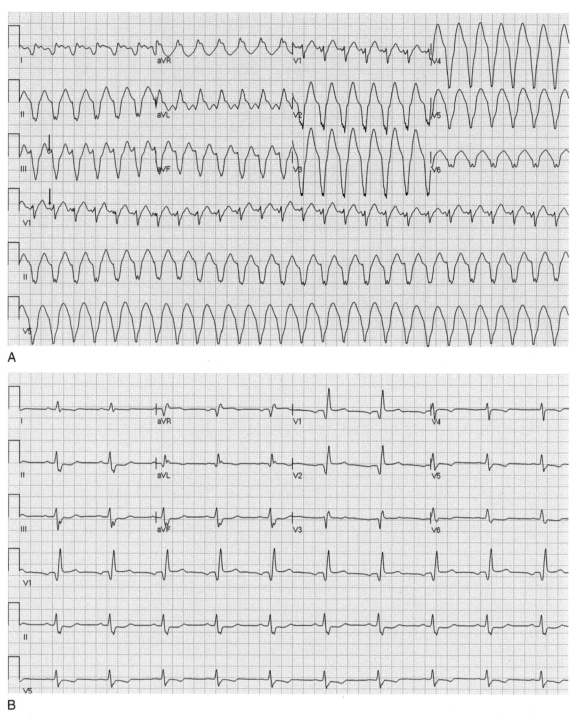

Fig. 10.19 Wide complex tachycardia in a 70-year-old man with a history of myocardial infarction. (A) Wide complex tachycardia has a QRS duration of 220 ms, northwest axis, negative precordial concordance of QRS, and a notch in the nadir of S wave in lead V1. All of these signs suggest ventricular tachycardia. Electrocardiogram also shows 1:1 ventriculoatrial conduction with retrograde P waves seen in lead III and V1 (*arrow*). (B) Baseline electrocardiogram shows anteroseptal Q waves resulting from a prior myocardial infarction. Ventricular tachycardia was mapped to the left ventricular apex.

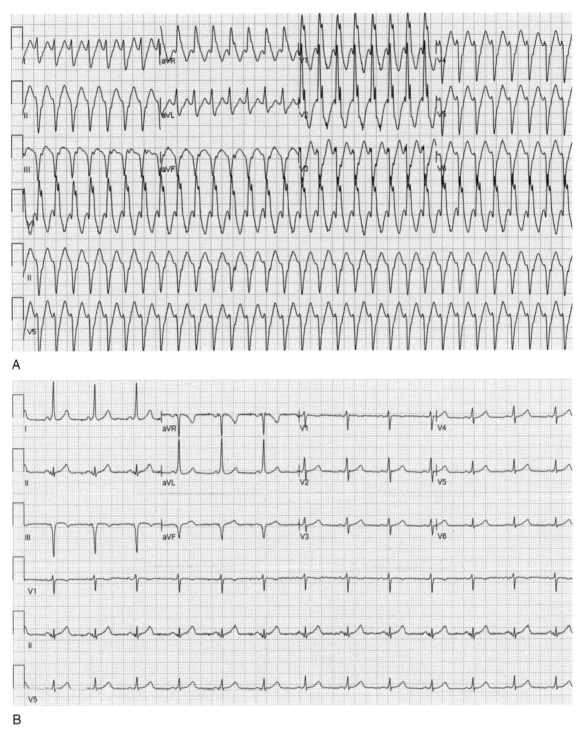

Fig. 10.20 (A) Wide complex tachycardia with retrograde (ventriculoatrial) conduction. Electrocardiogram (ECG) shows wide complex tachycardia with a QRS duration of 150 ms, atypical right bundle branch block pattern (double-peaked R in lead V1 with the amplitude of first peak higher than the second peak), a right superior (northwest) axis, and rS pattern in lead V6, suggestive of a ventricular tachycardia. ECG also demonstrates inverted (retrograde) P waves (*arrow*) in lead III, suggestive of 1:1 retrograde ventriculoatrial conduction. (B) Shows ECG of a patient with Wolff-Parkinson-White syndrome with right posteroseptal accessory pathway in sinus rhythm who later presented with wide complex tachycardia shown in (C). However, the wide complex tachycardia is not antidromic because QRS morphology does not correlate with delta waves shown in (A). This is an orthodromic tachycardia using same accessory pathway anterogradely with right bundle branch block aberrancy.

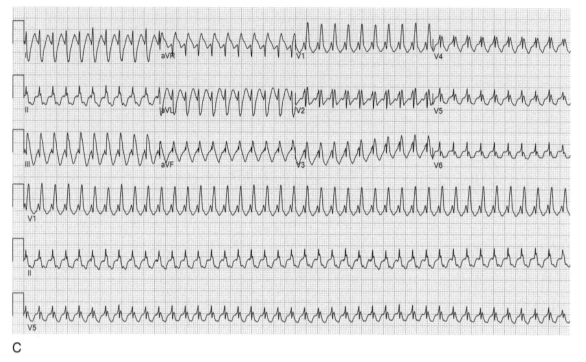

C

Fig. 10.20 (Continued).

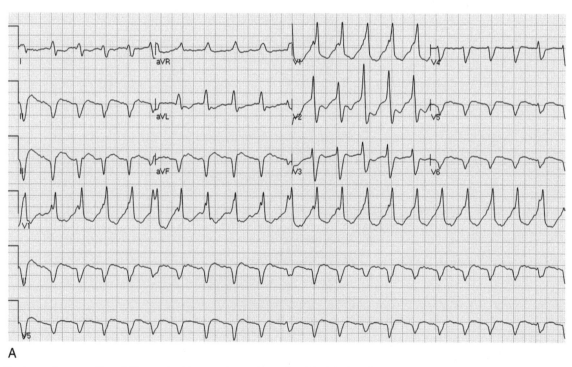

A

Fig. 10.21 Electrocardiograms (A and B) reveal wide complex tachycardia with right bundle branch block pattern, northwest axis, initial wide R wave in lead aVR, and V_i/V_t less than 1 in precordial leads, which is highly diagnostic of ventricular tachycardia in two separate patients.

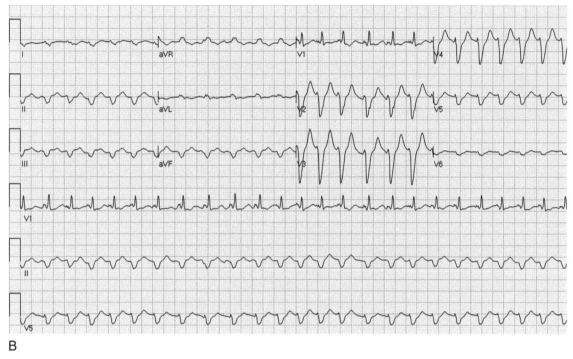

B

Fig. 10.21 (Continued).

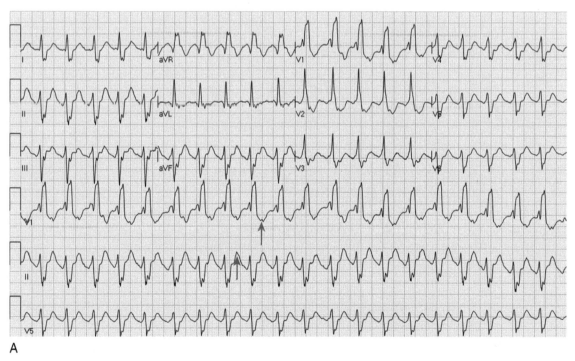

A

Fig. 10.22 Wide complex tachycardia (WCT) with typical right bundle branch block (RBBB) pattern. (A) Electrocardiogram shows a WCT with RBBB pattern, initial Q wave in lead aVR, Rs pattern with wide S wave in lead V6, and V_i/V_t greater than 1. There are notches in-between QRS waves in lead V1 and II suggestive of P waves (*arrow*); however, the interval between the two notches does not correlate with the tachycardia WCT cycle length. (B) With the use of atrioventricular nodal–blocking drugs, typical atrial flutter with a variable atrioventricular response and RBBB aberrancy is noted in electrocardiogram. Aberrancy is confirmed by the two narrow native QRS complexes that occur when RR interval lengthens.

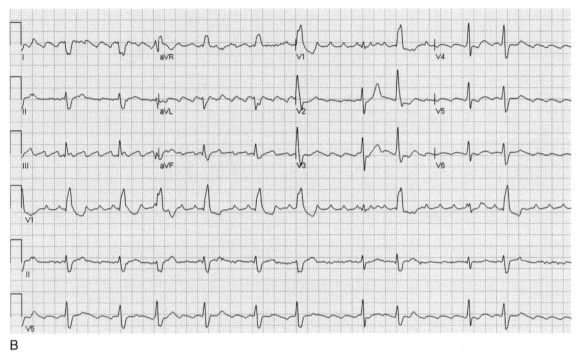

B

Fig. 10.22 (Continued).

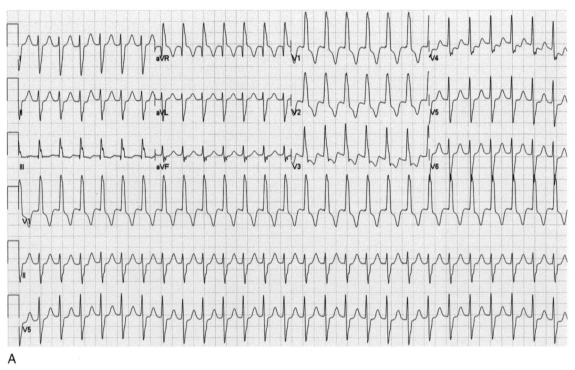

A

Fig. 10.23 Wide complex tachycardia in a patient with transposition of great arteries and Mustard surgery. These types of patients have a risk for ventricular tachycardia and supraventricular tachycardia. (A) Electrocardiogram depicts wide complex tachycardia with a QRS duration of only 124 ms with atypical right bundle branch block pattern (double-peaked R in lead V1 with the amplitude of initial peak higher than the second peak), a right inferior axis, and rS pattern in lead V6, suggestive of a supraventricular tachycardia. (B) Electrocardiogram of the same patient shows atrial flutter (arrows) with right bundle branch block and right axis deviation.

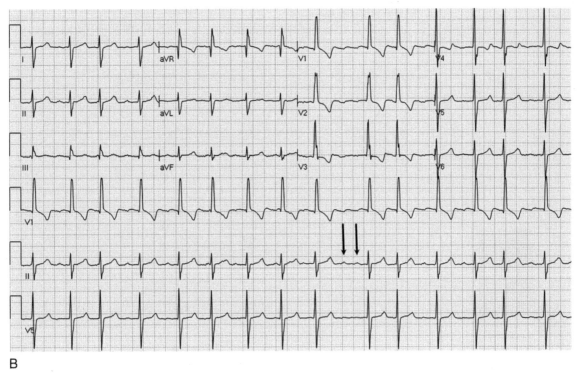

B

Fig. 10.23 (Continued).

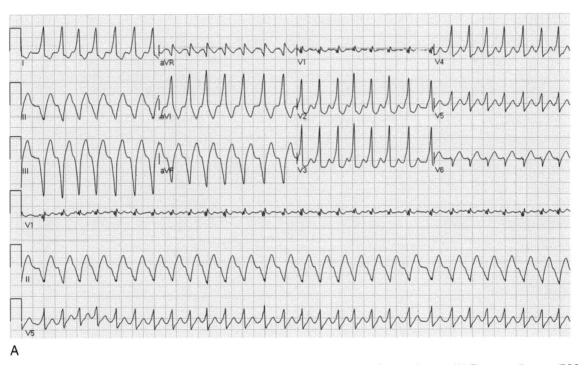

A

Fig. 10.24 Irregular wide complex tachycardia in a 69-year-old man without prior history of heart disease. (A) Electrocardiogram (ECG) depicts a wide complex tachycardia with atypical right bundle branch block and rS complex in lead V6 suggestive of ventricular tachycardia. However, the tachycardia cycle length has subtle variation, V_i/V_t in lead aVR is less than 1, and slurred upstroke in QRS in leads V2-V5, which suggests atrial fibrillation/atrial flutter with rapid conduction via a bypass tract. (B) ECG of the same patient later showed atrial fibrillation with obvious variation in cycle length with variation of QRS amplitude depending on the degree of preexcitation. (C) Baseline ECG of the patient after direct current cardioversion demonstrated positive delta waves in lead V1 and negative delta waves in inferior leads (*arrows*). The accessory pathway was mapped to the left posteroseptal region of the mitral annulus during the electrophysiology study.

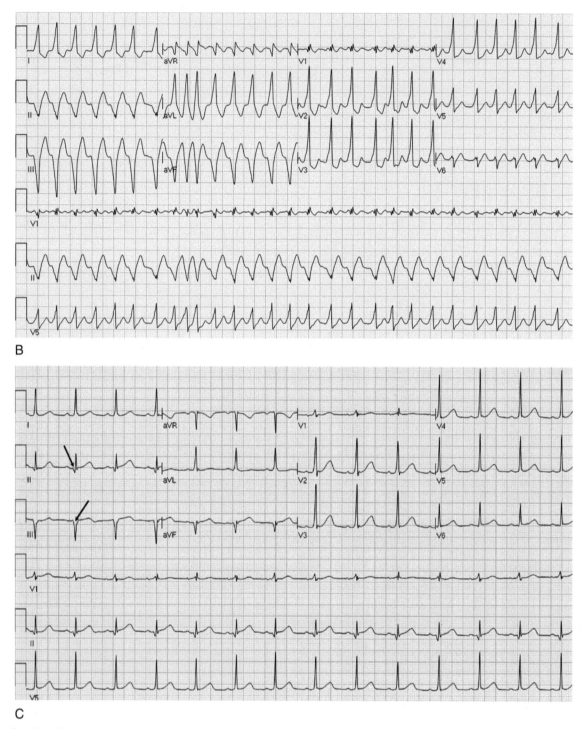

B

C

Fig. 10.24 (Continued).

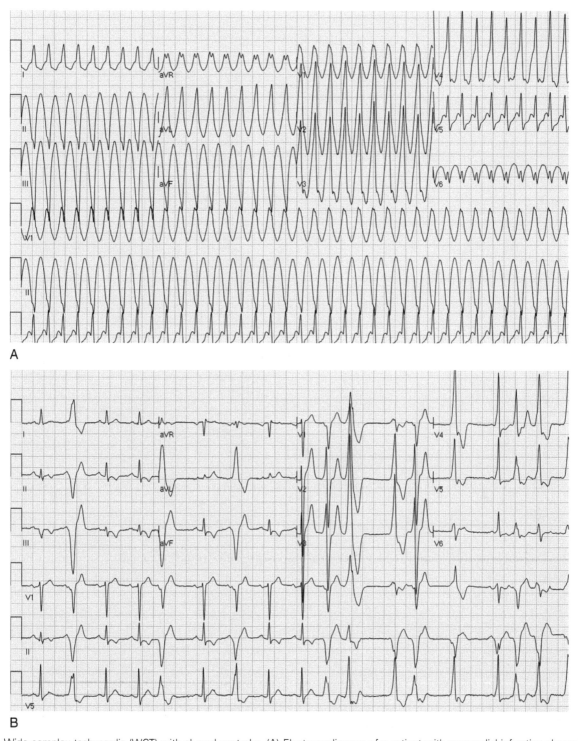

Fig. 10.25 Wide complex tachycardia (WCT) with slurred upstroke. (A) Electrocardiogram of a patient with myocardial infarction shows WCT with right bundle branch block pattern, QRS duration of 200 ms, QS pattern in lead V6, and slurred upstroke in precordial leads V1–V5. This appears to be Wolff-Parkinson-White syndrome with antidromic atrioventricular reentrant tachycardia; however, with the history of myocardial infarction, ventricular tachycardia (VT) should be ruled out. (B) Electrocardiogram after termination of the WCT showed frequent monomorphic premature ventricular complexes. Premature ventricular complex morphology is similar to the QRS morphology during WCT, confirming VT rather than antidromic atrioventricular reentrant tachycardia. This VT originated from the inferior basal left ventricle in the epicardium.

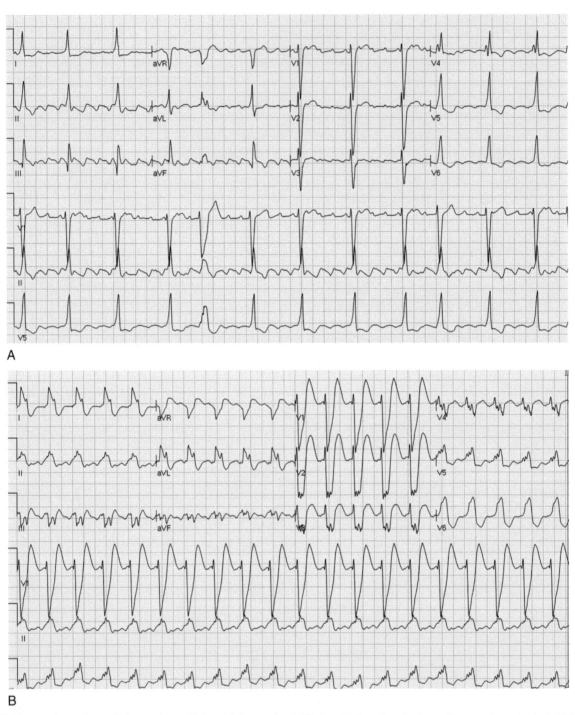

Fig. 10.26 Wide complex tachycardia in a patient with heart failure and atrial flutter. (A) Baseline electrocardiogram shows typical atrial flutter with a variable atrioventricular response. (B) Patient presented with a wide complex tachycardia with a markedly wide QRS (200 ms) at a rate of 119 bpm and V_i/V_t less than 1, suggestive of a ventricular tachycardia.

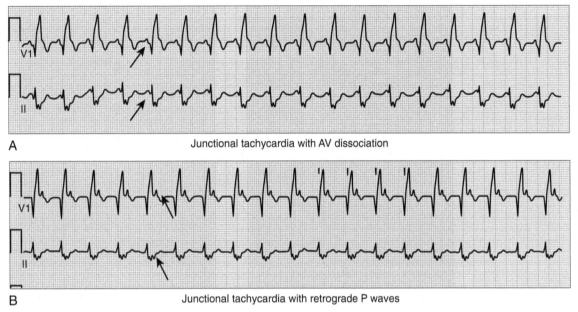

Fig. 10.27 Junctional tachycardia presenting as wide complex tachycardia. (A and B) Electrocardiograms show junctional tachycardia with atrioventricular (AV) dissociation in (A) and junctional tachycardia with retrograde ventriculoatrial conduction, respectively. (A) Wide complex tachycardia with isorhythmic AV dissociation. Electrocardiogram demonstrates junctional tachycardia with a very short P-R interval with upright P waves in the inferior leads and a subtle change in P-R interval suggestive of sinus tachycardia with isorhythmic AV dissociation. (B) Rhythm strips of (A) and (B) show anterograde versus retrograde P waves (*arrow*).

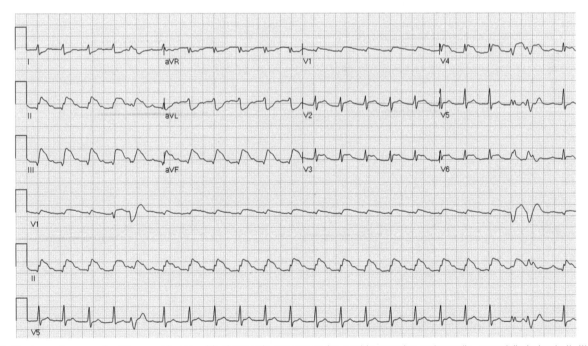

Fig. 10.28 Electrocardiogram of a 55-year-old man with chest pain appears to be a wide complex tachycardia, especially in leads II, III, aVF, and aVL. This is due to ST elevation during inferior acute myocardial infarction. A closer look reveals narrow QRS complexes in lead I and precordial leads.

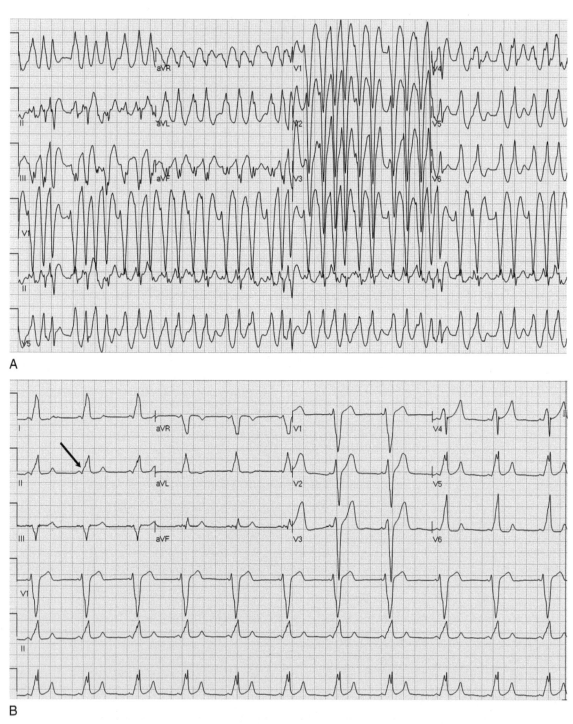

Fig. 10.29 Irregular wide complex tachycardia in a 26-year-old man presenting with sudden cardiac arrest who was resuscitated successfully with a direct-current shock. (A) Electrocardiogram shows irregular wide complex tachycardia, with varying QRS width and amplitude, but overall QRS axis remains the same. This is atrial fibrillation with a rapid ventricular response. (B) Electrocardiogram after cardioversion of the same patient revealed Wolff-Parkinson-White conduction over an accessory pathway (*arrow*). This bypass tract was mapped to the posterolateral tricuspid annulus and successfully eliminated with a single radiofrequency application.

11

Ventricular Tachycardia in the Absence of Structural Heart Disease

IDIOPATHIC VENTRICULAR TACHYCARDIA

Ventricular tachycardia (VT) in patients with structurally normal hearts is called *idiopathic VT*. Idiopathic VTs are of two types. The more common one is the focal VT caused by cyclic adenosine monophosphate—mediated triggered activity. This VT is sensitive to adenosine, beta blockers, and calcium channel blockers. The less common variety is a verapamil-sensitive reentrant left fascicular VT, which commonly originates from close to the left posterior fascicle of the left bundle branch and less commonly from the left anterior fascicle.[1]

Adenosine-Sensitive Idiopathic Ventricular Tachycardia

Adenosine-sensitive idiopathic VTs have various electrocardiogram (ECG) manifestations, ranging from frequent premature ventricular complexes (PVCs), ventricular couplets, and salvos of nonsustained VT or sustained VT (Fig. 11.1). This form of VT usually occurs at rest. In some patients it is exercise induced. Exercise testing reproduces VT in 25% to 50% of patients with clinical VT (Fig. 11.2). Idiopathic VT generally has a benign prognosis. However, rapid idiopathic VT can result in sudden cardiac death[2] (Fig. 11.3).

Sites of Origin of Idiopathic Ventricular Tachycardia

The most common form of idiopathic VT originates from the ventricular outflow tract. In approximately 75% to 80% of cases, VTs originate from the right ventricular outflow tract (RVOT), and the rest can originate anywhere in the ventricles, such as from the left ventricular outflow tract (LVOT), aortic coronary cusp, papillary muscle, and epicardial surface of the ventricles. The majority of epicardial VTs arise from the coronary sinus or great cardiac vein or the crux of the heart. These account for 15% of idiopathic VTs and PVCs.[3] Several algorithms have been proposed for ECG diagnosis for localization of VT origin by analyzing QRS morphology in different leads (Table 11.1)[4]:

1. **Bundle branch morphology (left bundle branch block [LBBB] vs. right bundle branch block [RBBB]):** In general, LBBB morphology of VT originates from the right ventricle and RVOT, however, VT originating from the septal LVOT or aortic cusp may also have LBBB morphology. RBBB morphology represents left ventricular origin.
2. **QRS axis (superior vs. inferior):** In general, superior axis represents inferior origin and inferior axis represents superior origin of the VT.
3. **Precordial transition of R wave (late vs. early):** QRS transition in precordial leads with change where R wave becomes greater than S wave (changes from Q-S or r-S pattern to R-S or R-s pattern) at or beyond lead V4 is defined as *late transition*. In RVOT, the QRS transition occurs at V3 or V4. Early transition (V1 or V2) may represent a supravalvular origin of the VT (aortic cusp, pulmonary artery, or epicardial).

4. **QRS morphology (Q waves, monophasic vs. notched R waves):** Q waves are usually present in leads representing the ventricular wall of origin of the VT. R waves are usually monophasic in septal VTs because of the simultaneous activation of both ventricles, whereas QRS is notched presumably because the two ventricles are activated in sequence.
5. **QRS duration (narrow vs. wide):** Septal VTs are relatively narrow (<140 ms), whereas free wall VTs tend to have wider QRS.
6. **Pseudo delta wave (i.e., delayed onset of the QRS appearing like the delayed QRS slurred upstroke in Wolff-Parkinson-White syndrome) and delayed intrinsicoid deflection (interval between the QRS onset to the peak of R wave) of QRS:** A pseudo delta wave of 34 ms or greater and delayed intrinscoid deflection time of 85 ms or greater in lead V2 (which results in a wider QRS) represent epicardial VT.[5] Epicardial VT originating from the midline (crux or anterior cardiac vein) tends to have less wide QRS.

However, these algorithms should serve only as a rough guide. QRS morphology and axis also depend on several other factors, such as direction of the exit of wavefront (endocardial vs. epicardial and rightward vs. leftward); position of heart in the thoracic cavity (horizontal vs. vertical and clockwise vs. counterclockwise rotation); shape of thorax; and, more important, ECG lead position.

Right Ventricular Outflow Tract Ventricular Tachycardia

RVOT VTs have LBBB morphology with precordial R wave transition in lead V3 or V4 and positive QRS complexes in inferior leads. RVOT can be divided into septal anterior, posterior, and lateral walls (Fig. 11.4).

1. **Anterior RVOT VT:** Most RVOT VTs originate from the anterosuperior aspect of the septum, just under the pulmonic valve. These VTs or PVCs have positive QRS complexes in inferior leads and large negative complexes in leads aVR and aVL. Lead I typically has an initial isoelectric or negative (Q or qR pattern) deflection and may also have multiphasic QRS complexes (Fig. 11.5).
2. **Septal RVOT VT:** The septal RVOT VT is associated with negative QRS complex in aVL. R waves are taller and monophasic in inferior leads (Fig. 11.6).
3. **Posterior RVOT VT:** VTs from posterior RVOT have a dominant R wave in lead I (no Q or qR pattern as seen in anterior RVOT VTs), QS or R wave in aVL, and an early precordial transition by lead V3 (Figs. 11.7 and 11.8).
4. **Free-wall (lateral) RVOT VT:** The lateral or free-wall RVOT VT is associated with positive QRS complexes in leads I and aVL. These VTs have wider and notched QRS complexes in the inferior leads and late precordial QRS transition (Fig. 11.9).

Pulmonary Artery Ventricular Tachycardia

VTs arising above the pulmonic valve have a greater R/S ratio in lead V2 and larger R wave amplitude in the inferior leads than those seen in RVOT

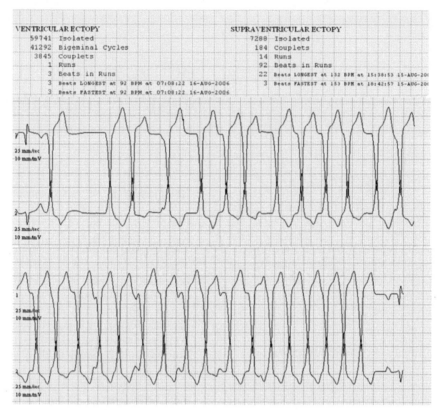

Fig. 11.1 Holter recording of a patient with idiopathic ventricular tachycardia showing frequent premature ventricular complexes, ventricular couplets, and several episodes of nonsustained ventricular tachycardia in salvos. Approximately 40% of total QRS complexes are ventricular complexes.

VTs. Furthermore, these VTs have a QS (or rS) pattern in lead I, and the Q wave amplitude in aVL is equal or greater to that of aVR (Fig. 11.10).

Right Septal Ventricular Tachycardia

Septal VTs have LBBB morphology with a relatively narrower QRS width (<140 ms). They have monophasic R waves and relatively lower amplitude of the QRS in the inferior leads (Fig. 11.11). In general, septal VTs have a QS complex in lead I, but as the site of origin moves rightward, either on the septum or on the free wall, R waves appear in lead I and become progressively dominant and the QRS axis becomes more leftward. Similarly, a QS amplitude in aVL greater than that in aVR suggests an origin on the left side of the RVOT; a QS amplitude in aVR greater than that in aVL suggests an origin on the right side.

Parahisian Ventricular Tachycardia

The characteristic ECG abnormalities for VTs arising from near the His bundle region include an R-RSR' pattern in aVL and taller R waves in leads I, V5, and V6. R waves are smaller in inferior leads, and lead V1 has QS pattern (Fig. 11.12).

Right Free Wall Ventricular Tachycardia

The QRS morphology of right free wall VT depends on the location of the VT focus. In general, they have a longer QRS duration with a triphasic RR' or Rr' waves. R waves have greater QRS amplitude in lead I, and there are no q waves in lead aVL. QRS axis is superior and leftward

in VTs originating from inferior/inferolateral right ventricular free wall and, lower or midseptum (Fig. 11.13).

Tricuspid Annular Ventricular Tachycardia

VTs arising from the tricuspid annulus have positive QRS polarity in leads I, aVL, V5, and V6. Tricuspid annular VTs have an rS or a QS pattern in lead aVR similar to an RVOT VT. These VTs have greater R wave amplitude without any negative component in the QRS in lead I and no positive QRS polarities in any of the inferior leads.

Left-Sided Ventricular Tachycardias

Left-sided idiopathic VTs commonly originate from the LVOT. Other left-sided sites include left mitral annulus, aortic cusps, aortomitral continuity, interventricular septum, papillary muscle, and epicardial sites mostly in the region of the coronary sinus and cardiac veins (Fig. 11.14).

Left Ventricular Outflow Tract Ventricular Tachycardias

The LVOT region can be divided anatomically as anteromedially septal, anterolateral free wall, posterolateral, and aortomitral continuity. Aortic cusps are also a source of VT. The absence of an S wave in leads V5 or V6 suggests an aortic cusp location, whereas the presence of S waves in these leads indicates an infravalvular location.

1. **Septal LVOT VT:** Both RVOT and septal LVOT VTs have LBBB morphology. The absence of an R wave in lead V1 or late precordial R wave transition (lead V4 or beyond) predicts RVOT

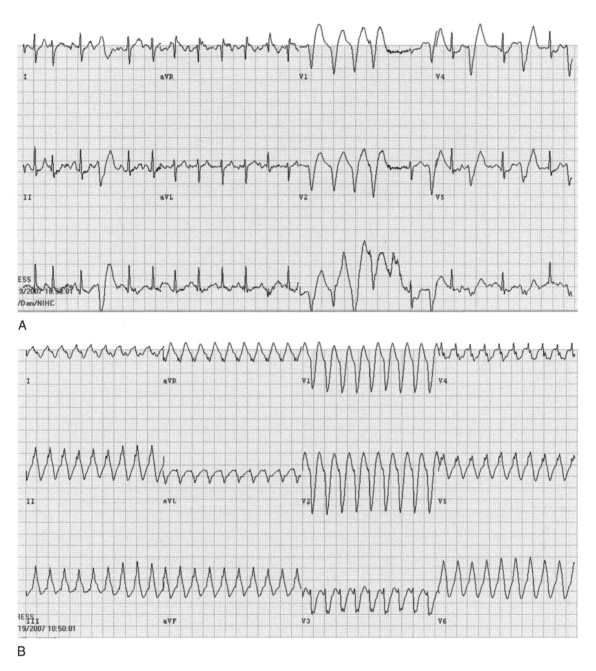

Fig. 11.2 Electrocardiogram during exercise in a patient with idiopathic ventricular tachycardia (VT) initially shows frequent premature ventricular complexes and nonsustained VT (A), which is followed by sustained VT (B) that responded to intravenous adenosine.

origin of the VT, whereas the presence of an R wave in leads V1 or V2 and precordial R wave transition in leads V1 or V2 are characteristic of LVOT VT. Additionally, a QS complex in lead I is consistent with LVOT origin (Fig. 11.15).

2. **LVOT free wall VT:** LVOT free wall VTs have RBBB morphology with an early QRS transition and persistent dominant R wave across the precordium, with a small or absent S wave in V5-V6 (Fig. 11.16).

3. **VT from the aortomitral continuity:** VT from the aortomitral continuity has RBBB morphology and broad monophasic R waves across the precordial leads. There is a qR pattern in V1 as a result of the left fibrous trigone deflecting initial electrical activation leftward (Fig. 11.17).

Mitral Annular Ventricular Tachycardia

VT in the anterior mitral annulus has RBBB and inferior axis. VT arising from anterolateral mitral annulus shows positive precordial concordance with an RBBB configuration in V1 and usually with late notching in the inferior leads (Fig. 11.18). As the VT focus moves

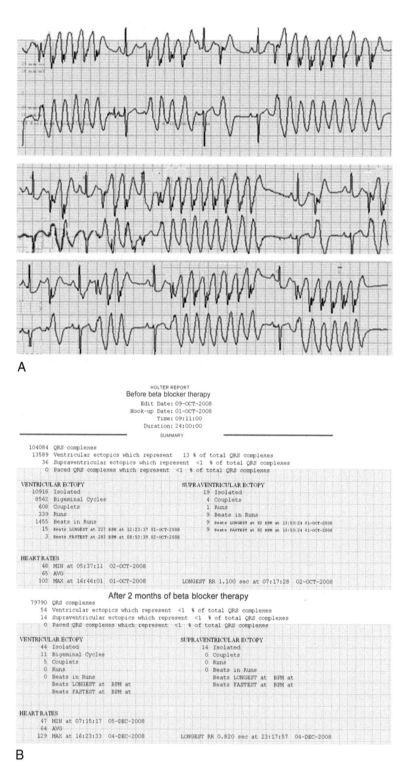

A

HOLTER REPORT
Before beta blocker therapy
Edit Date: 09-OCT-2008
Hook-up Date: 01-OCT-2008
Time: 09:11:00
Duration: 24:00:00
SUMMARY

104084 QRS complexes
 13589 Ventricular ectopics which represent   13 % of total QRS complexes
    36 Supraventricular ectopics which represent <1 % of total QRS complexes
     0 Paced QRS complexes which represent <1 % of total QRS complexes

VENTRICULAR ECTOPY		SUPRAVENTRICULAR ECTOPY	
10918	Isolated	19	Isolated
8562	Bigeminal Cycles	4	Couplets
608	Couplets	1	Runs
339	Runs	9	Beats in Runs
1455	Beats in Runs	9	Beats LONGEST at 82 BPM at 13:53:24 01-OCT-2008
15	Beats LONGEST at 227 BPM at 12:23:37 01-OCT-2008	9	Beats FASTEST at 82 BPM at 13:53:24 01-OCT-2008
3	Beats FASTEST at 283 BPM at 08:53:39 02-OCT-2008		

HEART RATES
    48 MIN at 05:37:11 02-OCT-2008
    65 AVG
   102 MAX at 16:46:01 01-OCT-2008   LONGEST RR 1.100 sec at 07:17:28 02-OCT-2008

After 2 months of beta blocker therapy
 79790 QRS complexes
    54 Ventricular ectopics which represent <1 % of total QRS complexes
    14 Supraventricular ectopics which represent <1 % of total QRS complexes
     0 Paced QRS complexes which represent <1 % of total QRS complexes

VENTRICULAR ECTOPY		SUPRAVENTRICULAR ECTOPY	
44	Isolated	14	Isolated
11	Bigeminal Cycles	0	Couplets
5	Couplets	0	Runs
0	Runs	0	Beats in Runs
0	Beats in Runs		Beats LONGEST at BPM at
	Beats LONGEST at BPM at		Beats FASTEST at BPM at
	Beats FASTEST at BPM at		

HEART RATES
    47 MIN at 07:15:17 05-DEC-2008
    64 AVG
   129 MAX at 16:23:33 04-DEC-2008   LONGEST RR 0.820 sec at 23:17:57 04-DEC-2008

B

Fig. 11.3 Malignant variety of idiopathic ventricular tachycardia (VT). (A) Holter recording of a patient without any structural heart disease and frequent presyncope and syncope revealed frequent monomorphic premature ventricular complexes (PVCs) followed by rapid nonsustained VT. (B) Holter recording of the same patient showed 13,500 PVCs in 24 hours. There are frequent nonsustained VT in salvos, which can be seen in patients with idiopathic adenosine-sensitive VT. PVCs burden reduced to 44 beats in 24 hours after beta blocker therapy in this patient.

TABLE 11.1 Electrocardiogram Diagnosis for Localization of Ventricular Tachycardia Origin by Analyzing QRS Morphology

LOCATION	BBB	QRS AXIS	I	V1	V6	PRECORDIAL TRANSITION	OTHER FEATURES
RVOT							
Septal	LBBB	Inf	−/±	rS	R	V3/V4	Negative QRS complexes in lead I
Posterior	LBBB	Inf		rS	R	V3	A dominant R wave in lead I, QS, or R wave in aVL
Anterior	LBBB	Inf		rR	R	V3/V4	Negative QRS complexes (QR/qR) in aVR and aVL
Lateral	LBBB	Inf		rS	R	V4/V5	Positive QRS complexes in leads I and aVL
							Wider and notched QRS complexes in inferior leads
Right septal	LBBB	Inf	−	rS	R		QRS width <140 ms
		Sup[a]					Monophasic R waves (lower amplitude in inferior leads)
							Right septal: QS amplitude in aVR >aVL
							Left septal: QS amplitude in aVL >aVR
Parahisian	LBBB	Inf	+	qS	R		R/RSR′ pattern in aVL
							Tall R wave in leads I, V5, and V6
							Small R waves in inferior leads
RV free wall	LBBB	Inf	+	R	RS		Wide QRS with a triphasic RR′ or Rr′ waves
		Sup[b]					No q waves in aVL
Pulmonary artery	LBBB	Inf	−			V1/V2	QS (or rS) pattern in lead I
							Q wave amplitude in aVL >aVR
Tricuspid annulus							
Posteromedial	LBBB	Inf	−	QS	R		Positive, isoelectric, or multiphasic in aVL in anteroseptal VT
		Sup[c]					
Anterolateral	LBBB	Inf	+	QS	R		Notching in limb leads, discordant forces in inferior leads in inferolateral tricuspid annular VT
		Sup[c]					
LVOT							
Septal	LBBB	L inf	+	rS	R	V1/V2	Rs in lead I
Free wall	RRRR	Inf				V1/V2	Persistent dominant R wave across the precordium
							Small or absent S wave in V5-V6
AMC	RBBB	Inf	−/±	qR	R	V1/V2	Broad monophasic R waves across the precordial leads
							No S in V6
Mitral annulus							
Anterolateral	RBBB	Inf	−	R	R	V3/V4	Wide QRS, Q wave in lead aVL
Posteromedial	RBBB	Sup	+	R	R		Negative/biphasic QRS in inferior leads
Right coronary cusp	LBBB	Inf	+	rS	RS	V1/V2	Atypical LBBB
							Broad R in V2
Left coronary cusp	LBBB	Inf	−/±	rS	RS	V1/V2	Atypical LBBB
							W- or M-shaped QRS in V1
							QS/RS in lead I
Papillary muscle							
Anterolateral	RBBB	Inf	−	rSR	RS	V4/V5	
Posteromedial	RBBB	Sup	+	rSR	RS	V4/V5	Late R to S transition
Epicardial							
LVOT	LBBB	Inf	−/±	R	R	V2 to V4	Relatively narrower QRS than other epicardial VTs
Crux	LBBB	Sup	−	rS	R	V1-V3	MDI >0.55, slurred intrinsicoid deflection
AIV/GCV	LBBB	Inf	−	rS	R		MDI >0.55
							R wave in V1 >85 ms
							Precordial pattern break with abrupt loss of R waves in V2
Anterior RV	LBBB	Inf	+	rS	R	V3	Q wave in lead I
							QS complexes in lead V2

AIV, Anterior interventricular vein; *AMC*, aortomitral continuity; *BBB*, bundle branch block; *GCV*, great cardiac vein; *Inf*, inferior; *LBBB*, left bundle branch block; *LVOT*, left ventricular outflow tract; *MDI*, maximum deflection index; *PA*, pulmonary artery; *RBBB*, right bundle branch block; *RV*, right ventricle; *RVOT*, right ventricular outflow tract; *Sup*, superior; *VT*, ventricular tachycardia; +, positive; −, negative.

[a]Left superior axis in inferoseptal/inferoapical.

[b]QRS axis is superior and leftward in VTs originating from inferior/inferolateral RV free wall and lower or midseptum.

[c]QRS axis is leftward superior in VT originating from posterior septal tricuspid annulus.

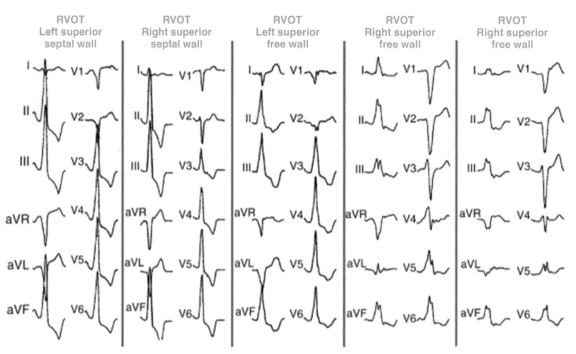

Fig. 11.4 Electrocardiogram of premature ventricular complexes from the right ventricular outflow tract (*RVOT*). (Issa ZF, Miller JM, Zipes DP, eds. *Clinical Arrhythmology and Electrophysiology*. Philadelphia, PA: Elsevier; 2012, chapter 23, p. 568).

laterally along the mitral annulus, the R waves in lead I and in the inferior leads decrease in amplitude and Q wave appears in lead aVL.

Idiopathic Ventricular Tachycardia Originating From the Papillary Muscles

Idiopathic VT can arise from the papillary muscles of the left ventricle and rarely can arise from the right ventricle. VTs arising from the anterolateral papillary muscle of the left ventricle have RBBB and right inferior axis, whereas VTs arising from the posteromedial papillary muscle have RBBB and right superior axis (Figs. 11.19 and 11.20).

Aortic Cusp Ventricular Tachycardia

Aortic cusp VTs arise from right and left coronary cusps and have LBBB morphology with an inferior axis (Figs. 11.21–11.24).[6] The noncoronary cusp, which usually does not have ventricular muscle strands, is rarely a source of an idiopathic VT. This is because the base of the noncoronary cusp is composed of fibrous tissue, given that it is in continuity with the mitral annulus. An earlier precordial transition (right cusp: V2/V3, left cusp: V1/V2) and a broad R wave duration in lead V1 or V2 (R wave duration index $\geq$ 50% and R/S ratio $\geq$ 30% in lead V1/V2) differentiate VT originating from coronary cusps and high left septum. This is unlike RVOT VT wherein the precordial transition is in lead V3/V4. The left coronary cusp is often associated with a W- or M-shaped pattern in lead V1 and a QS or rS complex in lead I, whereas

right aortic cusp VTs have greater R wave amplitude in lead I based on the anatomic position of the valve in relation to the chest wall.

Epicardial Ventricular Tachycardia

VTs in this region arise mainly from perivascular myocardial tissue associated with the coronary venous system, particularly at the junction of the great cardiac vein and anterior interventricular vein but also from other epicardial sites. Epicardial foci have a relatively slower conduction of the impulse from the origin toward the endocardium, and therefore have pseudo delta waves (duration $\geq$ 34 ms), a delayed intrinsicoid deflection (interval between the QRS onset to the peak of R wave) of 85 ms or greater, and a wider QRS (shortest precordial RS complex $\geq$ 121 ms).[4] Anterolateral or apical superior VTs have a Q wave in lead I, whereas the basal inferior or inferoapical VTs have a Q wave in inferior leads.

Epicardial Left Ventricular Outflow Tract Ventricular Tachycardia

A precordial maximum deflection index, which is defined as the shortest time to maximal positive or negative deflection in any precordial lead divided by the QRS duration, is helpful in identifying an epicardial focus.[4] A cutoff value of 0.55 has a high sensitivity and specificity in discriminating between epicardial foci and other outflow tract sites of origin. These VTs also show precordial "pattern break" or R wave

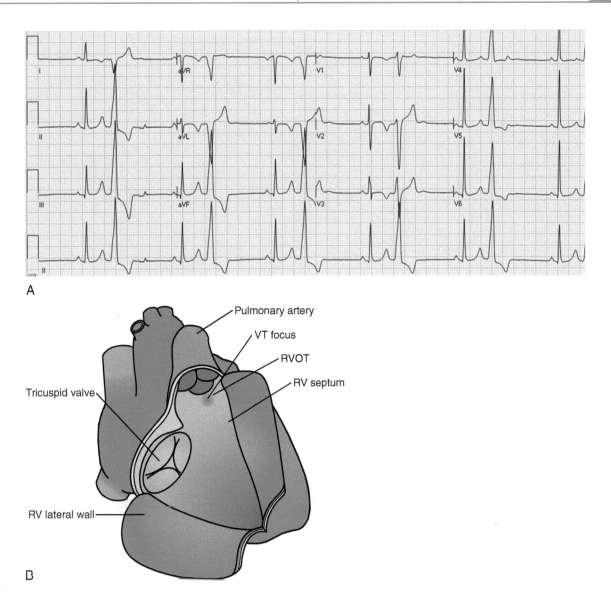

Fig. 11.5 (A) This patient had symptomatic premature ventricular complexes (PVCs). The electrocardiogram shows that the PVC has left bundle branch block—like morphology, inferior axis with monophasic, tall R waves in inferior leads, and late precordial transition of R wave. (B) During electrophysiology study, the PVC was mapped originating from the anteroseptal right ventricular outflow tract (*RVOT*) and was successfully ablated. *RV*, Right ventricle; *VT*, ventricular tachycardia.

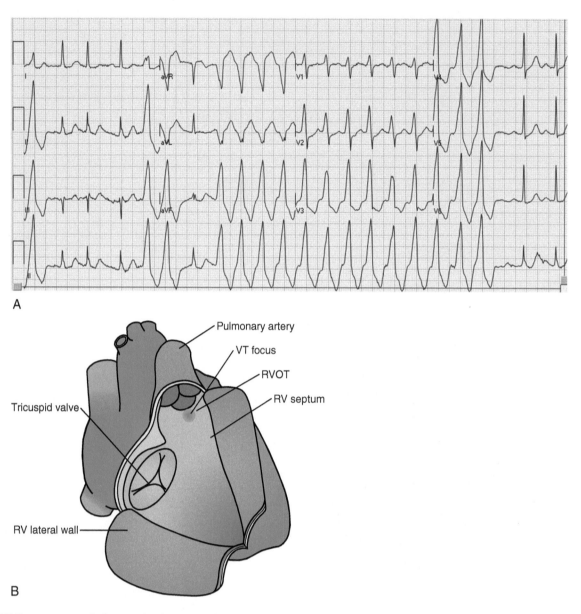

Fig. 11.6 (A) Premature ventricular complex has an atypical left bundle branch block morphology, inferior axis with monophasic, tall R waves in inferior leads, and the lead aVL has QS complex. (B) During electrophysiology study, the ventricular tachycardia (*VT*) was mapped originating from the septal right ventricular outflow tract (*RVOT*) just below the pulmonary valve and was successfully ablated. *RV*, Right ventricle.

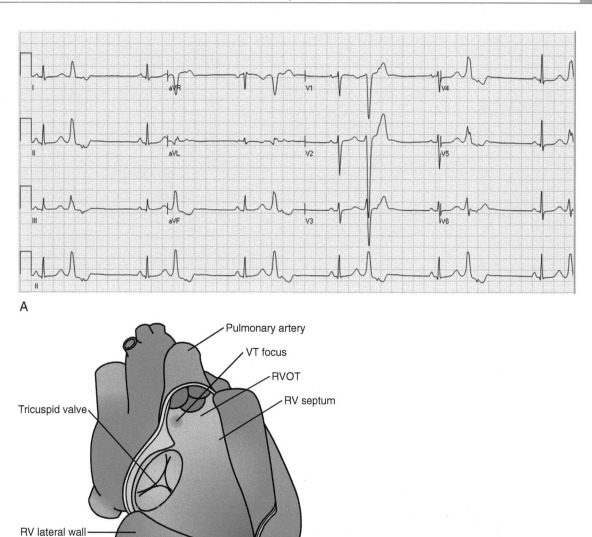

Fig. 11.7 Posterolateral right ventricular outflow tract (*RVOT*) ventricular tachycardia (*VT*). (A) Premature ventricular complex has left bundle branch block, inferior axis with notched, tall R waves in inferior leads, and the lead aVL has qR complex. (B) During electrophysiology study, the VT was mapped originating from the septal RVOT and was successfully ablated. *RV*, Right ventricle.

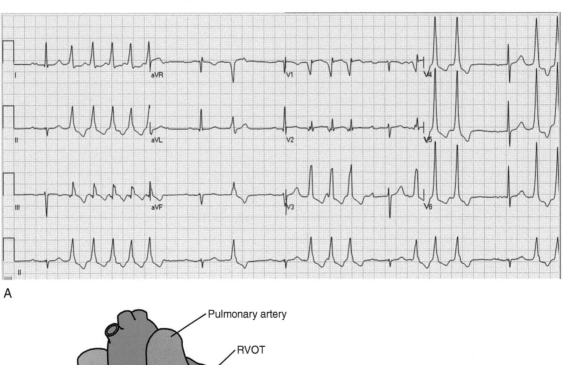

A

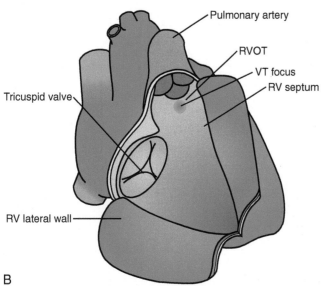

B

Fig. 11.8 Posteromedial right ventricular outflow tract (*RVOT*) ventricular tachycardia (*VT*). (A) VT has left bundle branch block, inferior axis with notched, tall R waves in inferior leads, and the lead aVR has qR complex, and lead aVL has positive QRS complex. During electrophysiology study, the VT was mapped originating from the posteromedial RVOT (B) and was successfully ablated. *RV*, Right ventricle.

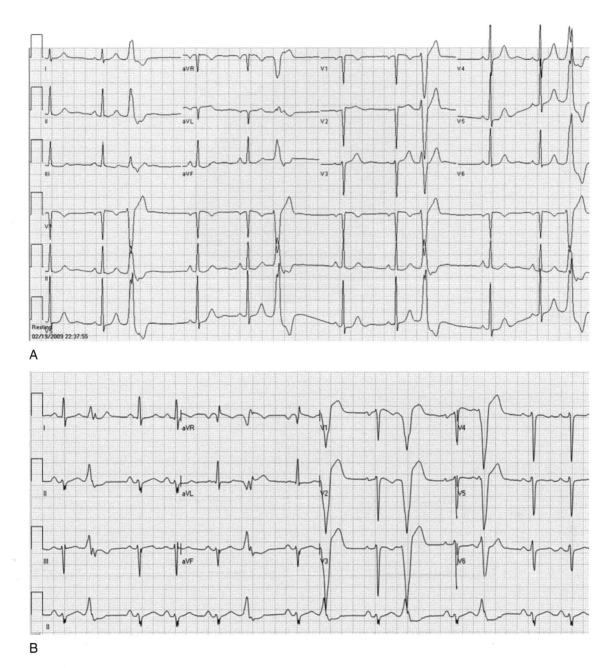

Fig. 11.9 Right ventricular outflow tract (*RVOT*) free wall premature ventricular complex (PVC). PVC has left bundle branch block, inferior axis with wide notched R waves in leads I and aVL (A and B). Inferior leads also have notched QRS complex and late precordial transition of R wave (in B only). (C) During electrophysiology study, these PVCs were mapped originating from the lateral (free wall) RVOT and were successfully ablated. *RV*, Right ventricle; *VT*, ventricular tachycardia.

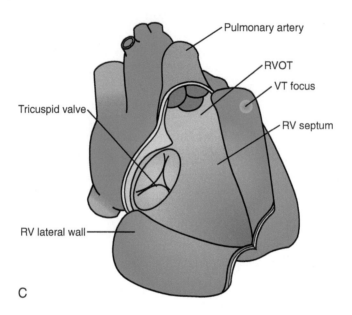

Fig. 11.9 (Continued).

regression/progression, in which there is an abrupt loss of R wave in V2 followed by resumption in R waves from V3 to V6.

Epicardial Ventricular Tachycardias Originating From the Coronary Sinus and Cardiac Veins

VT morphology has an RBBB pattern when it is originating from the proximal portion of the great cardiac vein. When the focus is in the distal great cardiac vein or anterior coronary vein, the VT has LBBB morphology with a broader (> 75 ms) R wave in V1 without the S wave as compared with the R wave of VTs originating from aortic cusps[2] (Figs. 11.25–11.27). VTs from the anterior coronary vein often have a characteristic precordial pattern break with abrupt loss of R waves in V2 with broad R waves in leads V3 through V6.

Epicardial Ventricular Tachycardias Originating From the Crux of the Heart

Epicardial idiopathic VTs arising from the crux of the heart in the pyramidal space adjacent to the posterior descending artery have a precordial transition at or before V2 in addition to a left superior axis and an maximum deflection index greater than 0.55. The inferior leads have deeply negative QS complexes with slurred intrinsicoid deflections. The QRS morphology is very similar to the pattern of maximal preexcitation seen with manifest posteroseptal pathways that share a similar ventricular insertion into the pyramidal space.

Right Ventricular Epicardial Ventricular Tachycardia

Anterior right ventricular epicardial sites have LBBB configuration with inferior axis and initial Q waves in lead I. There are QS complexes in lead V2 with precordial transition around V3.

Verapamil-Sensitive Idiopathic Fascicular Ventricular Tachycardia

Idiopathic ventricular fascicular VT results from reentry involving altered Purkinje fibers on the left ventricle. The VT is verapamil sensitive and adenosine insensitive. Because of the rapid access of the wavefront to the Purkinje system, the QRS duration is less than 140 ms and RS duration is 60 to 80 ms; therefore it can be mistaken for a supraventricular tachycardia. The VT rate is approximately 150 to 200 bpm and frequently exhibits cycle length alternans. There are three sites of the circuit:

1. **Left posterior fascicular VT:** This is the most common fascicular VT and involves a part of the left posterior fascicle with an exit at the inferoapical left ventricular septum. This displays an RBBB configuration, and the R/S ratio is less than 1 in leads V1 and V2. VTs arising more toward the middle, at the region of the posterior papillary muscle, have a left superior axis and RS in leads V5 and V6. Those arising closer to the apex have a right superior axis with a tiny r and deep S (or even QS) in leads V5 and V6. There may be loss of these late precordial R waves in cases with more apical exits (Figs. 11.28 and 11.29).
2. **Left anterior fascicular VT:** A minority of VTs are caused by reentry involving the left anterior fascicle. The VT has RBBB morphology with right axis deviation.
3. **Left upper septal fascicular VT:** This is a very rare VT that involves the proximal left bundle branch. It is remarkable for its narrow QRS complex with normal or rightward axis.

   Idiopathic VT arising from posteromedial and anterolateral papillary muscles can mimic left fascicular VT because of proximity to the left posterior and anterior fascicles, respectively.[7] However, there are few distinctions (Table 11.2).

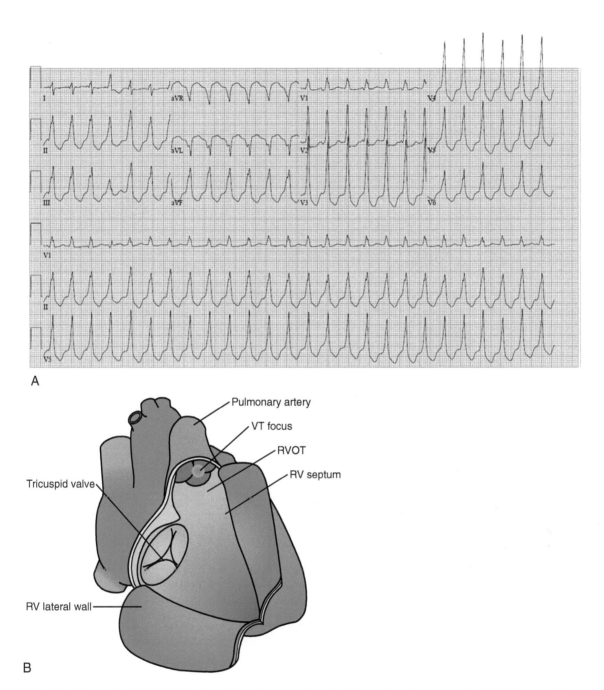

Fig. 11.10 Ventricular tachycardia (*VT*) originating from the pulmonary artery just above the pulmonary valve. (A) VT has positive concordance, suggestive of possible supravalvular origin. The QS pattern in lead aVL is equal to aVR in amplitude, which suggests midline origin of the focal VT. (B) During electrophysiology study, the VT was mapped to originate from the pulmonary artery just above the pulmonary valve and was successfully ablated. *RV*, Right ventricle; *RVOT*, right ventricular outflow tract.

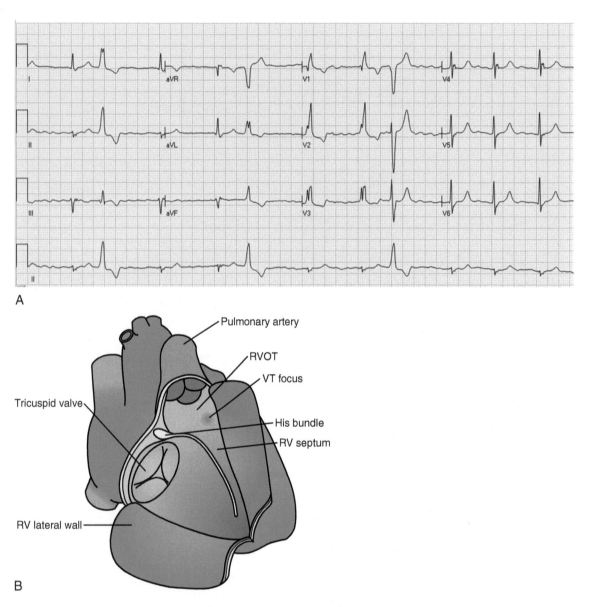

Fig. 11.11 Premature ventricular complex (PVC) originating from the ventricular septum near right ventricular outflow tract (*RVOT*). (A) PVC has left bundle branch block, inferior axis with narrow QRS complexes (QRS duration: 120 ms), and notched R waves in leads I and aVL. Inferior leads also have monophasic QRS complexes. (B) During electrophysiology study, the PVC was mapped originating from the ventricular septum near the RVOT and was successfully ablated. *RV*, Right ventricle; *VT*, ventricular tachycardia.

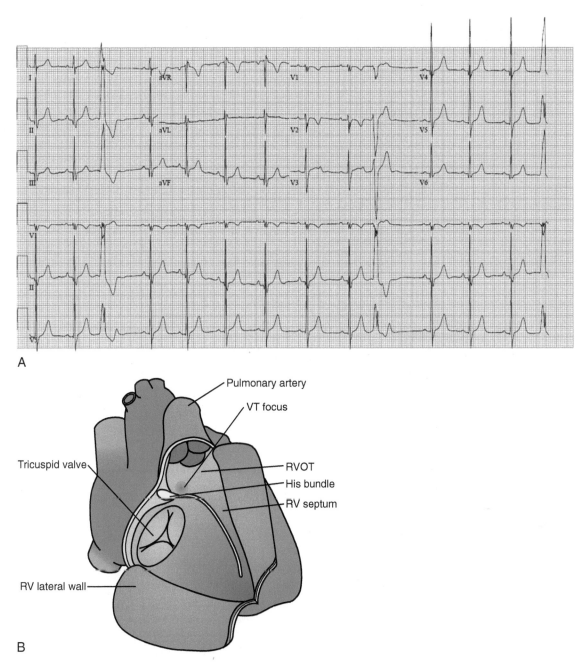

Fig. 11.12 Parahisian ventricular tachycardia (*VT*) and premature ventricular complexes (PVCs). (A) The PVC in a 9-year-old boy has left bundle branch block, inferior axis with narrow QRS complexes (QRS duration: 120 ms), and notched R waves in lead I. Inferior leads also have notched QRS complexes. (B) During electrophysiology study, the PVC was mapped to originate from the ventricular septum just above the proximal His bundle and was successfully ablated. *RV,* Right ventricle; *RVOT,* right ventricular outflow tract.

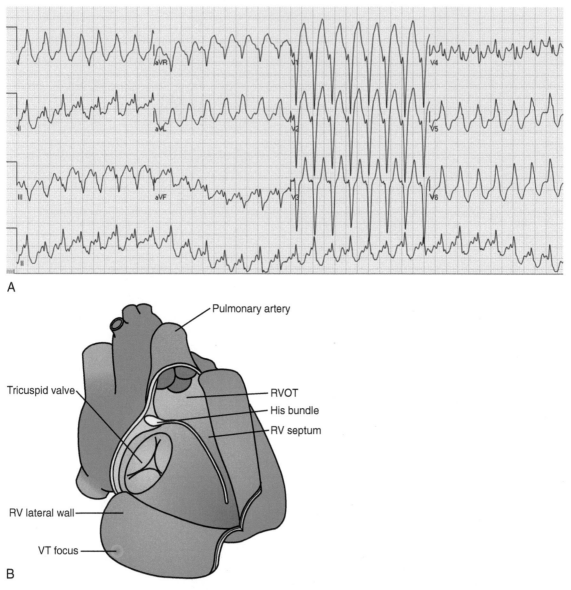

Fig. 11.13 Ventricular tachycardia (*VT*) originating from the right ventricle (*RV*) free wall. The VT has left bundle branch block, left superior axis. QRS complexes are prolonged and multiphasic in the inferior leads with a late precordial progression of R wave (A). Lead aVR is negative, whereas leads I and aVL are positive. (B) During electrophysiology study, the VT was mapped to originate from the right ventricular free wall and was successfully ablated. *RVOT*, Right ventricular outflow tract.

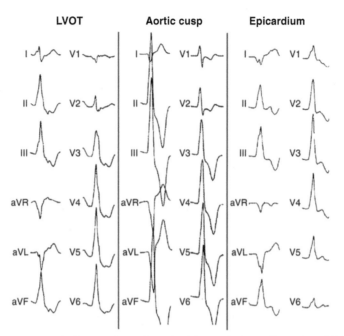

Fig. 11.14 Electrocardiograms of premature ventricular complexes from the left ventricular outflow tract (*LVOT*), aortic cusp, and epicardium. (Issa ZF, Miller JM, Zipes DP, eds. *Clinical Arrhythmology and Electrophysiology*. Philadelphia, PA: Elsevier; 2019, Chapter 23).

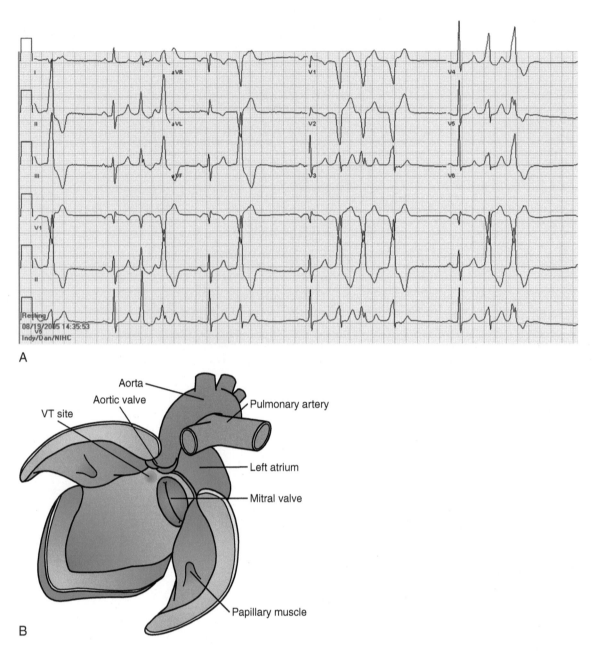

Fig. 11.15 Left septal left ventricular outflow tract (LVOT) ventricular tachycardia (*VT*) in a patient with tachycardia-induced cardiomyopathy. VT has left bundle branch block morphology, and unlike most of the septal LVOT VTs, the precordial transition of R wave is in lead V3. Negative deflection in lead I suggests LVOT rather than right ventricular outflow tract origin of the VT (A). During electrophysiology study, the VT was mapped to originate from the ventricular septum near the LVOT (B) and was successfully ablated.

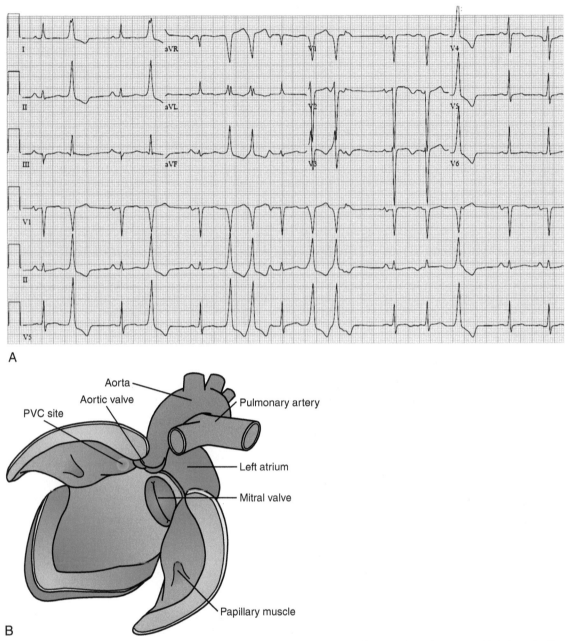

Fig. 11.16 Left ventricular outflow tract free wall premature ventricular complexes has left bundle branch block and inferior axis. The precordial R wave transition is in lead V3 with an R wave in lead V2 onward (A). During electrophysiology study, the premature ventricular complexes were mapped to originate from the lateral left ventricular outflow tract (B) and were successfully ablated.

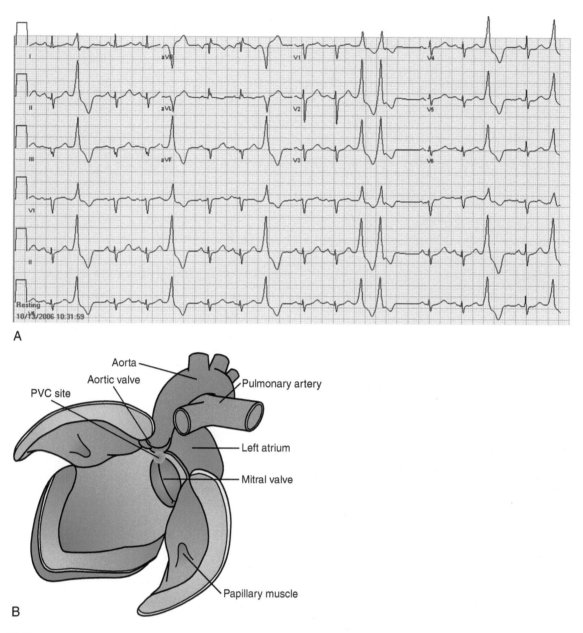

Fig. 11.17 (A) The premature ventricular complexes have has right bundle branch block morphology with precordial transition in lead V1 with monophasic R waves from lead V1 to V6. (B) During electrophysiology study, the premature ventricular complexes were mapped originating from the aortomitral continuity and was successfully ablated.

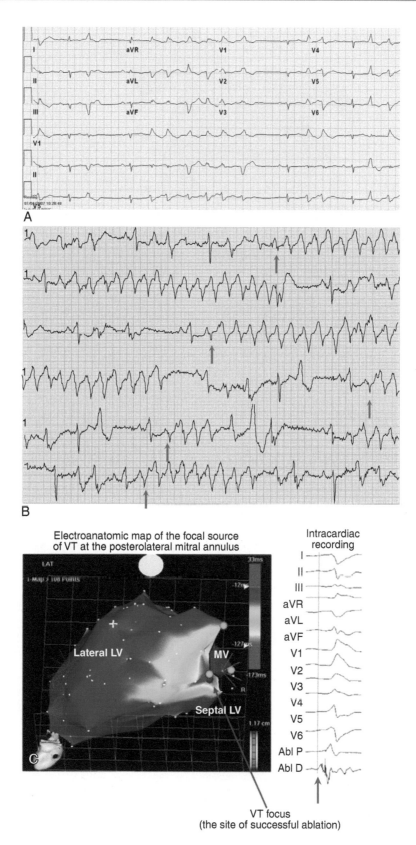

Fig. 11.18 Idiopathic ventricular tachycardia (*VT*) originating from the posterolateral mitral annulus. (A) The electrocardiogram comes from a morbidly obese (400 lb) patient with structurally normal heart who presented with recurrent syncope. It shows frequent predominantly monomorphic premature ventricular complexes (PVCs) with a right bundle branch block morphology and nonsustained VT. (B) Holter recording revealed numerous runs of rapid nonsustained VT initiated by single monomorphic PVC (*arrows*). The PVC initiating the VT was mapped to the posteroseptal mitral annulus (C and D). The electroanatomic activation mapping (C) shows centrifugal activation from the focal site of origin (red being the site of origin in the left ventricle, and yellow, green, dark blue, and purple zones represent farther sites in chronological order). Intracardiac mapping shows the site of origin 30 ms earlier than surface QRS complexes (*arrow*). Catheter ablation of the focus eliminated the arrhythmia. *LV*, Left ventricle; *MV*, mitral valve.

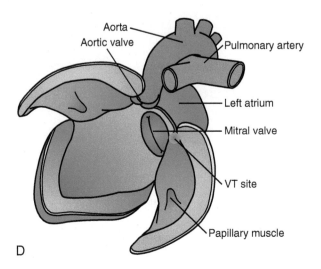

D

Fig. 11.18 (Continued).

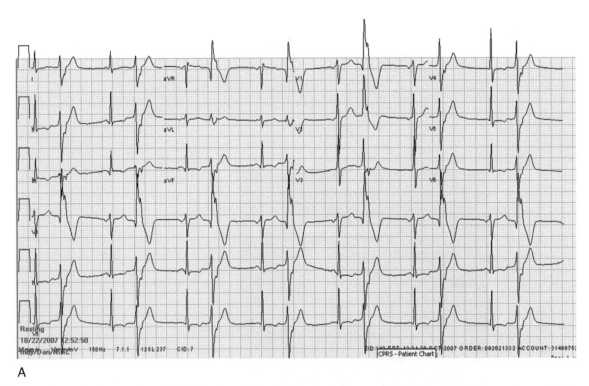

A

Fig. 11.19 Premature ventricular complexes originating from the anterolateral papillary muscle. (A) Electrocardiogram shows right bundle branch block, right superior axis morphology of the premature ventricular complex. The electroanatomic mapping with intracardiac ultrasound (B) reveals the site of successful catheter ablation at the anterolateral papillary muscle (C and D). *LV*, Left ventricle.

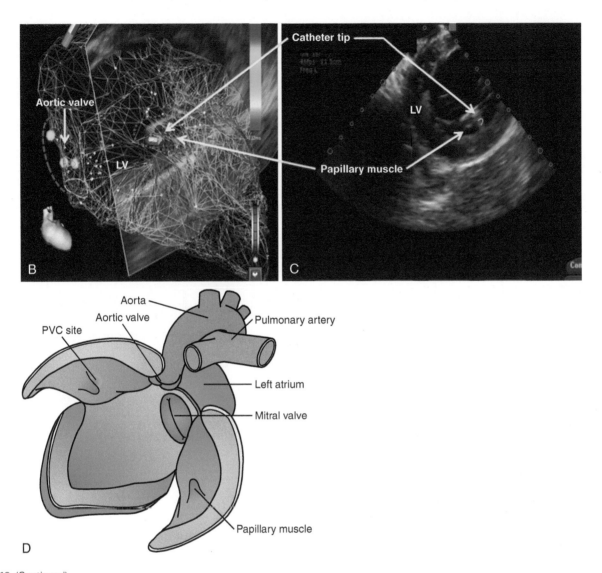

Fig. 11.19 (Continued).

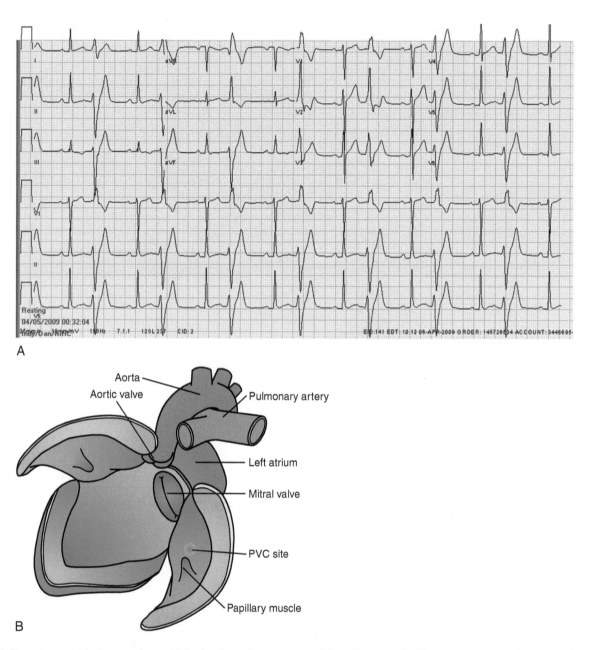

Fig. 11.20 Premature ventricular complexes originating from the posteromedial papillary muscle. The premature ventricular complex has right bundle branch block, left superior morphology (A), which was mapped at the body of the posteromedial papillary muscle (B).

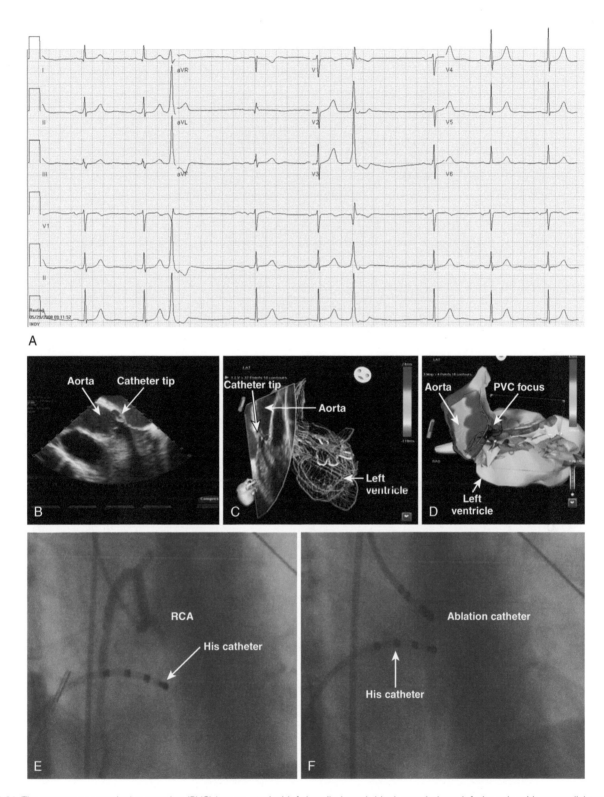

Fig. 11.21 The premature ventricular complex (PVC) has an atypical left bundle branch block morphology, inferior axis with precordial transition in lead V2 (A). PVC was mapped at the right coronary cusp. The electroanatomic mapping with intracardiac ultrasound and fluoroscopic guidance demonstrates the mapping catheter tip at the right coronary cusp (B–D). The intracardiac echocardiography shows the tip of the mapping/ablation catheter in aortic root in (B). In figure (C) the green network shows the left ventricular anatomy during endocardial mapping. The concomitant two-dimensional intracardiac echocardiography shows aortic root with the catheter tip at the site of origin of PVC, where it was successfully ablated. (D) The figure shows the activation mapping with earliest activation at the aortic root (*red*) with yellow, green, and blue being progressively late sites. The right coronary artery (*RCA*) angiography shows that the PVC focus is at least 8 mm away from the origin of the RCA (E and F).

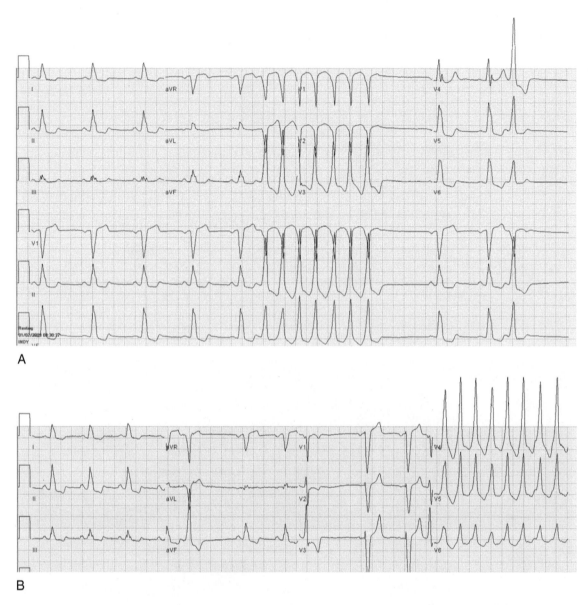

Fig. 11.22 Ventricular tachycardia (VT) originating from the right coronary cusp. The VT has left bundle branch block inferior axis (A and B). However, unlike the electrocardiogram of the patient in Fig. 11.21 with right coronary cusp VT, the precordial transition is later (lead V3). The precordial transition is similar to the right ventricular outflow tract (RVOT) VT. Up to one-fourth of aortic cusp VTs may have preferential conduction toward RVOT, and the electrocardiogram pattern may mimic that of an RVOT VT, with 20% of them having a late precordial transition (V3/V4). The VT was mapped at the right coronary cusp.

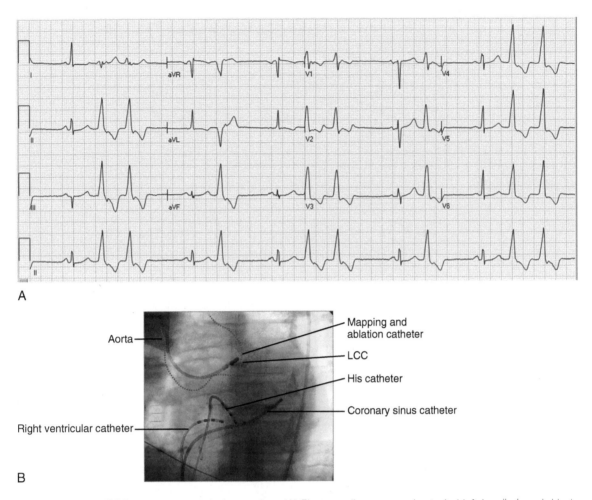

Fig. 11.23 Left coronary cusp (*LCC*) premature ventricular couplets. (A) Electrocardiogram reveals atypical left bundle branch block morphology, inferior axis premature ventricular complex (PVC) with early transition of R wave in the precordial lead (V1). Lead I has an rS pattern, and lead V1 has "M" pattern seen commonly in LCC ventricular tachycardia. (B) Fluoroscopic image (*left anterior oblique view*) depicts the mapping catheter placed at the earliest site of activation of the PVC at the base of LCC in the aortic sinus of Valsalva. During electrophysiology study, PVCs were mapped at the LCC of the aorta.

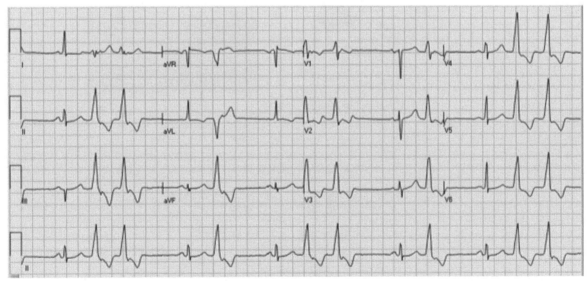

Fig. 11.24 Idiopathic premature ventricular complexes (PVCs) and ventricular couplets originating between right and left coronary cusp. Electrocardiogram shows atypical right bundle branch block morphology of the PVC with early transition in the precordial leads. During electrophysiology study, the PVC focus was mapped at the left coronary cusp of the aorta.

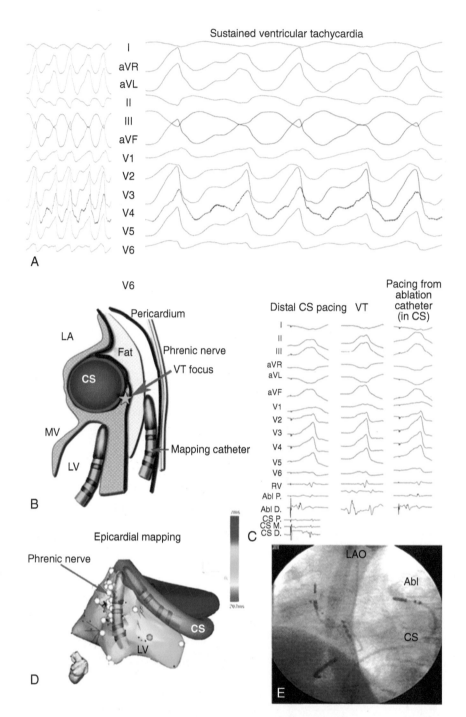

Fig. 11.25 Ventricular tachycardia (*VT*) originating from the great cardiac vein. Electrocardiogram shows a wide right bundle branch block, right inferior axis VT with a long intrinsicoid deflection (A). VT was initially mapped epicardially, where the mapping catheter tip is positioned at the site of VT focus that is adjacent to the phrenic nerve (B). The pacemap from the coronary sinus (*CS*) is identical with the VT. Catheter ablation could not be performed via the epicardial approach because of the presence of the adjacent left phrenic nerve, which was determined by stimulation during pacing from the site of earliest activation of the VT (C). Subsequently, the catheter ablation was performed successfully via the CS from where the intracardiac electrogram was recorded earliest during the activation mapping. The pacemapping from this site resulted in QRS complexes identical to VT complexes (D), which is shown in the fluoroscopic image in the left anterior oblique (*LAO*) view (E). The ablation catheter is placed in the coronary sinus adjacent to the site of origin of the VT. *Abl,* Ablation catheter; *D,* distal; *LA,* left atrium; *LV,* left ventricle; *M,* middle; *MV,* mitral valve; *P,* proximal; *RV,* right ventricle.

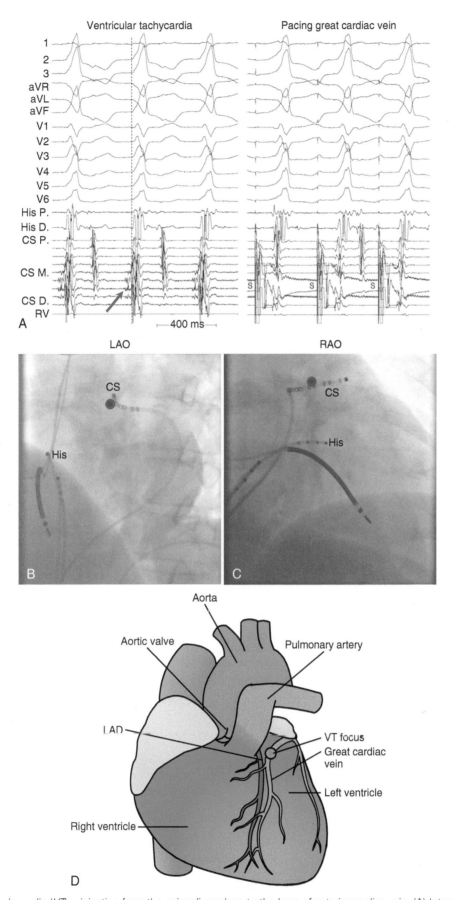

Fig. 11.26 Ventricular tachycardia (*VT*) originating from the epicardium close to the base of anterior cardiac vein. (A) Intracardiac recordings during the VT show earliest site of activation in the coronary sinus (*CS*) (distal) recordings (*red arrow*). CS recordings are from a decapolar catheter placed in the CS with its distal poles in the basal part of anterior branch of the great cardiac vein. Pacing from the same site demonstrated a perfect pacemap of QRS complexes in all leads (12/12). (B and C) The fluoroscopy images show the site of epicardial origin of VT (*red dot*) at the anterior cardiac vein (D). *D*, Distal; *His*, His bundle; *LAD*, left anterior descending artery; *LAO*, left anterior oblique view; *M*, middle; *P*, proximal; *RAO*, right anterior oblique view; *RV*, right ventricle; *S*, stimulation from one of the distal poles of the CS catheter.

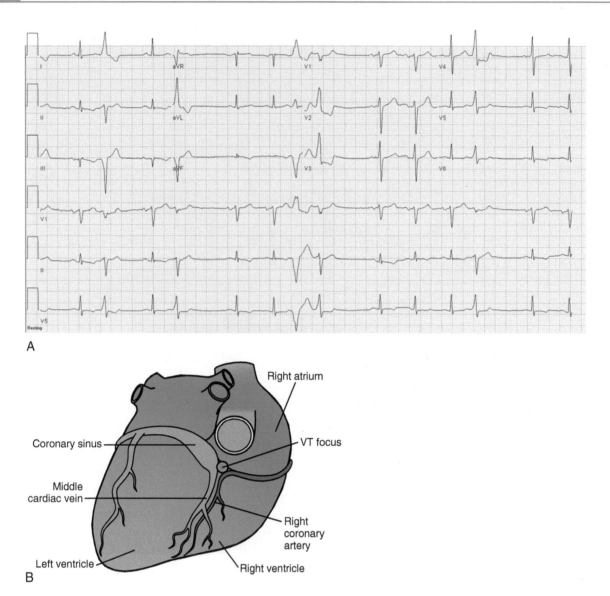

Fig. 11.27 Premature ventricular complex originating from the crux (inferoposterior basal epicardial surface) of the heart. (A) Electrocardiogram shows left bundle branch block pattern with R wave transition in lead V1 and slurred QS pattern in leads III and aVF. (B) The premature ventricular complex focus was mapped at the crux of the heart. *VT*, Ventricular tachycardia.

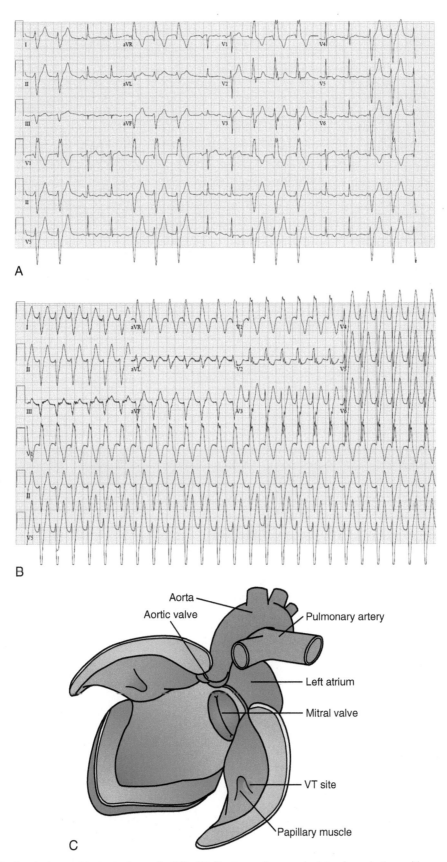

Fig. 11.28 Left ventricular fascicular ventricular tachycardia (*VT*). (A) Electrocardiogram depicts sinus rhythm with nonsustained VT (NSVT). The initial complex of three-beat runs of NSVT is a fusion complex. The QRS morphology (QRS duration: 140 ms) of NSVT and sustained VT (B) is right bundle branch block and right superior axis consistent with VT initiated from the posteromedial or midinferior left ventricular septum (C).

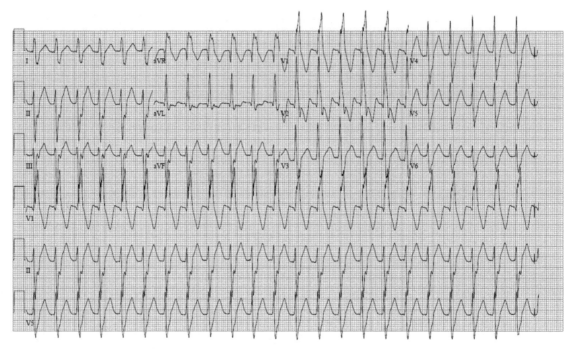

Fig. 11.29 Left ventricular fascicular ventricular tachycardia in another patient has right bundle branch block pattern with right superior axis. Ventricular tachycardia focus was mapped at the left ventricular inferior midseptum.

TABLE 11.2   **Distinctions Between Left Fascicular Ventricular Tachycardia and Papillary Muscle Ventricular Tachycardia[7]**

	LEFT FASCICULAR VT	PAPILLARY MUSCLE VT
Mechanism	Reentry	Focal
QRS duration	127 ± 11 ms	150 ± 15 ms
Lead V1	rsR′ pattern in all VTs	Monophasic R or qR
Q wave	Inferior leads (posterior VT) I, aVL (anterior VT)	None
Adenosine sensitivity	−	+
Verapamil sensitivity	+	+

VT, ventricular tachycardia.

REFERENCES

1. Killu AM, Stevenson WG. Ventricular tachycardia in the absence of structural heart disease. *Heart.* 2019;105:645−656.
2. Noda T, Shimizu W, Taguchi A, et al. Malignant entity of idiopathic ventricular fibrillation and polymorphic ventricular tachycardia initiated by premature extrasystoles originating from the right ventricular outflow tract. *J Am Coll Cardiol.* 2005;46:1288−1294.
3. Baman TS, Ilg KJ, Gupta SK, et al. Mapping and ablation of epicardial idiopathic ventricular arrhythmias from within the coronary venous system. *Circ Arrhythm Electrophysiol.* 2010;3:274−279.
4. Della Rocca DG, Gianni C, Mohanty S, Trivedi C, Di Biase L, Natale A. Localization of ventricular arrhythmias for catheter ablation: the role of surface electrocardiogram. *Card Electrophysiol Clin.* 2018;10:333−354.
5. Valles E, Bazan V, Marchlinski FE. ECG criteria to identify epicardial ventricular tachycardia in nonischemic cardiomyopathy. *Circ Arrhythm Electrophysiol.* 2010;3:63−71.
6. Daniels DV, Lu YY, Morton JB, et al. Idiopathic epicardial left ventricular tachycardia originating remote from the sinus of Valsalva: electrophysiological characteristics, catheter ablation, and identification from the 12-lead electrocardiogram. *Circulation.* 2006;113:1659−1666.
7. Good E, Desjardins B, Jongnarangsin K, et al. Ventricular arrhythmias originating from a papillary muscle in patients without prior infarction: a comparison with fascicular arrhythmias. *Heart Rhythm.* 2008;5:1530−1537.

Ventricular Tachycardia in Structural Heart Disease

Ventricular arrhythmias include single premature ventricular complexes (PVCs), ventricular couplets, nonsustained ventricular tachycardia (VT), sustained VT, ventricular flutter, and ventricular fibrillation (VF) (Table 12.1).

HISTORY, PHYSICAL EXAMINATION, AND BASELINE ECG

History (e.g., history of coronary artery disease [CAD] or cardiomyopathy, heart failure, cardiac surgery, cardiomegaly) and physical examination in patients presenting with sustained ventricular arrhythmias can be useful to establish the presence of structural heart disease. A baseline electrocardiogram (ECG) can help determine the underlying etiology by providing clues regarding the presence and type of structural heart disease, showing abnormal Q waves, fragmented QRS complexes (defined as the presence of two or more notches in the R wave or S wave without any bundle branch block [BBB]) in two contiguous leads. Fragmented wide QRS is defined as QRS duration greater than 120 ms with 2 or more notches in the R wave or the S wave in two contiguous leads, intraventricular conduction delay, and poor progression of R waves in the precordial leads. VTs arising from a normal myocardium typically have rapid initial forces, whereas VTs in structural heart disease have slurring of the initial forces. Slurring of initial forces is also encountered in epicardial VTs in structurally normal and abnormal hearts. VTs in structural heart disease have relatively lower amplitude and often have notching in the QRS complexes. The majority of VTs arise subendocardially but can arise epicardially (especially in nonischemic cardiomyopathy [NICM] and idiopathic VT) or in the mid myocardium. Mechanisms include reentry, triggered activity, and abnormal automaticity (Table 12.2).

SUSTAINED MONOMORPHIC VENTRICULAR TACHYCARDIA IN CORONARY ARTERY DISEASE

When ventricular tachyarrhythmias occur during acute myocardial infarction (MI), it is usually polymorphic VT or VF. Monomorphic VT typically occurs several years after MI and is mostly related to myocardial scar in the left ventricle (LV) (Fig. 12.1). It rarely arises from the right ventricle (RV). QRS duration is greater when the VT circuit is in the lateral LV rather than the septal LV. However, QRS duration also depends on the extent of myocardial scar and transmyocardial conduction delay and the presence of antiarrhythmic drug therapy that slows intramyocardial conduction. Q waves in the baseline ECG, BBB pattern, QRS axis, presence of QS complexes, precordial concordance (when all QRS complexes completely upright [positive] or completely downward [negative] in the precordial leads), and QRS duration during VT provide clues to the site of the VT circuit (Table 12.3). In general, QRS patterns are less accurate in

localizing the site of origin of post-MI reentrant VTs than they are for focal VTs in patients with normal hearts.[1] VT in patients with structural heart disease is mostly due to a reentrant mechanism. The VT wavefront passes slowly by way of the narrow corridor (isthmus) in the region of the myocardial scar and exits into the relatively healthy myocardium to depolarize the rest of the ventricle, giving rise to QRS waves.[2] The propagation of impulses from the site of origin to the remainder of the ventricle produces the sum of depolarizing vectors responsible for a particular QRS morphology during VT. QRS morphology during VT depends on several factors, including the location of the site of origin of the QRS, myocardial scar surrounding it, cardiac orientation (vertical heart vs. horizontal heart, or clockwise vs. counterclockwise rotation of the heart), and shape of the chest. Nevertheless, the ECG is capable of regionalizing the VT to areas smaller than 15 to 20 cm.

Therefore algorithms developed for recognizing the site of origin of VT in CAD have a predictive accuracy of 70% only. These algorithms use BBB morphology, QRS polarity, QRS axis, and eight different patterns of R wave progression in the precordium in addition to relationship with prior anterior or inferior MI (Figs. 12.2—12.4).

BASELINE ECG

Q waves, fragmented QRS, and persistent ST segment elevation (representing a ventricular aneurysm) in contiguous leads represent myocardial scar in the corresponding myocardial wall. Such findings provide valuable information regarding the site of VT (Fig. 12.5).

BUNDLE BRANCH BLOCK—LIKE PATTERN

In CAD, VTs with left bundle branch block (LBBB) patterns almost always arise from or close to the LV septum and rarely arise from the RV. Therefore the ECG has a high predictive accuracy for LBBB pattern VT. Right bundle branch block (RBBB) patterns virtually always arise in the LV, and the VT circuit can be present anywhere from the LV septum to the LV lateral wall and LV apex to the LV base. RBBB pattern VTs associated with inferior MIs are clustered in a small inferoposterior area of the LV region, whereas VTs associated with an anterior MI can arise from a wide area because of the relatively larger area (anterolateral) of myocardial scar. The ECG with an RBBB pattern VT does not have a good predictive accuracy.

QRS AXIS

QRS axis depends mainly on the exit site of the VT circuit. It also depends on the extent and site of myocardial scar through which the impulse travels after it leaves the exit site of the protected corridor of slow conduction. Therefore the axis may be misleading in the presence of large myocardial scarring found in patients with a large anterior wall scar (LBBB or RBBB pattern with a right or left superior axis).

TABLE 12.1   Classification of Ventricular Arrhythmia

Arrhythmia	Electrocardiogram Features	Comments
Premature ventricular complexes	Spontaneous ventricular depolarization independent of supraventricular impulse.	Usually benign but can cause tachycardia-induced cardiomyopathy and heart failure or precipitate VT/VF.
Nonsustained VT	≥3 Consecutive ventricular depolarizations at rate >100 bpm and <30 sec.	
Sustained VT	Repetitive ventricular depolarizations at rate >100 bpm for >30 sec or requiring termination <30 sec owing to hemodynamic instability.	
Monomorphic VT	Single stable QRS morphology from beat to beat. CL variation and QRS alternans can occur. Heart rate can be <100 bpm in the presence of antiarrhythmic drug therapy.	LBBB-like pattern has a predominantly negative QRS polarity in V1 (QS, rS, qrS). RBBB-like pattern has a predominantly positive QRS polarity in V1 (rs-R′, qR, R-R , R, R-S).
Polymorphic VT	Continuously changing or multiform QRS morphology (without a constant QRS morphology for >5 complexes). No clear isoelectric baseline between QRS complexes at rate >100 bpm or QRS complexes that have different morphologies in multiple simultaneously recorded leads.	Indicates a variable sequence of ventricular activation and/or no single site of origin.
Torsades de pointes	Polymorphic VT associated with a long QT interval. Twisting of the peaks of the QRS complexes around the isoelectric line.	Mostly drug-induced and in congenital long QT syndrome.
Bidirectional VT	A beat-to-beat alternation of the QRS frontal plane axis.	Associated with catecholaminergic VT and digitalis toxicity.
Ventricular flutter	Regular, rapid (300 bpm with a CL variability usually <30 ms) monomorphic ventricular arrhythmia without any isoelectric interval between successive QRS complexes.	Differentiation between a very rapid VT and ventricular flutter usually just of academic interest. Similarly, differentiation between rapid ventricular flutter and VF of academic interest only.
VF	A rapid (usually ≥300 bpm), grossly irregular ventricular rhythm with marked variability in QRS CL, morphology, and amplitude.	

CL, Cycle length; *LBBB*, left bundle branch block; *RBBB*, right bundle branch block; *VF*, ventricular fibrillation; *VT*, ventricular tachycardia.

TABLE 12.2   Ventricular Tachycardia in Structural Heart Disease

	Scar-Related VT	Focal VT	Bundle Branch Reentry VT	Endocardial	Epicardial
CAD	+	+	+	+	+
Nonischemic dilated CM	+	+	+	+	+
ARVC	+			+	+
Sarcoidosis	+				
Hypertrophic and restrictive CM	+				
Amyloidosis	+				
Valvular heart disease	+		+		
Congenital heart disease	+		+		

ARVC, Arrhythmogenic right ventricular cardiomyopathy; *CAD*, coronary artery disease; *CM*, cardiomyopathy; *VT*, ventricular tachycardia.

QRS CONCORDANCE

A positive concordance in the precordial leads (i.e., all QRS complexes positive) represents VT arising from basal LV (basal septum, mitral annulus, aortic annulus) or RV outflow region, whereas negative concordance (all QRS complexes negative in precordial leads) represents VT circuit at or near LV apex.

QS COMPLEXES DURING VENTRICULAR TACHYCARDIA

The presence of QS complexes in any ECG lead represents a wavefront propagating away from the myocardial site represented by that particular ECG lead. Therefore QS complexes in the inferior ECG leads suggest that the activation is originating in and moving away from the

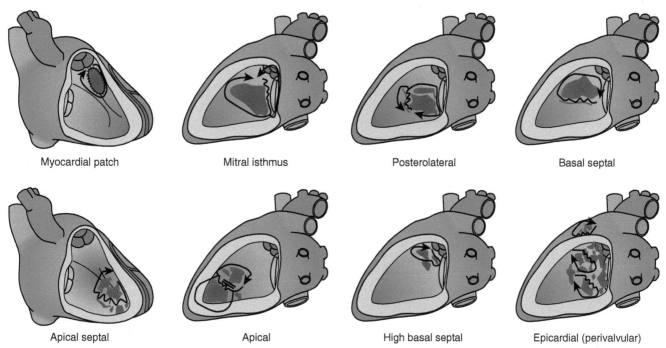

Myocardial patch   Mitral isthmus   Posterolateral   Basal septal

Apical septal   Apical   High basal septal   Epicardial (perivalvular)

Fig. 12.1 Different types and sites of ventricular tachycardia (VT) circuits in structural heart disease. VT can occur around the myocardial patch in patients with ventricular septal defect repair. Similarly, reentrant VTs can be seen around myocardial infarction scars, mostly in the left ventricle. Multiple epicardial or midmyocardial scars are present mainly around the cardiac valves in patients with nonischemic cardiomyopathy. Dark red color indicates myocardial scar.

TABLE 12.3 Electrocardiogram Morphology and the Site of Ventricular Tachycardia

Major ECG Pattern	QRS Axis QRS Morphology	Site of VT Circuit In LV	Comments
Baseline ECG Q wave, fragmented QRS, ST segment elevation	Inferior leads (II, III, aVF)	Inferior	
	Anterior/anterolateral leads (V1-V5)	Anterior	
	Lateral leads (I, aVL, V6)	Lateral	
Bundle branch block pattern	LBBB	Septum, rarely RV	
	RBBB	Anywhere in LV	Anywhere from apex or base or septum to lateral wall
QRS axis	Right inferior	Basal	VT can arise anywhere from septum to lateral wall
	Left inferior	Basal septum	Usually associated with inferoposterior MI
	Right superior	Apex	VT can arise anywhere from septum to lateral wall QS in inferior leads and QS or rS in leads V5 and V6
Precordial concordance	Positive	Basal	VT circuit can be located anywhere close to basal septum, in LVOT or RVOT, or around mitral annulus
	Negative	Apex	Mostly in anteroseptal MI
QS complexes	V2-V4	Anterior	
	V3-V5	Apical	
	Inferior leads	Inferior	
Q wave	With RBBB pattern in leads I, V1, V2, V6	Apex	Q waves are absent from VTs arising from inferobasal LV
	With LBBB pattern leads I and V6	Apical septal	

(Continued)

TABLE 12.3 Electrocardiogram Morphology and the Site of Ventricular Tachycardia—cont'd

Major ECG Pattern	QRS Axis QRS Morphology	Site of VT Circuit In LV	Comments
R wave	With RBBB or LBBB pattern in I, V1, V2, V6	Posterior	
	With LBBB pattern in leads I and V6	Inferobasal	
Anterior MI with LBBB	Left superior axis QS V1-V6 (negative concordance), Q in lead I and aVL	Anteroapical septum Anteroseptal	
	R wave in lead V1 and Q wave in lead aVL	Posterior septum (closure to middle third)	
	Right inferior axis arise close to the ventricular septum but occasionally can be off the septum	Upper half of the mid or apical septum	Occasionally may be away from the septum in LV
Anterior MI with RBBB	Right superior axis, qR, or monophasic R wave in lead V1, QS, or QR complex in leads V2, V3, and/or V4	LV apex	
	QS complex in leads I, II, and III; there is also a QS complex across the precordium from leads V2 through V6	LV apex	
Anterior MI with RBBB	Right inferior axis, negative deflection aVR and aVL	LV septum	VTs with LBBB or RBBB patterns and a marked inferior right axis arise superiorly on what usually is the edge of an anterior aneurysm
	Right superior axis, QS complexes in the lateral leads (V4-V6)	LV apex anywhere from septum to lateral wall	This pattern is less specific in localizing the VT site
	Right superior axis, the R wave in lead aVR >R wave in aVL	Distal posterolateral LV	Usually associated with large LV aneurysm
Anterior MI with LBBB or RBBB	Inferior axis	Base (superior part) of the LV aneurysm	
Posterolateral MI with RBBB	Right inferior axis, prominent R wave in leads V1-V4	Lateral or posterolateral LV	Left circumflex artery territory
Inferior MI with RBBB	Positive concordance in precordial leads (R waves V1-V6)	Posterior LV near base	When the VT originates near the posterior basal septum and when it arises more laterally (or posteriorly), there can be a decrease in the R wave amplitude across the precordium because the infarct can extend to the posterolateral areas
Inferior MI with LBBB	Left axis deviation	Inferobasal septum	The more the VT moves from the midline toward the lateral (i.e., posterior) wall, the more right or superior the axis will become
Inferoposterior MI with LBBB	rS in lead V1, R in V6, and left superior axis	Mitral isthmus (between the mitral annulus and inferior infarct scar)	This critical zone of slow conduction is activated parallel to the mitral annulus in either direction, resulting in two distinct bundle branch block morphologies
Inferoposterior MI with RBBB	R in lead V1, QS in lead V6, and right superior axis		

(Continued)

TABLE 12.3 Electrocardiogram Morphology and the Site of Ventricular Tachycardia—cont'd

Major ECG Pattern	QRS Axis QRS Morphology	Site of VT Circuit In LV	Comments
VT from peri-aortomitral continuity	RBBB, transition in lead VT, R wave V2-V6, mean QRS:165 ± 47 ms	Fibrous area between left coronary cusp and anterior mitral leaflet	Can occur in CAD (48%), NICM (33%), and valvular cardiomyopathy (19%)
Epicardial VT with RBBB	Pseudo delta wave (the earliest ventricular activation to the earliest fast deflection in any precordial lead) of ≥ 34 ms	Anywhere in epicardial LV	Sensitivity 83%, specificity 95%
	Intrinsicoid deflection time in V2 (earliest ventricular activation to the peak of the R wave in V2) of >85 ms		Sensitivity 87%, specificity 90%
	Shortest RS complex duration (the earliest ventricular activation to the nadir of the first S wave in any precordial lead) ≥ 121 ms QRS duration >200 ms		Sensitivity 76%, specificity 85%

CAD, Coronary artery disease; *ECG*, electrocardiogram, *LBBB*, left bundle branch block; *LV*, left ventricle; *LVOT*, left ventricular outflow tract; *MI*, myocardial infarction; *NICM*, nonischemic cardiomyopathy; *RBBB*, right bundle branch block; *RV*, right ventricle; *RVOT*, right ventricular outflow tract; *VT*, ventricular tachycardia.

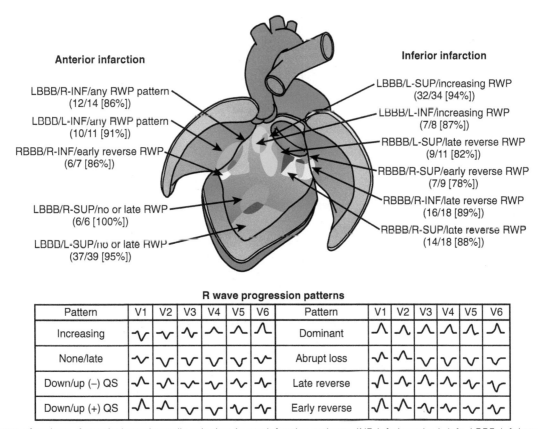

Anterior infarction
LBBB/R-INF/any RWP pattern (12/14 [86%])
LBBB/L-INF/any RWP pattern (10/11 [91%])
RBBB/R-INF/early reverse RWP (6/7 [86%])
LBBB/R-SUP/no or late RWP (6/6 [100%])
LBBB/L-SUP/no or late RWP (37/39 [95%])

Inferior infarction
LBBB/L-SUP/increasing RWP (32/34 [94%])
LBBB/L-INF/increasing RWP (7/8 [87%])
RBBB/L-SUP/late reverse RWP (9/11 [82%])
RBBB/R-SUP/early reverse RWP (7/9 [78%])
RBBB/R-INF/late reverse RWP (16/18 [89%])
RBBB/R-SUP/late reverse RWP (14/18 [88%])

R wave progression patterns

Pattern	V1	V2	V3	V4	V5	V6	Pattern	V1	V2	V3	V4	V5	V6
Increasing							Dominant						
None/late							Abrupt loss						
Down/up (−) QS							Late reverse						
Down/up (+) QS							Early reverse						

Fig. 12.2 Scheme of regions of ventricular tachycardia exit sites in postinfarction patients. *INF*, Inferior axis; *L*, left; *LBBB*, left bundle branch block pattern; *R*, right; *RBBB*, right bundle branch block pattern; *RWP*, precordial R wave progression pattern (diagrammed in table at bottom); *SUP*, superior axis.

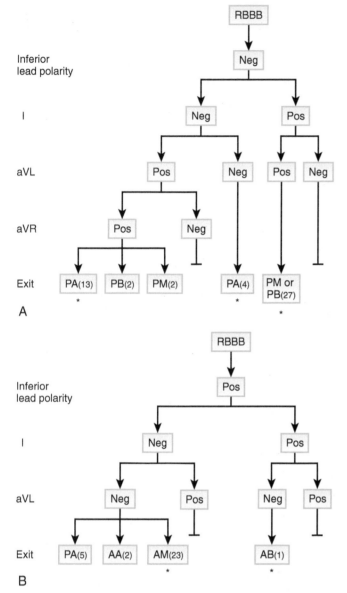

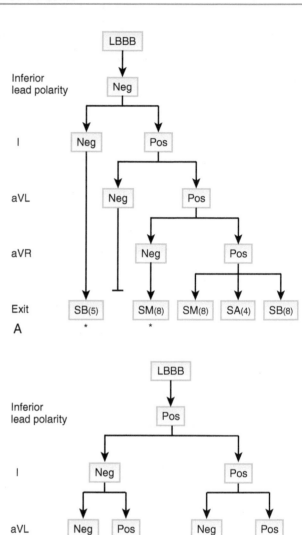

Fig. 12.3 Algorithm correlating 12-lead electrocardiogram (ECG) morphology of right bundle branch block (*RBBB*) ventricular tachycardia (VT) with exit site region, derived from retrospective analysis. (A) VT with negative (*Neg*) polarity in the inferior leads. (B) VT with positive (*Pos*) polarity in the inferior leads. A vertical line ending a horizontal bar indicates that no VT with this ECG pattern was identified. Exit sites with positive predictive value equal to or greater than 70% are marked by *asterisks*. The numbers of VTs for each ECG pattern and exit site region identified in retrospective analysis are shown in brackets. *AA,* Anteroapical; *AB,* anterobasal; *AM,* midanterior; *PA,* posteroapical; *PB,* posterobasal; *PM,* midposterior. (From Segal OR, Chow AW, Wong T, et al. A novel algorithm for determining endocardial VT exit site from 12-lead surface ECG characteristics in human, infarct-related ventricular tachycardia. *J Cardiovasc Electrophysiol.* 2007;18:161.)

Fig. 12.4 Algorithm correlating 12-lead electrocardiogram (ECG) morphology of left bundle branch block (*LBBB*) ventricular tachycardia (VT) with exit site in the heart, derived from retrospective analysis. (A) VT with negative (*Neg*) polarity in the inferior leads. (B) VT with positive (*Pos*) polarity in the inferior leads. A vertical line ending with a horizontal bar indicates that no VT with this ECG pattern was identified. Exit sites with positive predictive value equal to or greater than 70% are marked by *asterisks*. Numbers of VT for each ECG pattern and exit site region identified in retrospective analysis are shown in brackets. *SA,* Anteroseptal; *SB,* basal septum; *SM,* midseptum. (From Segal OR, Chow AW, Wong T, et al. A novel algorithm for determining endocardial VT exit site from 12-lead surface ECG characteristics in human, infarct-related ventricular tachycardia. *J Cardiovasc Electrophysiol.* 2007;18:161.)

inferior wall, whereas QS complexes in the precordial leads suggest activation originating in and moving away from the anterior wall; QS complexes in leads V2 to V4 suggest anterior wall origin, QS complexes in leads V3 to V5 suggest apical location, and QS complexes in leads V5 to V6 suggest lateral wall location. The presence of Q waves in leads I, V1, V2, and V6 are seen in VTs with RBBB pattern originating near the apex but not in those originating in the inferobasal parts of the LV.

R waves in leads I, V1, V2, and V6 are specific for VTs with RBBB or LBBB pattern of posterior origin. Additionally, the presence of Q waves in leads I and V6 in VTs with an LBBB pattern is seen with an apical septal location, whereas the presence of R waves in leads I and V6 are

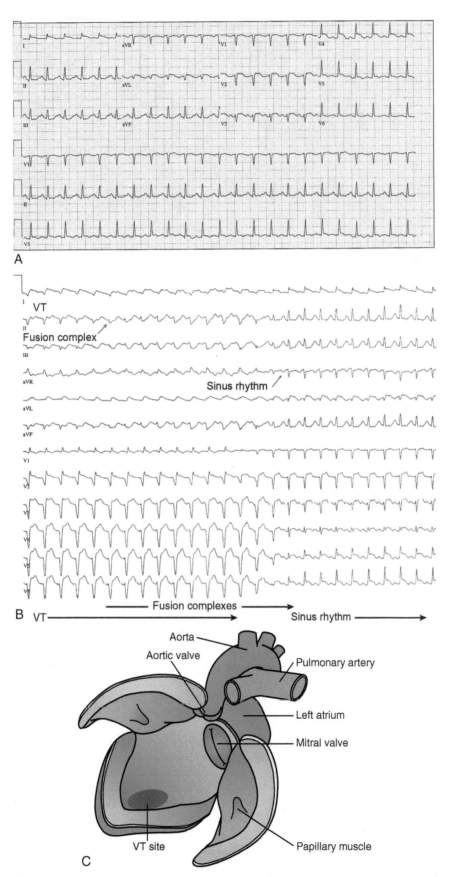

Fig. 12.5 Ventricular tachycardia (*VT*) in the setting of acute anterolateral myocardial infarction. (A) Sinus rhythm with ST segment elevation in anterolateral leads. (B) VT with right bundle branch block and right superior axis with QS pattern in precordial leads is suggestive of VT arising from the inferoapical area. The VT terminates spontaneously. There are fusion complexes (sixth beat onward) followed by sinus tachycardia. The initiation the fusion complexes (there are subtle changes in QRS complexes such as initial r wave in lead II, which was not present during VT) are marked with *red arrow* and initiation of pure sinus complexes are marked with *blue arrow*. (C) VT circuit was mapped at the inferoapical area of the left ventricle.

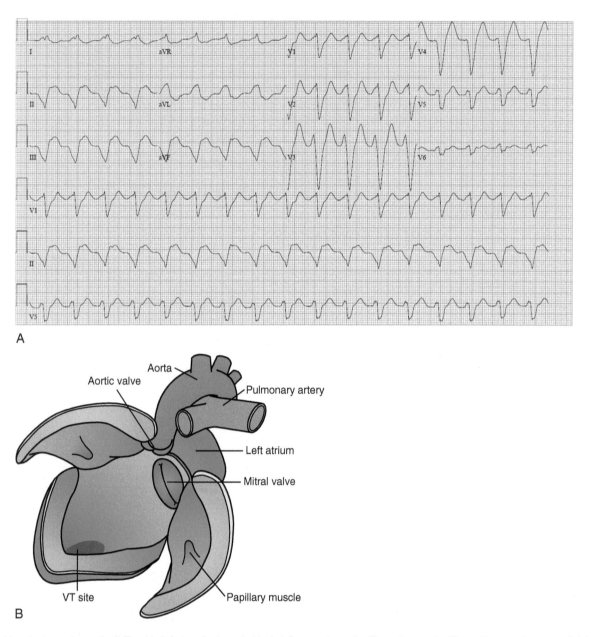

Fig. 12.6 Ventricular tachycardia (*VT*) with left bundle branch block left superior axis. There is no significant R wave in precordial leads (A), suggesting that VT is originating from the left ventricular apex close to the interventricular septum. Rarely, VT of similar morphology can originate from the right ventricular apex close to the septum. VT circuit was mapped at the inferoapical area of the left ventricle (B).

associated with inferobasal septal locations. Endocardial and epicardial reentrant VTs of different morphologies mapped during catheter ablation have been shown in Figs. 12.6 to 12.28.

FOCAL MONOMORPHIC VENTRICULAR TACHYCARDIA IN CORONARY ARTERY DISEASE

A focal mechanism (automatic, triggered, or microreentry) is present in up to 9% of monomorphic VTs in patients with CAD. Although not

definitive, the following characteristics help differentiate focal VT from macroreentrant VT in patients with CAD[3]:

1. Occurrence of spontaneous bursts of VT as opposed to prolonged episodes of sustained VT is more consistent with a focal mechanism (Figs. 12.29 and 12.30).

2. Focal VTs in CAD are adenosine insensitive unless idiopathic VT coexists with CAD. In a series of focal VT in CAD, only one of nine patients had adenosine-sensitive VT, suggesting a specific mechanism.

3. Requirement of isoproterenol for initiation or maintenance of VT is more consistent with a focal mechanism and is rarely helpful in

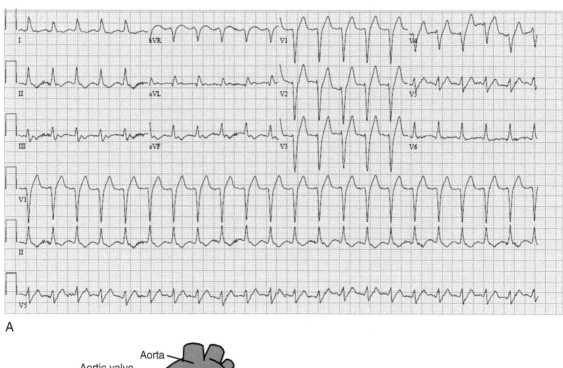

A

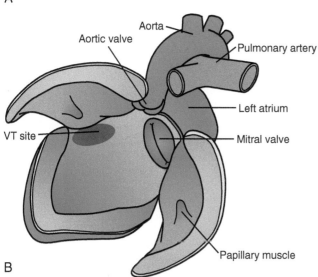

B

Fig. 12.7 Ventricular tachycardia (*VT*) with relatively narrow QRS (septal VT). (A) The VT is a relatively narrow complex because of septal origin with simultaneous left and right ventricular activation. The poor progression of R wave in precordial leads suggest that VT originates from the anterior septum (positive QRS in inferior leads). VT circuit was mapped at the anterior midseptum of the left ventricle, close to the apex (B).

ventricular macroreentry. The focal VT originates from relatively healthy myocardium or from the scar border zone. In contrast, macroreentrant VT has a critical isthmus in a region of myocardial scar or its border zone.

4. Focal VTs predominantly originate from the basal or midcavity (within 3 cm of valve annuli) of the LV.[3]

POLYMORPHIC VENTRICULAR TACHYCARDIA AND VENTRICULAR FIBRILLATION IN CORONARY ARTERY DISEASE

Frequent polymorphic VT or VF occurs in the setting of acute MI or in chronic CAD remote from MI. The ECG usually has no diagnostic feature for the origin of the arrhythmia in the majority of cases. However, in a few cases single monomorphic PVCs trigger polymorphic VT or VF. Mapping and catheter ablation of the PVCs can eliminate the arrhythmia (Fig. 12.31). Therefore attention should be paid to the monomorphic PVCs on the rhythm strip and 12-lead ECG.

BUNDLE BRANCH REENTRANT VENTRICULAR TACHYCARDIA

Bundle branch reentrant ventricular tachycardia (BBR-VT) is seen in patients with underlying disease of the His-Purkinje system and usually cardiomegaly. It accounts for approximately 6% of all patients with inducible sustained monomorphic VT who undergo programmed electrical stimulation for VT induction. In patients with NICM and in patients with prior valve surgery, approximately one-third of inducible

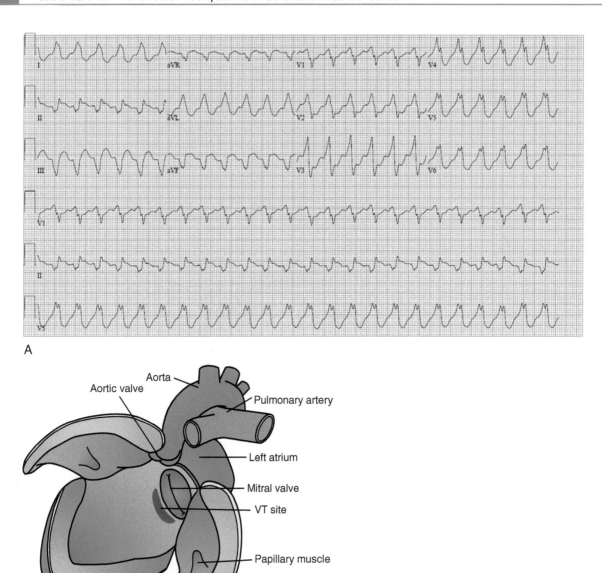

Fig. 12.8 Ventricular tachycardia (*VT*) with left bundle branch block left superior axis morphology. VT has positive concordance in the precordial leads indicating basal septal origin. VT morphology similar to this is encountered in the inferoposterior myocardial infarction with the VT origin at the inferior septum or the mitral annulus close to the septum (A). This VT was mapped at the mitral annulus close to the septum (B).

sustained VTs are BBR-VTs.[4] The unique electrophysiologic properties of rapid conduction and long refractory periods ordinarily prevent sustained reentry within the His-Purkinje system. However, in conditions in which the conduction in the His-Purkinje system is prolonged because of disease or drugs, sustained reentry within the bundle branches is facilitated. Three types of BBR-VT (Table 12.4) have been described. Type A (Fig. 12.32) and type C are the classic BBR-VTs of counterclockwise and clockwise circuits, respectively. Type B is interfascicular reentry characterized by reentry within the fascicles of the left bundle. Initiation of interfascicular reentry occurs when an atrial or ventricular premature depolarization conducts over the healthy fascicle, giving rise to a QRS identical to that in sinus rhythm, and then reenters the blocked fascicle in the retrograde direction to induce and sustain reentrant VT.

A resting ECG in these patients often reveals conduction abnormalities in the form of a prolonged P-R interval, nonspecific intraventricular conduction delay, incomplete or complete BBB, and occasionally complete atrioventricular heart block. Usually, these are rapid VTs with a typical BBB pattern. VT caused by interfascicular reentry (type B) is most commonly seen in patients with an anterior wall infarction and either left anterior or posterior hemifascicular block.

VENTRICULAR TACHYCARDIA IN NONISCHEMIC CARDIOMYOPATHY

All types of ventricular tachyarrhythmias occur in patients with NICM. Frequent PVCs, ventricular couplets, and nonsustained VT can cause a

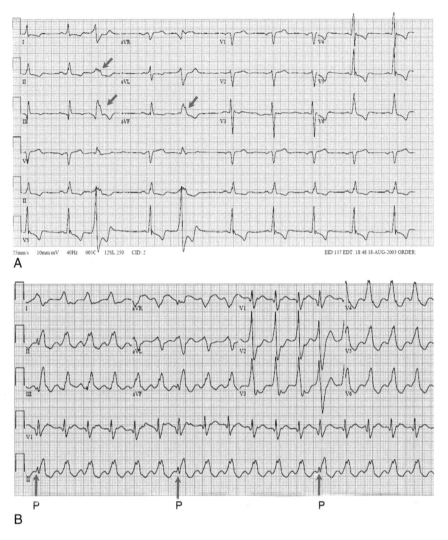

Fig. 12.9 Ventricular tachycardia (*VT*) with left bundle branch block, inferior axis. (A) Baseline electrocardiogram of a patient with history of myocardial infarction shows sinus rhythm with fragmented QRS complexes (shown with arrows) in leads II, aVF, and V3-V4, suggesting inferior and anterior myocardial scar. (B) Positive precordial concordance with inferior QRS axis signifies left ventricular anterior basal VT I. There are three premature ventricular complexes with fusion complexes (*red arrows*). VT was mapped in the anterior basal area of the left ventricle approximately 1 cm lateral to the septum.

reversible tachycardia-induced cardiomyopathy and can be indistinguishable from NICM. Suppression or cure of the arrhythmia results in improvement of LV function. In patients presenting with NICM of unclear etiology with a PVC burden greater than 20% to 25%, catheter ablation of the PVCs is appropriate before consideration of an implantable cardioverter-defibrillator (implantation for primary prevention of sudden death). The majority (90%) of VTs in NICM originate from myocardial scars located near the superior and lateral perivalvular aortic and mitral valve region and from aortomitral continuity (Figs. 12.33–12.36; see also Table 12.3).

EPICARDIAL VENTRICULAR TACHYCARDIA IN NONISCHEMIC CARDIOMYOPATHY

Nearly one-third of VTs in NICM and 70% of VTs in Chagas cardiomyopathy have epicardial or subepicardial reentrant circuits that require epicardial ablation. The prior published criteria for epicardial

VT (Q wave in lead I and no Q waves in inferior leads and interval criteria: pseudo delta wave ≥ 34 ms, intrinsicoid deflection time > 85 ms, shortest R-S complex ≥ 121 ms, and maximum diastolic index ≥ 0.55) were revisited in 14 patients with NICM by Vallès and associates by pacemapping endocardially and epicardially during electrophysiology study.[5] They suggested a four-step algorithm for identifying epicardial origin from basal superior and lateral LV in the setting of NICM (Figs. 12.37–12.40).

VENTRICULAR TACHYCARDIA IN ARRHYTHMOGENIC RIGHT VENTRICULAR DYSPLASIA/CARDIOMYOPATHY

Arrhythmogenic right ventricular dysplasia/cardiomyopathy (ARVD/C) is an inherited cardiomyopathy characterized by progressive fibrofatty replacement of the right ventricular myocardium. This disorder usually involves the RV, but the LV and septum can also be affected.

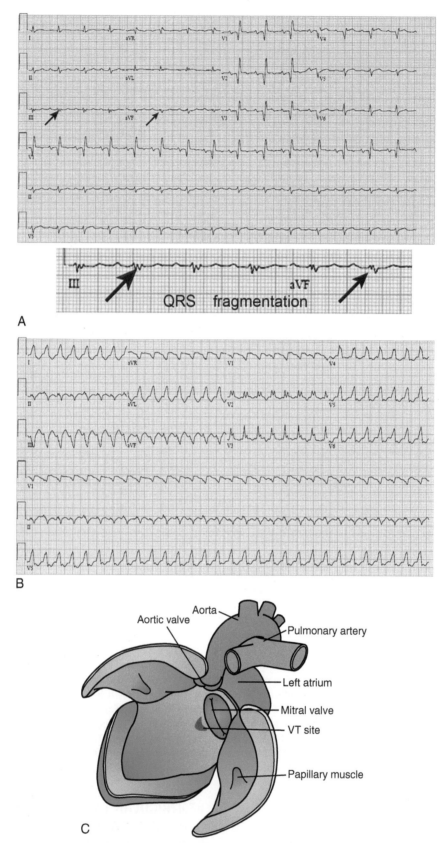

Fig. 12.10 Ventricular tachycardia (*VT*) originating from mitral isthmus. (A) Baseline electrocardiogram depicts Q waves in leads V1 to V4, indicating anteroseptal myocardial infarction and fragmented QRS (*arrows*) in inferior leads (enlarged view below), suggesting an old inferior wall myocardial infarction. (B) The same patient has VT with left bundle branch block, left superior axis morphology. VT circuit was mapped between the inferoposterior left ventricular scar and the mitral annulus (mitral isthmus) (C). VT was successfully treated by catheter ablation between the posterior mitral valve and the scar.

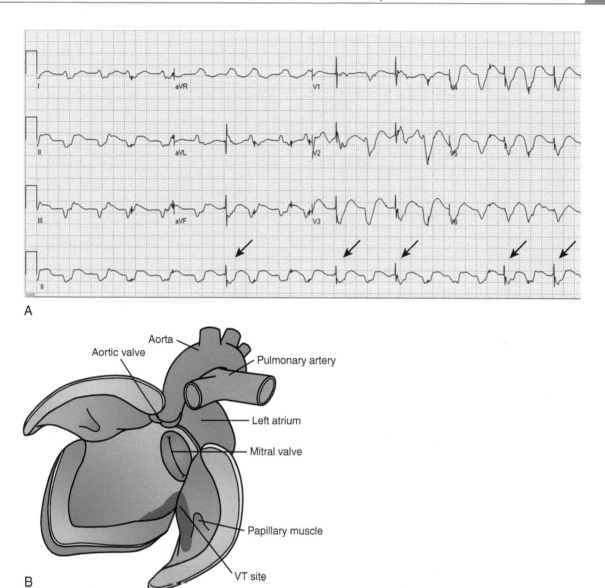

Fig. 12.11 (A) Ventricular tachycardia (*VT*) with left bundle branch block—like morphology with right axis deviation originating from the left ventricle apex near the septum. QS complexes in the inferior leads suggest VT location at the inferior part of the apical septum (B). VT was mapped at the inferior apical septum. There are five pacing artifacts because of undersensing (*arrows*) of ventricular impulses by the implantable cardioverter-defibrillator.

Fibrofatty replacement of the myocardium produces "islands" of scar regions that can lead to reentrant LBBB morphology VTs. Approximately 40% to 50% of patients with ARVD/C have a normal ECG at presentation.[6] However, by 6 years of disease presence, almost all patients have one or more of several findings related to RV depolarization and repolarization abnormalities on baseline ECG (Table 12.5).[6] There are several major and minor criteria for the diagnosis of ARVD/C. Epsilon waves and QRS duration greater than 110 ms in leads V1, V2, or V3 are major criteria, whereas T wave inversion (lead V_2-V_3 age >12 years in the absence of RBBB) is a minor criterion. The "epsilon waves" are "postexcitation" electrical potentials of small amplitude that occur in the ST segment after the end of the QRS complex and are seen in 33% of patients (Fig. 12.41). The terminal activation duration is the longest value in V1 to V3, from the nadir of the S wave to the end of all depolarization deflections, thereby including not only the S wave upstroke but also both late fractionated signals and epsilon waves (Fig. 12.41). It represents delayed activation of the RV

owing to myocardial scar and fatty replacement. Fig. 12.41 shows incomplete RBBB and inverted T waves in lead V2. However, increasing the sweep speed to 500 mm/sec and amplitude to 0.05 mV/mm clearly unmasks the epsilon waves (arrows) in leads V1 and V2 with QRS fragmentation in lead V1.

A terminal activation duration of 55 ms or greater, VT with LBBB morphology and superior axis, and multiple VT morphologies are all highly specific for ARVD/C (Figs. 12.42—12.44). In addition, late potentials on signal-averaged ECG recordings are the counterpart of these depolarization abnormalities and are considered a minor criterion.

VENTRICULAR TACHYCARDIA LATE AFTER REPAIR OF CONGENITAL HEART DISEASE

VT accounts for 38% of wide complex tachycardias in patients with congenital heart disease. Supraventricular tachycardias include atrial

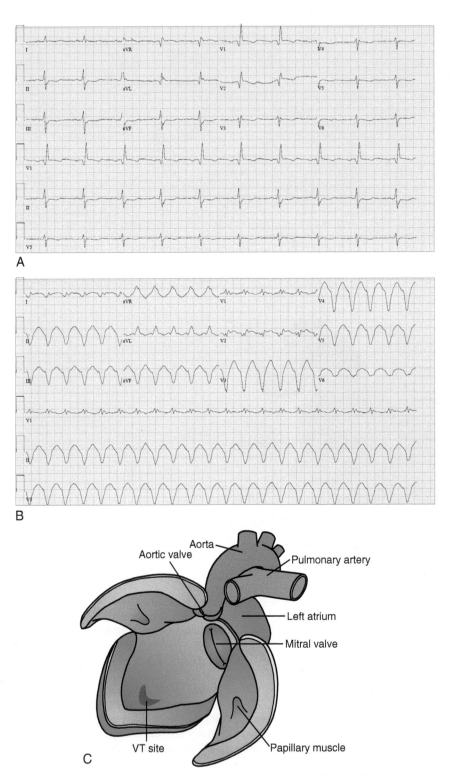

Fig. 12.12 Right bundle branch block superior axis ventricular tachycardia (*VT*). Patient has history of anterior wall myocardial infarction with Q wave in leads V1 and V2 (A). VT has right bundle branch block with QS pattern in inferior leads, as well as in precordial leads V2-V6 (B). VT was mapped at the inferior septum close to the left ventricular apex (C).

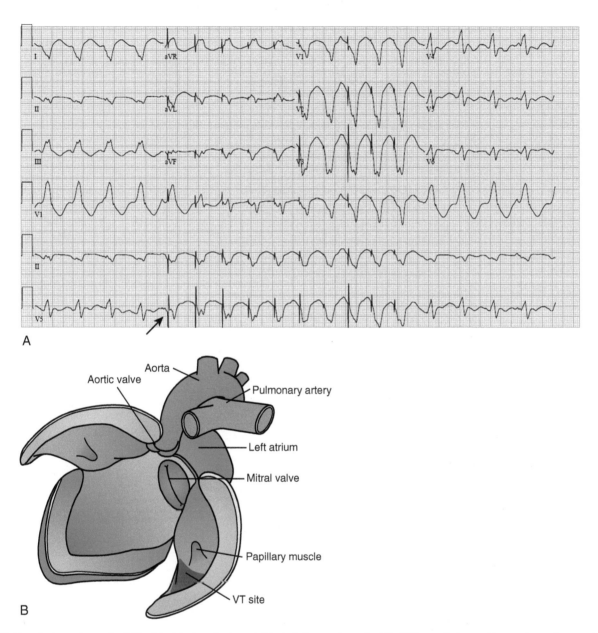

Fig. 12.13 Ventricular tachycardia (*VT*) with right bundle branch block, left superior axis. (A) QRS morphology with prominent R wave in lead V1 with progressively decreasing amplitude in precordial leads V4-V6 and negative complexes in lead I and lead II suggests the VT origin at the inferolateral left ventricle, close to the base. Pacing spikes followed by a different QRS morphology (left bundle branch block) (*arrow*) is caused by ventricular capture during antitachycardia pacing by the implantable cardioverter-defibrillator. The antitachycardia pacing failed to terminate the VT. VT originated from the apical lateral area (B).

flutter, atrial tachycardia, atrioventricular reentrant tachycardia, atrioventricular nodal reentrant tachycardia, and ventricular arrhythmias late after repair of congenital heart disease occur predominantly in those with tetralogy of Fallot and ventricular septal defect repair. (Fig. 12.45; see also Fig. 12.1). Independent predictors of sustained VT include QRS duration of 180 ms or greater, increase in QRS duration after surgical repair, increased dispersion of QRS duration (QRS duration is defined as the difference between the longest and the shortest QRS duration within a 12-lead ECG), increased Q-T interval dispersion (QT dispersion is simply defined as the difference between the longest and the shortest QT intervals within a 12-lead ECG), high-grade ventricular ectopy on Holter monitoring, complete heart block, older age at surgery (>10 years), presence of a transannular right ventricular outflow tract (RVOT) patch, increased RV systolic pressures, RVOT aneurysm, and pulmonic and tricuspid regurgitation. VT originating from the RVOT is related to prior right ventriculotomy or reconstruction of the RVOT, and VT originating from the RV inflow tract septum is related to closure of the ventricular septal defect. The VT is most commonly monomorphic and macroreentrant, rotating clockwise or counterclockwise around myotomy scars or surgical patches that determine the ECG morphology during VT. Most commonly, an LBBB or an RBBB and right inferior axis morphology is seen during clockwise rotation around the scar. Less commonly, LBBB and left axis morphology can occur. VT and VF can also occur in various other cardiac anomalies related to severe LV dysfunction or in Ebstein anomaly with multiple accessory pathways causing VT.

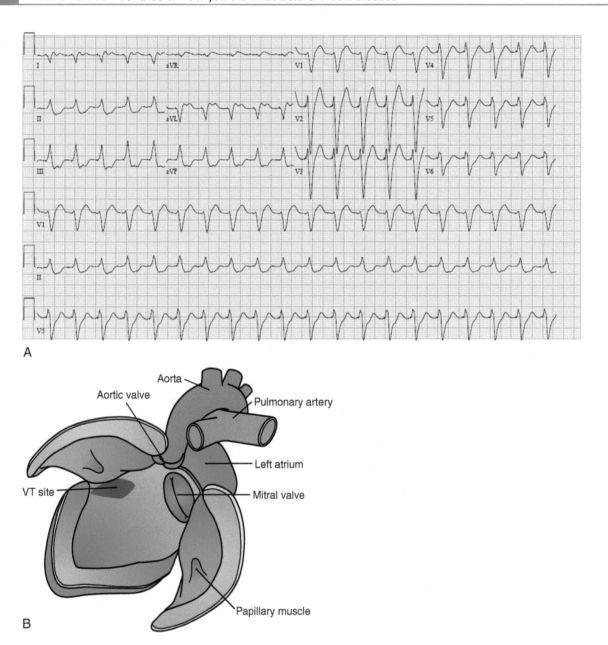

Fig. 12.14 Ventricular tachycardia (*VT*) with left bundle branch block, right inferior axis originating from midanterior septum. (A) VT has inferior QRS axis and negative QRS complexes in leads aVR and aVL, as well as relatively narrow QRS complexes, suggesting septal origin. The relatively lower amplitude of R waves in precordial leads suggest a more apical site (B). VT was mapped at the anterior apical septum area.

VENTRICULAR TACHYCARDIA IN PATIENTS WITH LEFT VENTRICULAR ASSIST DEVICES

Ventricular arrhythmias in patients with left ventricular assist devices (LVADs) are not uncommon owing to significant underlying structural heart disease. De novo monomorphic VT can also occur after an LVAD is implanted; 60% of patients suffer from monomorphic VT after implantation of an LVAD. The majority of these VTs have an exit site close to the region of the inflow cannula at the LV apex[7] (Fig. 12.46).

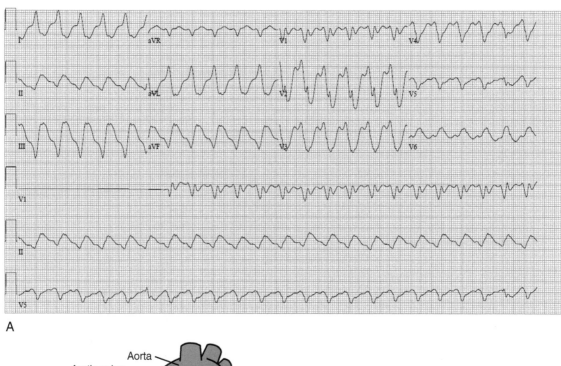

A

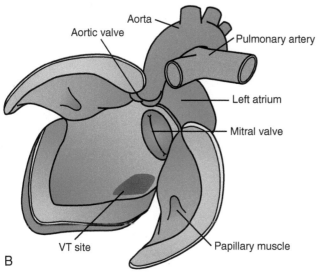

B

Fig. 12.15 Ventricular tachycardia (*VT*) with left bundle branch block, left superior axis. Electrocardiogram shows precordial reversal of R waves in leads V4-V5 and QS pattern in inferior leads (A). VT originated from the inferior midseptum in the left ventricle (B).

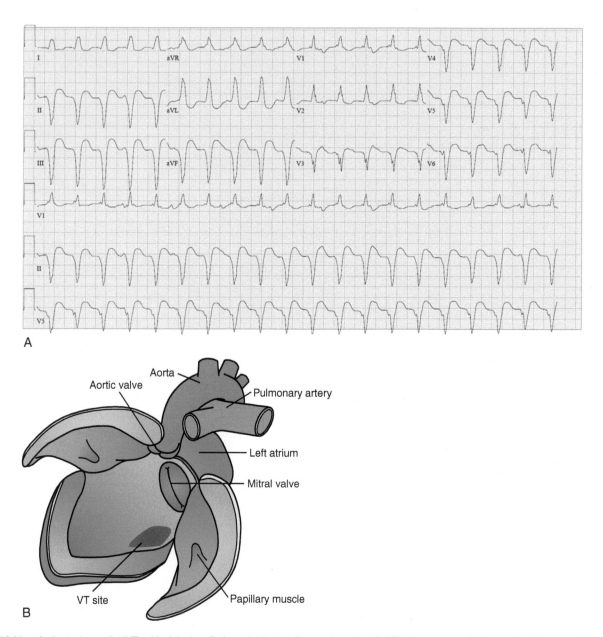

Fig. 12.16 Ventricular tachycardia (*VT*) with right bundle branch block, left superior axis. (A) VT shows precordial reversal of R waves in lead V4-V5 and QS pattern in inferior leads. This right bundle branch block morphology VT originated from the inferior midseptum in the left ventricle (B), at the same site from where the left bundle branch block morphology VT originated in the patient in Fig. 12.15.

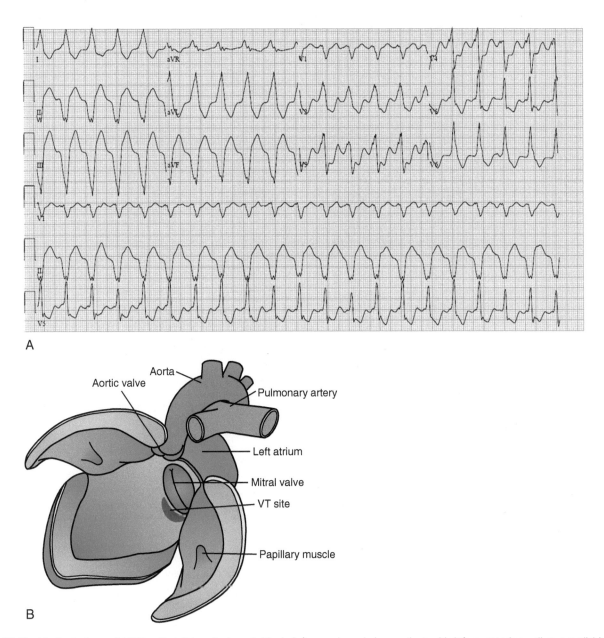

Fig. 12.17 Ventricular tachycardia (*VT*) with left bundle branch block, left superior axis in a patient with inferoposterior wall myocardial infarction. (A) Electrocardiogram reveals an early transition of QRS, suggesting a basal origin, and the left superior QRS axis suggests inferoposterior left ventricle of the VT. VT was mapped in the posterior left ventricle, with the VT isthmus being between the myocardial scar and the mitral annulus at 6 o'clock position (B).

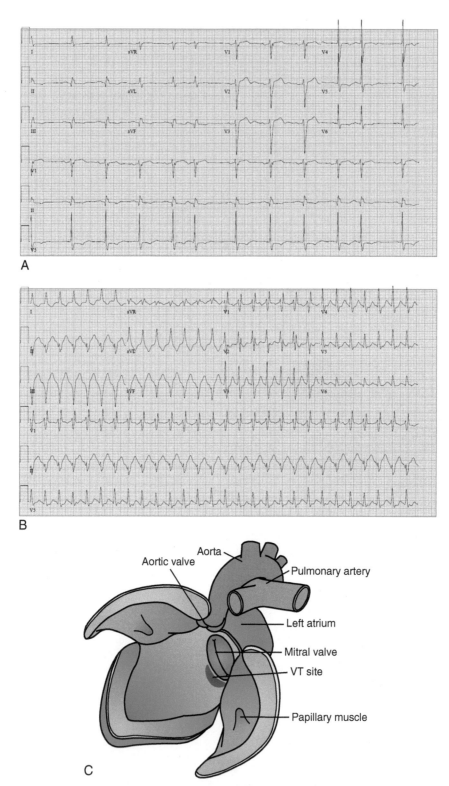

Fig. 12.18 Ventricular tachycardia (*VT*) with right bundle branch block, left superior axis in a patient with inferior wall myocardial infarction. (A) Baseline electrocardiogram depicts Q waves in inferior leads owing to an old inferior wall myocardial infarction. The positive concordance of QRS during VT suggests a basal origin, and the left superior QRS axis suggests inferoposterior left ventricle location of the VT circuit (B). VT was mapped in the inferoposterior left ventricle, with the VT isthmus being between the myocardial scar and the mitral annulus at 6 o'clock position (C). The patient in Fig. 12.17 had the VT origin in the same area, but the VT had left bundle branch block morphology and superior axis.

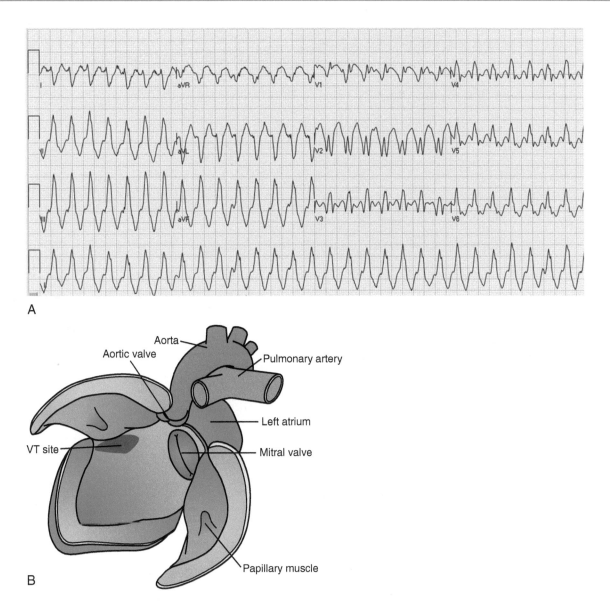

Fig. 12.19 Ventricular tachycardia (*VT*) with left bundle branch block, right inferior axis. (A) Progression of R wave from precordial leads V3 onward with positive QRS complexes in inferior leads suggests midanterior left ventricular origin of the VT. Negative QRS complexes in leads aVR and aVL suggest septal origin. (B) VT was mapped at the anterior septum.

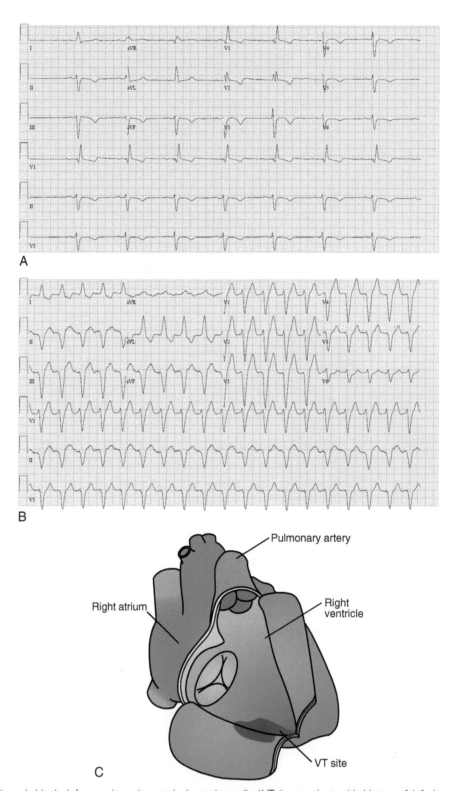

Fig. 12.20 Left bundle branch block, left superior axis ventricular tachycardia (*VT*) in a patient with history of inferior myocardial infarction and coronary artery bypass graft. (A) Baseline electrocardiogram shows poor progression of R wave and no abnormal Q waves. (B) This VT morphology is most consistent with VT origin from left ventricular apex, but VT was mapped to right ventricle close to the interventricular septum, midway between apex and base (C), and successfully ablated.

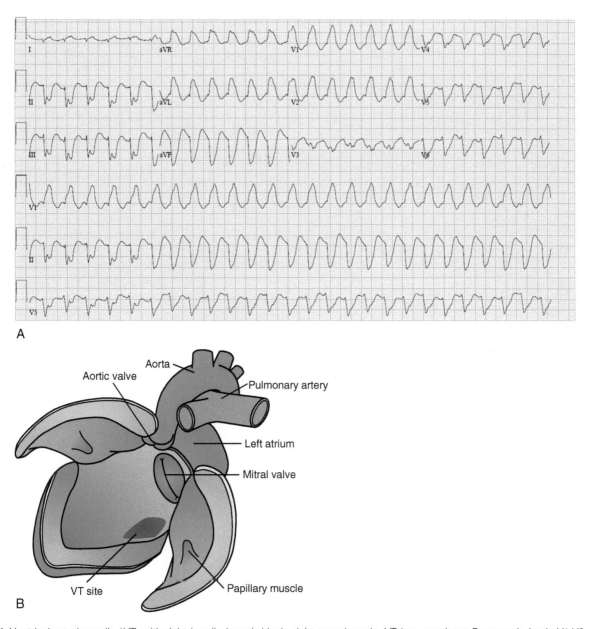

Fig. 12.21 Ventricular tachycardia (*VT*) with right bundle branch block, right superior axis. VT has prominent R waves in leads V1-V2 with early reversal of R wave in precordial leads with right superior axis (A). VT isthmus was mapped in the inferior mid left ventricular wall (B).

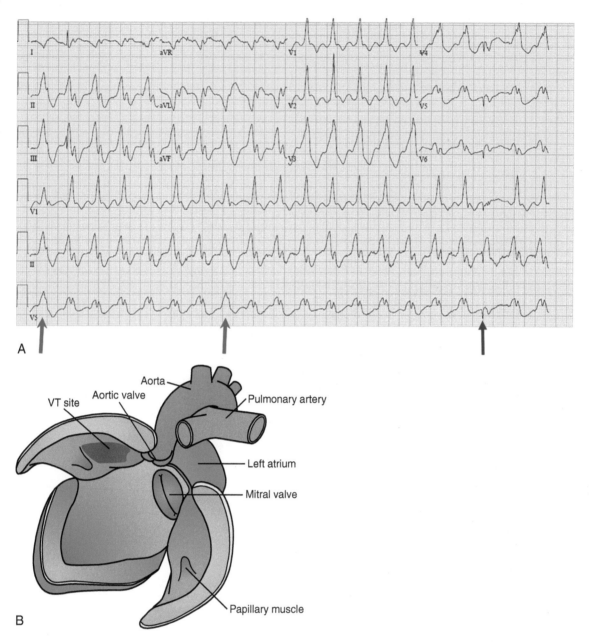

Fig. 12.22 Ventricular tachycardia (*VT*) with right bundle branch block, inferior axis, originating from anterolateral basal left ventricle. (A) A different VT in the same patient as in Fig. 12.17. VT has positive concordance in precordial leads, which suggests basal location, and negative QRS complexes in leads I and aVL suggest lateral location, whereas inferior axis suggests anterior left ventricular origin of the VT. VT was mapped originating from anterolateral basal left ventricle (B). First and eighth beats are fusion complexes (*red arrows*) and the third from last beat is a fusion complex of VT beat and the ventricular paced (*blue arrow*) beat, due to undersensing.

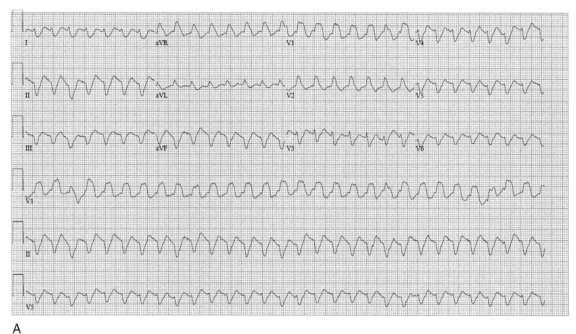

A

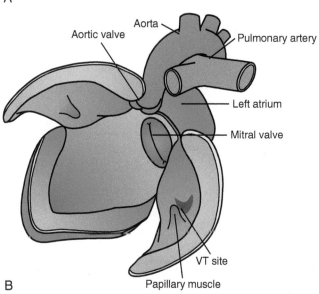

B

Fig. 12.23 Ventricular tachycardia (*VT*) with right bundle branch block, right superior axis. (A) VT has right superior axis with early reversal of R wave in lead V3, which suggests mid left ventricular cavity. (B) VT was mapped at the mid inferior left ventricle.

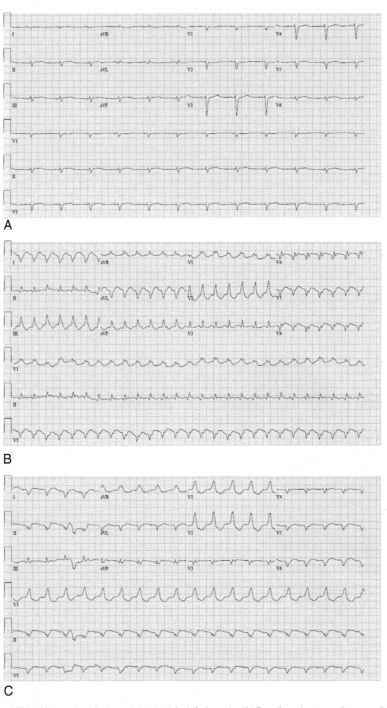

Fig. 12.24 Ventricular tachycardias (*VTs*) with right bundle branch block, right inferior axis. (A) Baseline electrocardiogram of a patient with severe three-vessel disease with recent myocardial infarction caused by left circumflex artery occlusion. The low-voltage electrocardiogram was attributed to obesity. (B) VT morphology is right bundle branch block with right inferior axis. There is reverse transition of the R wave in the precordial leads V5-V6. VT originated from the mid anterolateral left ventricle. (C) In the same patient, another VT of different morphology was recorded after amiodarone therapy, owing to the different exit site of the VT circuit in the left ventricle. This VT originated from the inferolateral wall in the mid left ventricle (QS pattern in leads II and aVF and reversal of R wave in lead V3 onward) in the left circumflex artery distribution. (D) Site of origin of the VT.

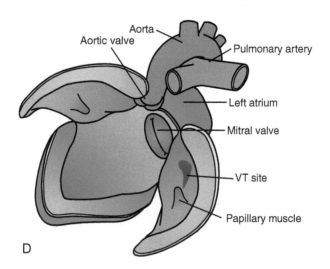

D

Fig. 12.24 (Continued).

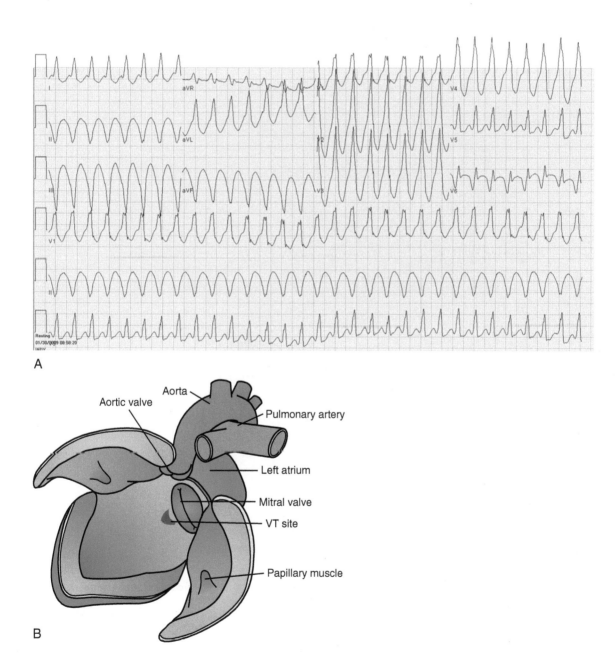

A

B

Fig. 12.25 Right bundle branch block, left superior axis ventricular tachycardia (*VT*). (A) VT in this patient with inferior myocardial infarction has right bundle branch block pattern with a positive precordial concordance (except for lead V6), indicating basal origin. QS pattern in inferior leads suggests inferior wall origin. Leads I, aVL, and aVR have positive QRS complexes, which suggests VT origin is closer to the interventricular septum. (B) VT was mapped at the inferoseptal aspect of mitral valve.

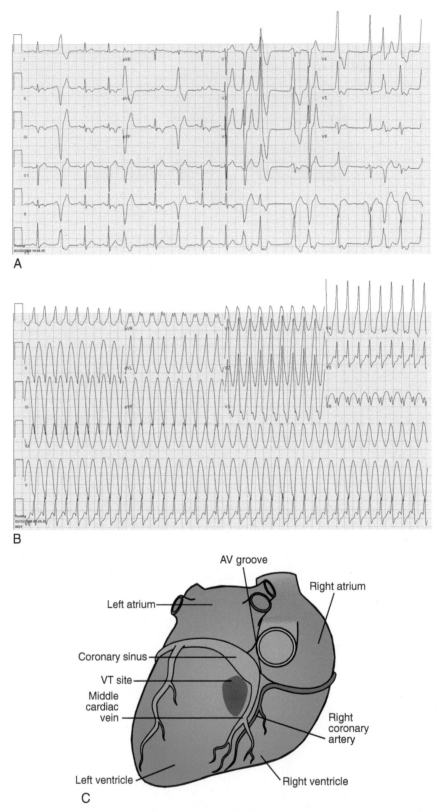

Fig. 12.26 Post—myocardial infarction epicardial ventricular tachycardia (*VT*). (A) Baseline electrocardiogram shows sinus rhythm with frequent premature ventricular complexes and a three-beat run of nonsustained VT. (B) Patient later had sustained monomorphic VT with right bundle branch block morphology and left superior axis. There are slurred upstrokes in leads V1-V4, suggesting possible epicardial origin. During epicardial mapping, the VT was mapped at the inferior basal left ventricle close to the interventricular septum (C). *AV*, Atrioventricular.

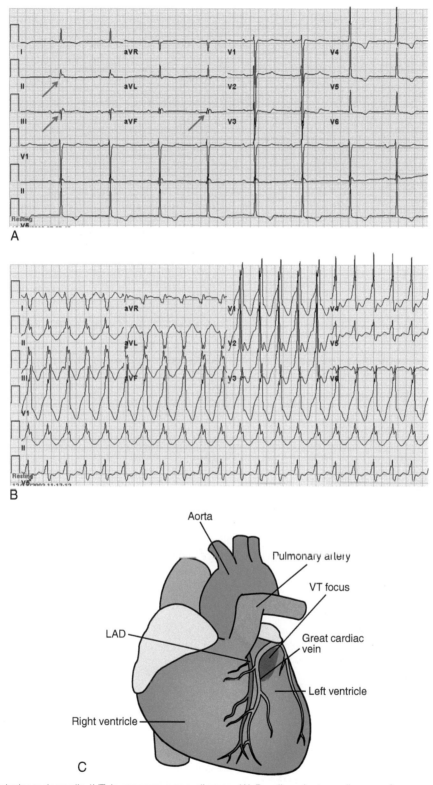

Fig. 12.27 Epicardial ventricular tachycardia (*VT*) in coronary artery disease. (A) Baseline electrocardiogram of a man with history of anterior and inferior wall myocardial infarction. The inferior leads have fragmented QRS (*arrows*). (B) VT without any antiarrhythmic therapy has right bundle branch block, right inferior axis. Positive precordial concordance of QRS (except lead V6) suggests basal left ventricular origin of the VT. Lead aVR has QS pattern, and lead aVL has rS (predominantly negative) pattern, suggesting that the VT origin is closer to the interventricular septum. The delayed intrinsicoid deflection in precordial leads suggests epicardial origin of the VT. The epicardial focus of the VT was mapped to basal anterior left ventricle (C). *LAD*, Left anterior descending artery.

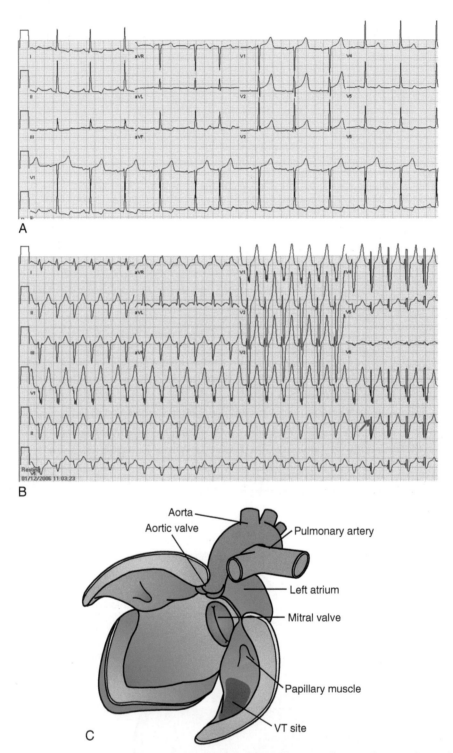

Fig. 12.28 (A) Sinus rhythm shows early repolarization abnormalities in leads V2-V4. Electrocardiogram shows early repolarization abnormality with J point elevation in leads V2-V3. (B) Patient developed ventricular tachycardia (*VT*) that was unresponsive to amiodarone and was cardioverted successfully. VT has a relatively narrow QRS (120 msec) with right superior axis (unlikely to be a supraventricular tachycardia), most likely originating from the left ventricle. Last four beats have pacing spikes of antitachycardia pacing (*arrow*) by the implantable cardioverter-defibrillator. VT was mapped originating from the left ventricle inferior apex (C).

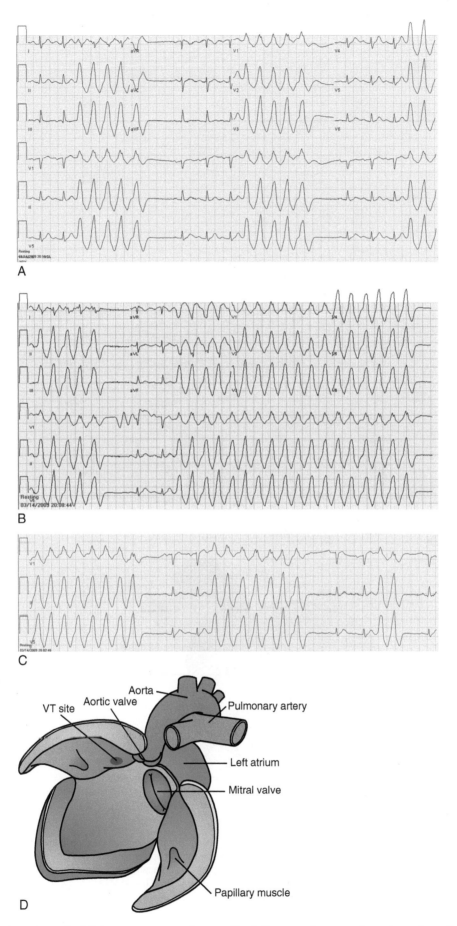

Fig. 12.29 Focal ventricular tachycardia (*VT*) in coronary artery disease. (A–C) Electrocardiograms of a patient who suffered frequent premature ventricular complexes and nonsustained and sustained VT within 24 hours of acute myocardial infarct. Three electrocardiograms are shown to demonstrate frequent repetitive ventricular arrhythmia. (D) VT was mapped to the base of anterior left ventricle.

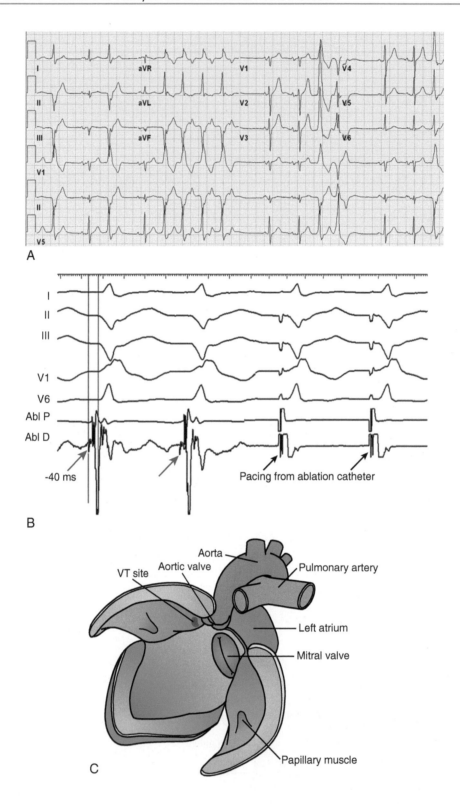

Fig. 12.30 (A) Electrocardiogram of a patient with history of myocardial infarction depicts frequent predominantly monomorphic premature ventricular complexes and nonsustained ventricular tachycardia (*VT*). (B) The activation map (*red arrows*) with the ablation catheter (*Abl D*) from the site of VT focus is 40 ms earlier than the surface QRS on the electrocardiogram. The pacemap (*black arrows*) with the ablation catheter (*Abl D*) from that site revealed QRS morphology identical to the VT in all 12 leads (leads I, II, III, V1, and V6 are shown). (C) VT origin was mapped at the anterior mitral annulus. *Abl D*, Ablation distal pole; *Abl P*, ablation proximal pole.

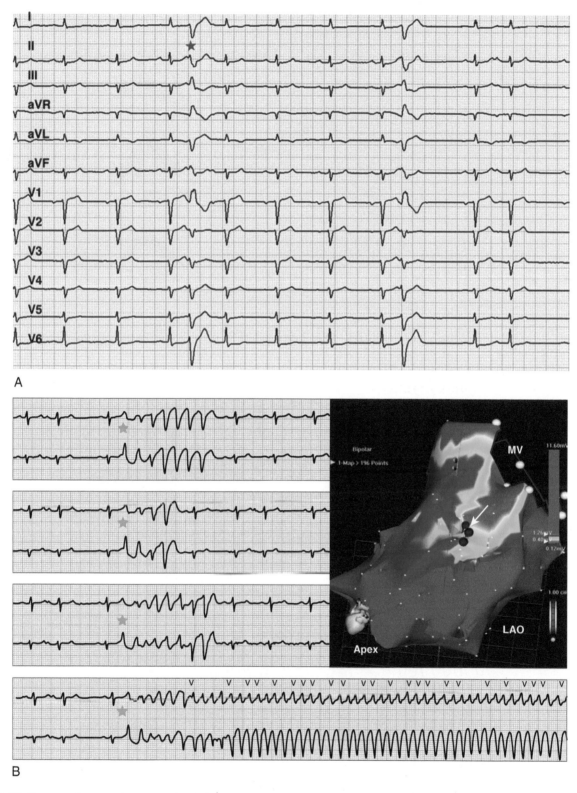

Fig. 12.31 (A) Electrocardiogram of a man who had frequent nonsustained and sustained polymorphic ventricular tachycardia during acute myocardial infarction initiated by R on T, that is, a QRS complex arriving during the T wave of the previous QRS complex. Electrocardiogram shows frequent monomorphic premature ventricular complexes (PVCs) that have right bundle branch block, inferior axis morphology (marked by blue stars). (B) Rhythm strip shows nonsustained and sustained polymorphic ventricular tachycardia and ventricular fibrillation initiated by a single PVC (*blue stars*). The electroanatomic activation map (*inset*) shows a focal activation (*white arrow*) of the PVC originating from the posterolateral mitral annulus. The red zone in the electroanatomic activation map represents myocardial scar, and green and blue color represent scar border zone. The purple color represents healthy myocardium. The arrhythmia was eliminated after ablation of the PVC. *LAO,* Left anterior oblique; *MV,* mitral valve.

TABLE 12.4   Types of Bundle Branch Reentry Ventricular Tachycardia

Type	Retrograde Conduction	Anterograde Conduction	Diagram	VT Morphology
A	Left bundle	Right bundle		LBBB
B	Anterior or posterior left fascicle	Contralateral fascicle		RBBB
C	Right bundle	Left bundle		RBBB

LAF, Left anterior fascicle; *LB*, left bundle; *LBBB*, left bundle branch block; *LPF*, left posterior fascicle; *RB*, right bundle; *RBBB*, right bundle branch block; *VT*, ventricular tachycardia.

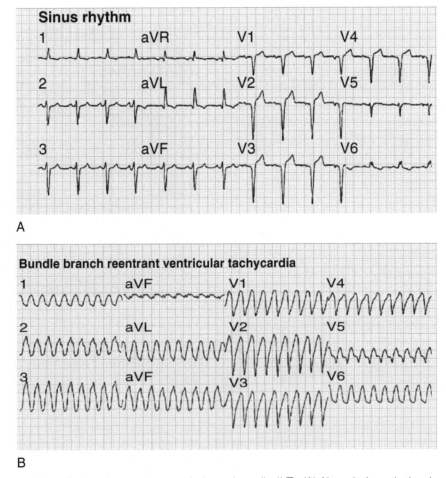

Fig. 12.32 Electrocardiogram of bundle branch reentrant ventricular tachycardia (*VT*). (A) Normal sinus rhythm baseline with intraventricular conduction delay resembling left bundle branch block. (B) Bundle branch reentrant VT. Note typical-appearing complete left bundle branch block in this rapid VT. (Issa ZF, Miller JM, Zipes DP, eds. *Clinical Arrhythmology and Electrophysiology.* 3rd ed. Philadelphia, PA: Saunders; 2019:897–906.)

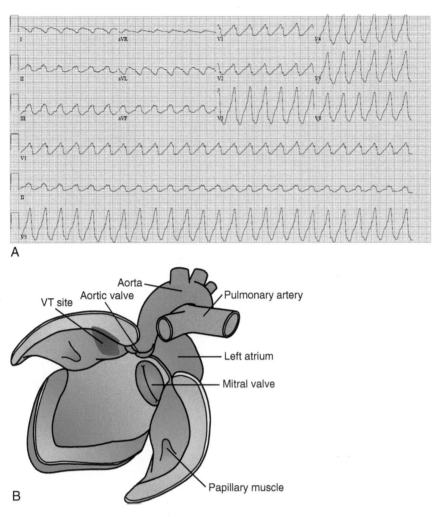

A

B

Fig. 12.33 Ventricular tachycardia (*VT*) in nonischemic cardiomyopathy. VT morphology is right bundle branch block, right inferior axis with a positive concordance in precordial leads suggesting basal origin in the left ventricle (A). Positive QRS complexes in inferior leads and negative complexes in leads I and aVL suggest anterolateral location of the VT circuit. VT was mapped to the anterolateral perimitral area (B).

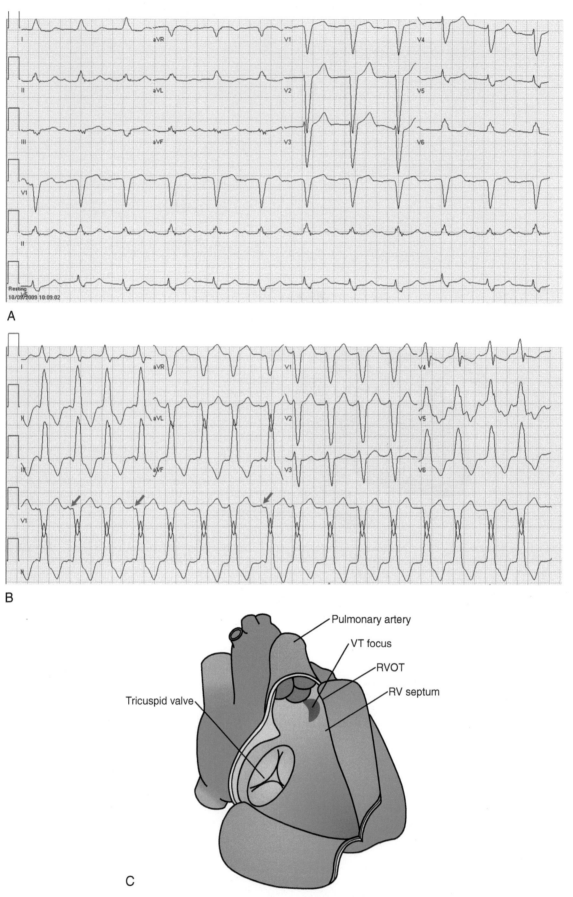

Fig. 12.34 Electrocardiograms (ECGs) of patients with nonischemic cardiomyopathy. (A) ECG reveals sinus rhythm with left bundle branch block at 70 bpm, first-degree atrioventricular block. (B) ECG shows left bundle branch block, left inferior axis ventricular tachycardia (*VT*) (100 bpm) and atrial tachycardia (106 bpm) with atrioventricular dissociation, which was confirmed by intracardiac ECGs recorded during implantable cardioverter-defibrillator interrogation on the same patient. The upright P waves in lead 2 (arrows) suggest that it is not retrogradely conducted P waves due to VT. (C) VT was mapped in the right ventricular outflow tract (*RVOT*). *RV*, Right ventricle.

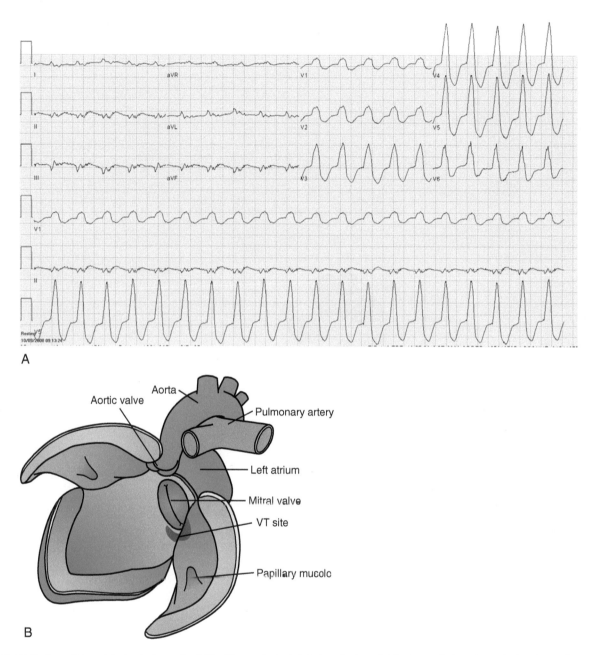

Fig. 12.35 (A) Endocardial ventricular tachycardia (*VT*) with an atypical right bundle branch block morphology in nonischemic cardiomyopathy. In contrast to epicardial VT, the VT has Q waves in inferior leads and no Q wave in lead I. The maximum deflection index is calculated as follows: earliest time to maximum deflection in any precordial lead divided by the total QRS duration. A maximum deflection index larger than 0.55 was related to epicardial origin remote from the sinus of Valsalva compared with other sites of origin with a sensitivity of 100% and specificity of 98.7%.[8] (B) VT circuit was mapped in the inferobasal left ventricle.

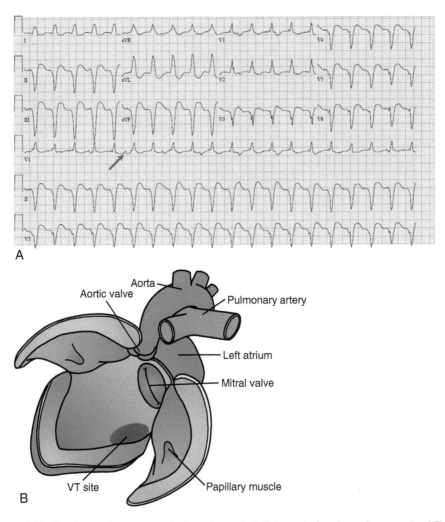

Fig. 12.36 Right bundle branch block, left superior axis ventricular tachycardia (*VT*) in nonischemic cardiomyopathy. VT has QS pattern in inferior leads with abrupt loss of R wave progression after lead V2. Atrioventricular dissociation is demonstrated (the *red arrow* shows P wave) in lead V1 (A). VT was mapped on the inferior septum in the mid left ventricle (B).

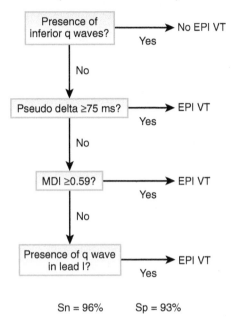

Probable Epicardial Origin
(based on interval criteria)

Fig. 12.37 The four-step diagnosis criteria for epicardial (*EPI*) ventricular tachycardia (*VT*) in nonischemic cardiomyopathy. The three top steps have a high specificity, and the last step is the most accurate. The total sensitivity (*Sn*) and specificity (*Sp*) of the algorithm are 96% and 93%, respectively.[5] *MDI*, Maximum diastolic index.

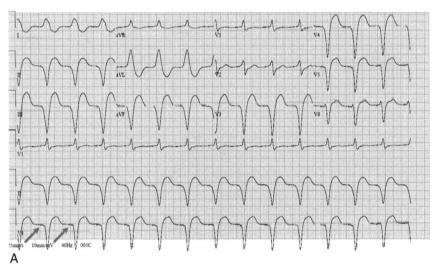

A

Fig. 12.38 Electrocardiogram of a patient with nonischemic cardiomyopathy with epicardial ventricular tachycardia (*VT*). (A) Baseline electrocardiogram shows atrial paced rhythm. *Arrows* point to P waves. (B) Right bundle branch block, right inferior axis VT. VT has a wide slurred upstroke with a maximum diastolic index that is greater than 0.6. Maximum diastolic index is defined as the interval measured from the earliest ventricular activation to the peak of the largest amplitude deflection in each precordial lead (taking the lead with shortest QRS initiation to QRS peak time) divided by the QRS duration. The slurred upstroke or pseudo delta wave (defined as the interval from the earliest ventricular activation to the onset of the earliest fast deflection in any precordial lead) is 120 ms in lead V3, and Q waves are present in lead I and absent in inferior leads. It is consistent with an epicardial VT. (C) The second VT in the same patient also meets the criteria for epicardial VT. (D) These epicardial VTs were mapped on the left lateral side of the basal left ventricle. *LAD*, Left anterior descending artery.

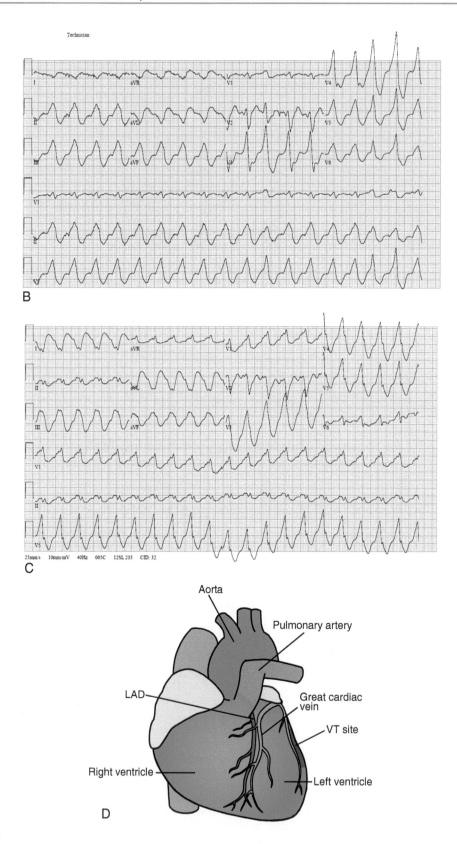

Fig. 12.38 (Continued).

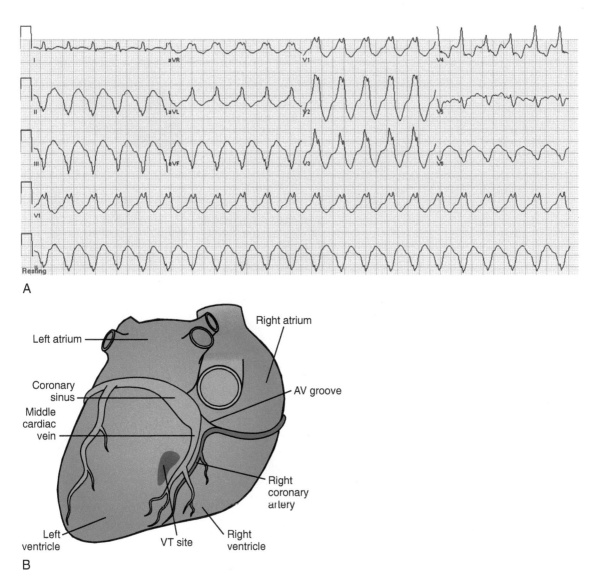

Fig. 12.39 Electrocardiogram of a patient with nonischemic cardiomyopathy with epicardial ventricular tachycardia (*VT*). (A) Right bundle branch block, left superior axis VT. VT has a wide slurred upstroke with maximum diastolic index greater than 0.6. There are slurred upstrokes of QRS in leads V1 to V4, and slurred downslopes with QS pattern in inferior leads. It is consistent with an epicardial VT. (B) VT circuit was mapped in the inferior mid left ventricle close to the interventricular septum. *AV*, Atrioventricular.

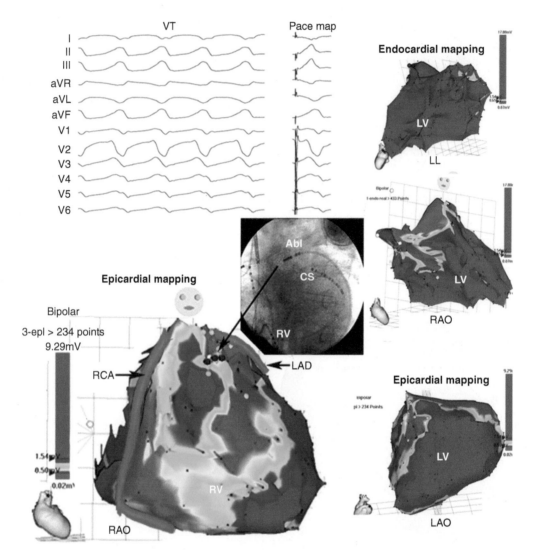

Fig. 12.40 Endocardial and epicardial bipolar voltage mapping using an electroanatomic mapping system in a patient with dilated cardiomyopathy with sustained monomorphic ventricular tachycardia (*VT*). Endocardial mapping recorded minimal basal scar regions in the left ventricle (*LV*), whereas the epicardial mapping revealed extensive LV basal scars and scar on right ventricle (*RV*). The tachycardia was hemodynamically unstable. Pace mapping revealed an exit site medial to the proximal left anterior descending artery (*LAD*), which was ablated successfully. LAD and right coronary arteries (*RCA*s) are drawn by mapping the coronary artery locations during coronary angiography. The fluoroscopic position of the catheter is shown in the left anterior oblique (*LAO*) view. *Abl*, Ablation catheter; *CS*, coronary sinus; *LL*, left lateral view; *RAO*, right anterior oblique view. The purple color in the map represents normal endocardial voltage whereas the red color represents myocardial scar. The blue, green, and yellow colors are present between the healthy myocardium (*purple*), and scar (*red*) represents relatively unhealthy myocardium in decreasing magnitude.

TABLE 12.5 **Electrocardiogram During Sinus Rhythm and During Ventricular Tachycardia in Arrhythmogenic Right Ventricular Dysplasia/Cardiomyopathy**

Rhythm		Electrocardiogram Abnormalities	Task Force Criteria
Sinus rhythm	Depolarization abnormalities	Epsilon waves in leads V1-V3 (*arrow*)	Major
		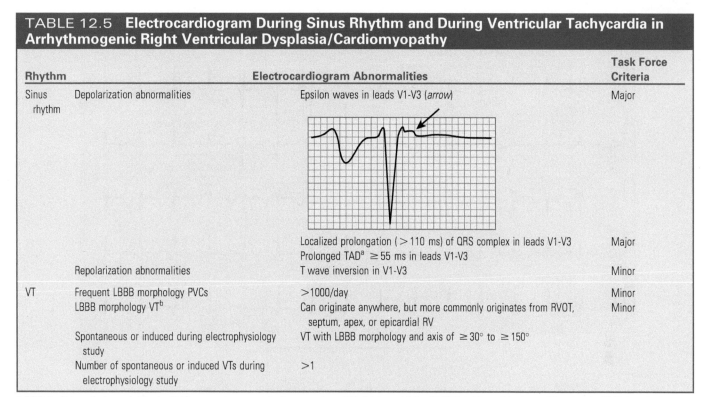	
		Localized prolongation (>110 ms) of QRS complex in leads V1-V3	Major
		Prolonged TAD[a] ≥55 ms in leads V1-V3	
	Repolarization abnormalities	T wave inversion in V1-V3	Minor
VT	Frequent LBBB morphology PVCs	>1000/day	Minor
	LBBB morphology VT[b]	Can originate anywhere, but more commonly originates from RVOT, septum, apex, or epicardial RV	Minor
	Spontaneous or induced during electrophysiology study	VT with LBBB morphology and axis of ≥30° to ≥150°	
	Number of spontaneous or induced VTs during electrophysiology study	>1	

LBBB, Left bundle branch block; *PVC*, premature ventricular complex; *RV*, right ventricle; *RVOT*, right ventricular outflow tract; *TAD*, terminal activation duration; *VT*, ventricular tachycardia.

[a]TAD is the longest value in V1-V3, from the nadir of the S wave to the end of all depolarization deflections, thereby including not only the S wave upstroke but also both late fractionated signals and epsilon waves.

[b]RBBB with a peritricuspid circuit can occur.

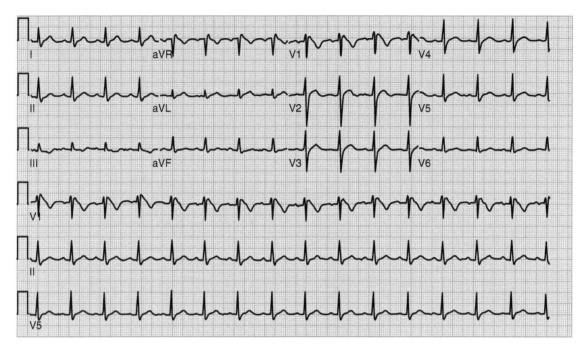

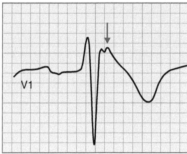

Fig. 12.41 Baseline electrocardiogram of a patient with arrhythmogenic right ventricular dysplasia depicts notching on the ST segment after J point (epsilon wave shown by the arrow) in lead V1.

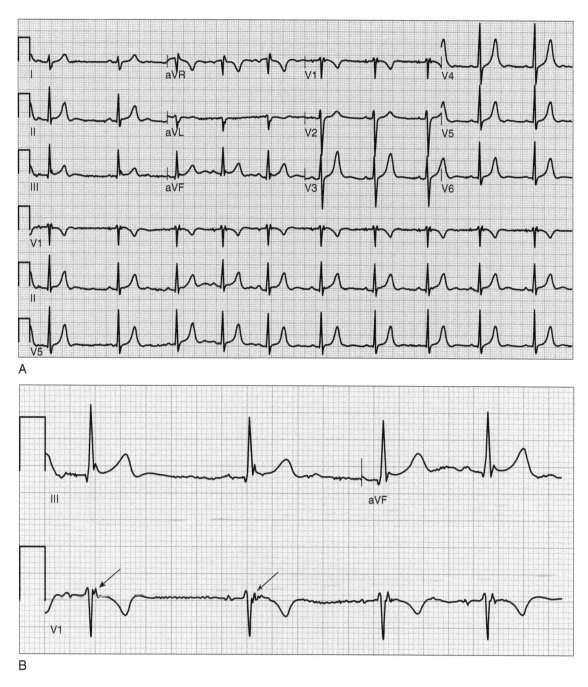

Fig. 12.42 (A) QRS fragmentation in inferior leads and lead V1 in a patient with arrhythmogenic right ventricular dysplasia. (B) Enlargement shows fragmentation of QRS complexes in lead V1, which may also qualify for epsilon waves (*arrows*).

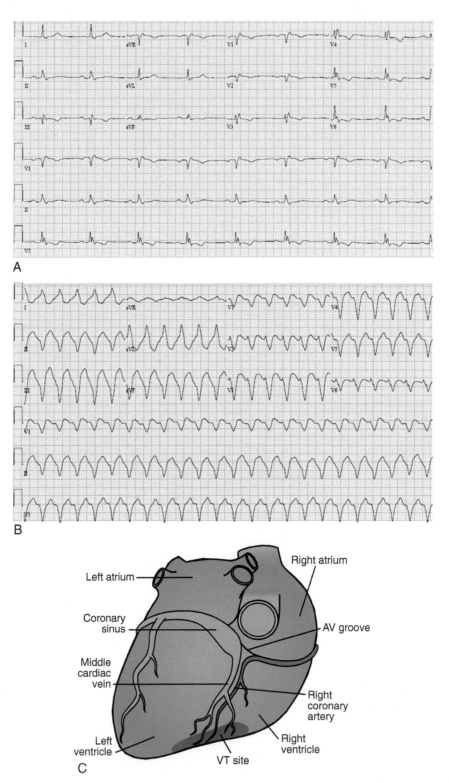

Fig. 12.43 (A) Baseline electrocardiogram of a patient with arrhythmogenic right ventricular dysplasia reveals incomplete right bundle branch block and T wave inversion in leads V1-V3. (B) Ventricular tachycardia (*VT*) in the same patient has left bundle branch block morphology with left superior axis. (C) The circuit was located in the inferolateral right ventricle close to the right ventricular apex. This is not a common site for VT in coronary artery disease or nonischemic cardiomyopathy. *AV,* Atrioventricular.

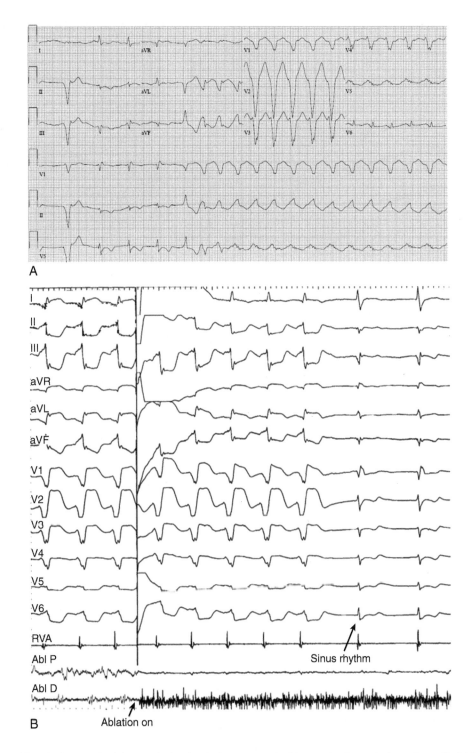

Fig. 12.44 This patient with arrhythmogenic right ventricular dysplasia presented with sustained ventricular tachycardia (*VT*). (A) Electrocardiogram shows right bundle branch block, T wave inversion in leads V1-V3. Spontaneous VT began with a single premature ventricular complex. VT morphology is left bundle branch block, inferior axis with a slurred upstroke, suggestive of epicardial origin. VT was mapped endocardially and epicardially. (B) VT was successfully ablated epicardially in the right ventricular outflow tract (RVOT) area (*arrow*). (C) Radiologic image shows the catheter placement at the successful site of ablation over the RVOT and implantable cardioverter defibrillator area (epi: epicardial, endo: endocardial position of ablation catheter). Electroanatomic voltage mapping revealed a scar in the peritricuspid annulus, RVOT, and inferior right ventricular wall. *Abl P*, Ablation catheter proximal; *Abl D*, ablation catheter distal; *LAD*, left anterior descending artery; *RCA*, right coronary artery; *RV*, right ventricle; *RVA*, right ventricular apex. (Issa ZF, Miller JM, Zipes DP, eds. *Clinical Arrhythmology and Electrophysiology*. Philadelphia, PA: Saunders; 2019:942–967.)

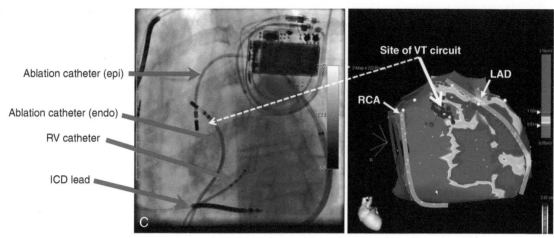

Fig. 12.44 (Continued).

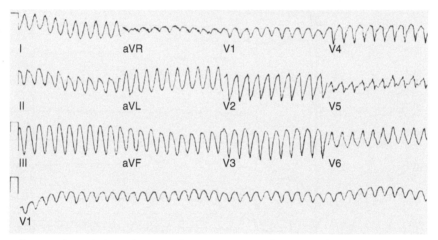

Fig. 12.45 Surface electrocardiogram of ventricular tachycardia after surgical repair of tetralogy of Fallot. Note the left bundle branch block pattern and left superior axis morphology characteristic of clockwise macroreentry around the right ventriculotomy scar. (Issa ZF, Miller JM, Zipes DP, eds. *Clinical Arrhythmology and Electrophysiology.* 3rd edition, Philadelphia, PA: Saunders; 2019.)

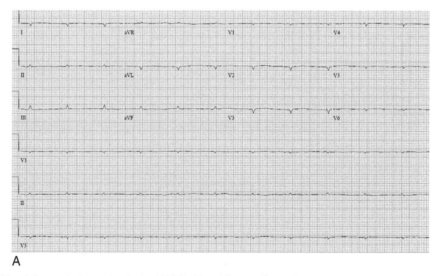

A

Fig. 12.46 This patient with a left ventricular assist device (*LVAD*), HeartMate, suffered from recurrent sustained ventricular tachycardias (VTs) of three different morphologies. (A) Baseline electrocardiogram shows sinus rhythm with generalized low voltage caused by severe cardiomyopathy. (B) Patient had a fast VT with right bundle branch block, right superior axis morphology. (C) The second VT in the same patient has right bundle branch block, right superior axis morphology, and is probably the same VT at a slower rate, owing to antiarrhythmic drug therapy. (D) Electrocardiogram shows the third VT with left bundle branch block morphology; VT terminates with antitachycardia pacing but reinitiates after one sinus beat. The antitachycardia pacing resumes shown with *arrows*. (E) Electroanatomic map reveals scar in the septal aspect of the LVAD. The posteroanterior view radiograph shows the location of the LVAD cannula at the apical region of the left ventricle.

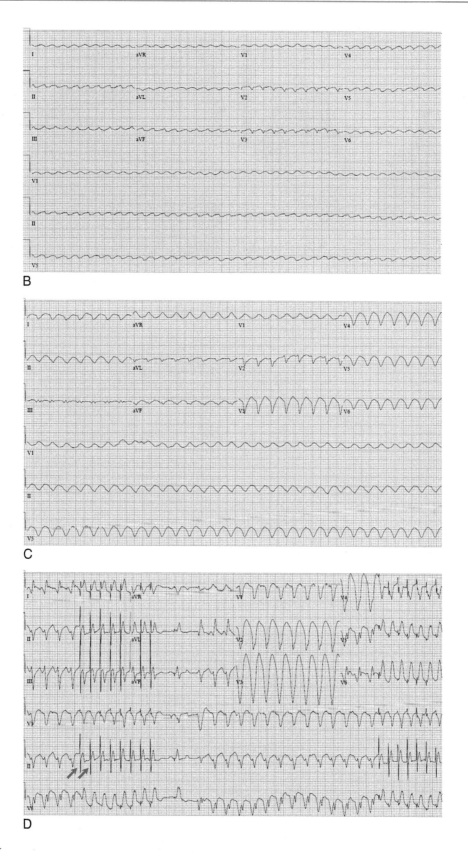

Fig. 12.46 (Continued).

Right anterior oblique   Left anterior oblique

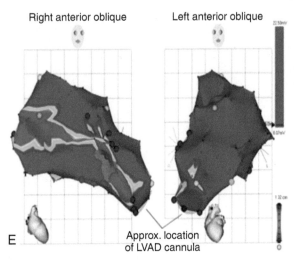
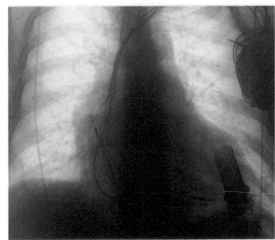

Approx. location
of LVAD cannula

Fig. 12.46 (Continued).

REFERENCES

1. Guandalini GS, Liang JJ, Marchlinski FE. Ventricular tachycardia ablation: past, present, and future perspectives. *JACC Clin Electrophysiol.* 2019;5: 1363–1383.

2. Shivkumar K. Catheter ablation of ventricular arrhythmias. *N Engl J Med.* 2019;380:1555–1564.

3. Das MK, Scott LR, Miller JM. Focal mechanism of ventricular tachycardia in coronary artery disease. *Heart Rhythm.* 2010;7:305–311.

4. Blanck Z, Sra J, Akhtar M. Incessant interfascicular reentrant ventricular tachycardia as a result of catheter ablation of the right bundle branch: case report and review of the literature. *J Cardiovasc Electrophysiol.* 2009;20: 1279–1283.

5. Vallés E, Bazan V, Marchlinski FE. ECG criteria to identify epicardial ventricular tachycardia in nonischemic cardiomyopathy. *Circ Arrhythm Electrophysiol.* 2010;3(1):63–71.

6. Gandjbakhch E, Redheuil A, Pousset F, Charron P, Frank R. Clinical diagnosis, imaging, and genetics of arrhythmogenic right ventricular cardiomyopathy/dysplasia: JACC state-of-the-art review. *J Am Coll Cardiol.* 2018;72:784–804.

7. Dandamudi G, Ghumman WS, Das MK, Miller JM. Endocardial catheter ablation of ventricular tachycardia in patients with ventricular assist devices. *Heart Rhythm.* 2007;4:1165–1169.

8. Daniels DV, Lu YY, Morton JB, et al. Idiopathic epicardial left ventricular tachycardia originating remote from the sinus of Valsalva: electrophysiological characteristics, catheter ablation, and identification from the 12-lead electrocardiogram. *Circulation.* 2006;113:1659–1666.

Polymorphic Ventricular Tachycardia and Ventricular Fibrillation in the Absence of Structural Heart Disease

Polymorphic ventricular tachycardia (VT) and ventricular fibrillation (VF) more commonly occur in patients with structural heart disease but can occur in the presence of structurally normal hearts as a result of primary electrical instability of the heart. *Polymorphic VT* is defined as a ventricular rhythm greater than 100 bpm with frequent variations of the QRS axis, morphology, or both. The majority of these arrhythmias are inherited and can be initiated by one or more premature ventricular complexes (PVCs). Polymorphic VT in the setting of prolonged QT interval is called *torsades de pointes* (TdP) (Table 13.1).[1] Polymorphic VT with variations in morphology can take the form of a progressive, sinusoidal, cyclic alteration of the QRS axis. The peaks of the QRS complexes appear to "twist" around the isoelectric line of the recording. Therefore it was named TdP, or "twisting of the points." In TdP, usually the ventricular rate is 160 to 250 bpm, and the QRS axis cycles through 180 degrees every 5 to 20 beats. TdP is most commonly initiated by short-long R-R intervals and is usually repetitive, short-lived, and terminates spontaneously (Fig. 13.1). However, these episodes can recur in rapid succession, potentially degenerating to VF and sudden cardiac arrest.

INHERITED AND ACQUIRED LONG QT SYNDROME AND TORSADES DE POINTES

QT interval signifies the duration of cardiac repolarization beginning from the onset of ventricular systole to the end of the T wave. In normal physiologic states, repolarization is longer at slower heart rates and shorter at higher heart rates. The corrected QT interval is used to normalize the QT interval to a heart rate of 60 bpm. Several formulas exist to do this, and none of them are considered perfect. The Bazett formula is commonly used to correct the QT interval (QTc) by dividing the QT interval in milliseconds by the square root of the R-R interval in seconds (QTc = QT in ms/ $\sqrt{RR}$ in sec). A QTc interval longer than 460 ms for men and longer than 470 ms for women is generally considered abnormal. Other formulae, such as Fridericia correction, is calculated as the QT/RR1/3, whereas the Framingham correction is calculated as QT + 0.154 (1 − RR). The long QT syndrome (LQTS) can be both acquired and inherited with acquired more common than inherited. LQTS is associated with polymorphic VT. Polymorphic VT in the presence of long QT duration is known as TdP. These patients may present with syncope caused by a self-terminating TdP (Fig. 13.2), or they may present with sudden cardiac death (SCD) as a result of TdP and VF (Fig. 13.3). *Congenital LQTS* refers to a group of inherited disorders caused by mutations of genes encoding the structure of cardiac K^+, Na^+, and Ca^+ ion channels and membrane-anchoring proteins.

Phenotypically, two hereditary variants of LQTS have been recognized since 1975: the autosomal dominant Romano-Ward syndrome, and the autosomal recessive Jervell and Lange-Nielsen syndrome, which is associated with sensorineural deafness (Figs. 13.4 and 13.5). A recessive form of the Romano-Ward syndrome has been described in one family of individuals homozygous for mutations in the *KVLQT1* gene. Presently, 12 types of LQTS have been described (Table 13.2).[7] Up to 11% of patients with the LQTS gene mutation have a normal QTc, and a genetic study is needed to diagnose these cases. The autosomal dominant trait is the most common form of LQTS. Of LQTS cases, 75% are caused by mutations in three genes (35% to *KCNQ* [LQTS1], 30% to *KCNH2* [LQTS2], and 10% to *SCN5A* [LQTS3]). Episodes of TdP in patients with LQTS can be precipitated by emotional or physical stress. Genotype-phenotype correlations have been observed and include swimming- or exertion-provoked TdP in LQTS1, auditory triggers or postpartum period TdP in LQTS2, and sleep- or rest-associated TdP in LQT3. LQTS4 to LQTS12, which also include Andersen-Tawil syndrome (LQTS7) and Timothy syndrome (LQTS8), are much less prevalent. Sinus bradycardia and sinus pauses can occur in LQTS3. In addition, 2:1 atrioventricular (AV) block can also be present in LQT1, LQT3, and Andersen-Tawil syndrome. Macroscopic T wave alternans can appear before TdP in patients with LQTS. Patients with QTc greater than 500 ms, LQTS3 genotype, Jervell and Lange-Nielsen syndrome, LQTS with syndactyly, male sex during childhood, and history of syncope or near-syncope are considered to be at high risk for SCD, whereas the family history of SCD is not a significant risk factor for SCD.

Clinical diagnosis of LQTS can be made using the diagnostic criteria based on a point system (Table 13.3). A score of less than 1 point is associated with low probability of LQTS, a score of greater than 1 to 3 points is associated with intermediate probability of LQTS, and a score of 3.5 or more points is associated with a high probability of LQTS.

Gene-specific electrocardiogram (ECG) patterns of repolarization have been identified. Patients with LQT1 tend to have smooth, broad-based T waves (Fig. 13.5), whereas patients with LQT2 frequently have low-amplitude and notched T waves (Figs. 13.6 and 13.7). Emotional stress and sudden loud noises can cause a rapid increase in heart rate from sympathetic discharge, which acutely prolongs the action potential before subsequent shortening by a slowed enhancement of I_{Ks}. This acute prolongation of the action potential enhances transmural repolarization heterogeneity and triggers TdP in patients with reduced I_{Kr}. Bradycardia reduces I_{Kr}, delays repolarization, and increases transmural dispersion. Therefore both sudden catecholamine surge and bradycardia can trigger arrhythmias in LQT2. Patients with LQT3 have a more distinctive pattern characterized by a prolonged JT segment (late onset of T wave; Figs. 13.8–13.11). However, T wave morphologies are not specific for a particular LQTS and may vary even within families (Figs. 13.12 and 13.13). ECG analysis in identifying the genetic substrate is as high as 85% and 83% in LQTS1 and LQTS2, respectively, but unsatisfactory for LQT3 (43%). LQTS4 is associated with marked sinus node dysfunction, sinus bradycardia or junctional escape rhythm, and episodes of atrial fibrillation. Sudden death occurs after physical exertion or emotional stress. LQTS5 is shown in Fig. 13.14.

TABLE 13.1	Ventricular Tachycardia and Ventricular Fibrillation in Structurally Normal Heart	
Inheritance	Disease	Comments
Inherited disorders	Congenital long QT syndrome	Acquired form (more common)
	Congenital short QT syndrome	Risk for ventricular and atrial arrhythmias
	Brugada syndrome	Brugada-pattern electrocardiogram can be acquired
	Catecholaminergic polymorphic VT	Exercise induced, beta blocker sensitive
Noninherited (?)	Idiopathic VF	Early repolarization abnormalities occur in one-third of patients
	Pause-dependent TdP	Occurs in the setting of bradycardia or heart block
	Short-coupled TdP	Verapamil sensitive
	Acquired long QT syndrome	? Ion channel polymorphism

TdP, Torsades de pointes; *VF*, ventricular fibrillation; *VT*, ventricular tachycardia.

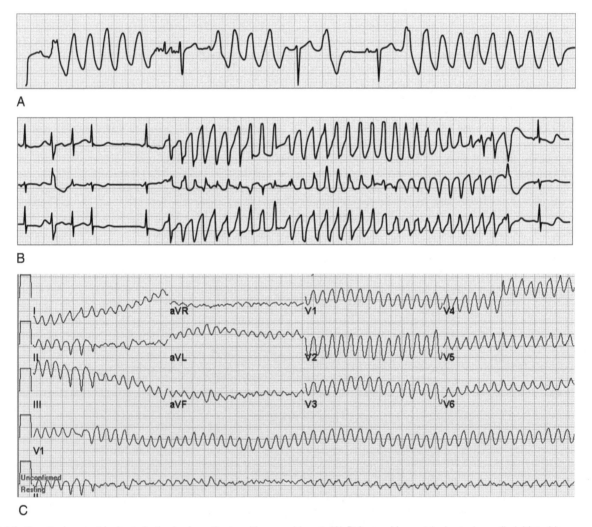

Fig. 13.1 Life-threatening ventricular arrhythmias in patients with normal heart. (A) Polymorphic ventricular tachycardia initiated by monomorphic premature ventricular complexes with a short coupling interval (360 ms). (B) Polymorphic ventricular tachycardia in the presence of long QT (torsades de pointes). (C) Ventricular fibrillation.

Long QT Syndrome 7 (Andersen-Tawil Syndrome)

Andersen-Tawil syndrome results from a mutation of the *KCNJ2* gene (Fig. 13.15). It is an autosomal dominant or sporadic disorder characterized by periodic paralysis and dysmorphic features. ECG findings include mild QTc interval prolongation but marked prolongation of the QUc interval (interval between the initiation of Q wave to end of U wave); prolongation of the T wave downslope; wide T-U junction; and high-amplitude, broad U waves. Arrhythmias associated with LQTS7 include frequent PVCs, bidirectional VT, and polymorphic VT[13] (Fig. 13.16).

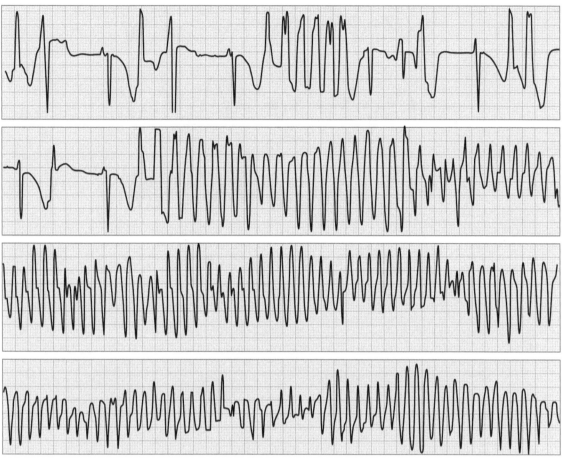

Fig. 13.2 Nonsustained and sustained torsades de pointes. Sinus rhythm with prolonged QT interval and frequent premature ventricular complexes on the T waves resulted into a six-beat run of polymorphic ventricular tachycardia followed by a sustained torsades de pointes.

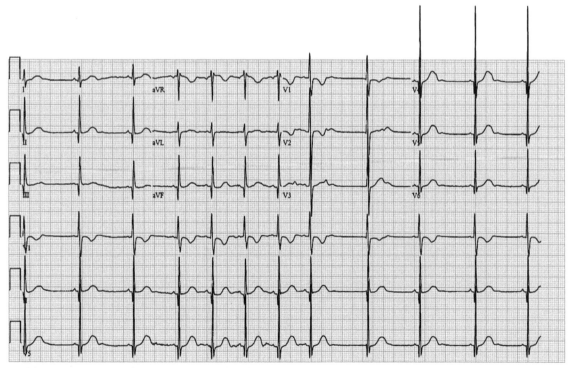

Fig. 13.3 Long QT syndrome with deafness (Jervell and Lange-Nielsen syndrome). Electrocardiogram of a 2-year-old boy with long QT syndrome, deafness, and syncope shows a five-beat run of atrial tachycardia. QTc at baseline is 431 ms and during the atrial tachycardia at 100 bpm is 520 ms.

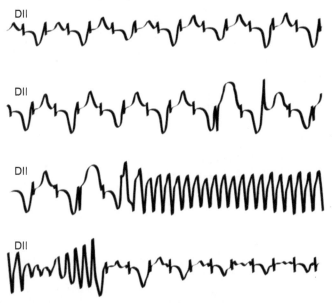

Fig. 13.4 Tracing recorded from a 5-year-old patient with Jervell and Lange-Nielsen syndrome during a syncopal episode. T wave alternans precedes the onset of torsades de pointes; the torsade event is not preceded by a pause. (From Pernot C. Le syndrome cardio-auditif de Jervell et Lange-Nielsen. Aspects electrocardiographiques. *Proc Assoc Europ Paediatr Cardiol.* 1972;8:28—36.)

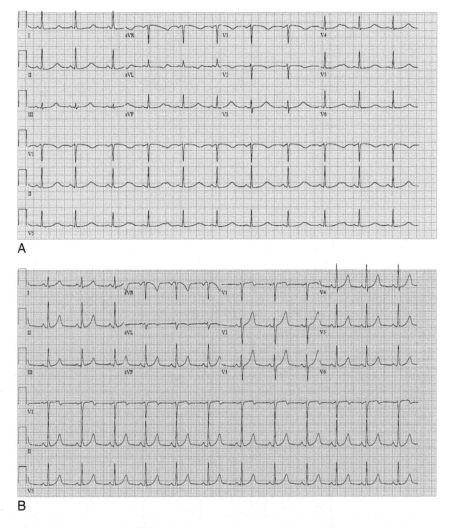

Fig. 13.5 Genetically proven long QT syndrome 1 (LQTS1). (A) Electrocardiogram of 48-year-old woman with history of multiple presyncope and syncope with QT/QTc intervals of 626/656 ms. The T wave is broad and smooth, which is commonly seen in LQTS1. (B) Electrocardiogram of a 34-year-old woman with LQTS1 and QT/QTC of 416/461 ms. She underwent genetic testing after her two daughters were diagnosed with LQTS1.

TABLE 13.2 Gene Mutations Associated With Inherited Cardiac Arrhythmia Syndromes

Channel Dysfunction[2,3]	Gene Mutation	Ion Current	Protein/Aliases	Gene Locus	GAIN-OF-FUNCTION MUTATION[2]			LOSS-OF-FUNCTION MUTATION[2]			
					Clinical Syndrome	Inheritance	Drugs to Reduce Risk of VT/VF	Locus	Clinical Syndrome	Inheritance	Drugs to Reduce Risk of VT/VF
Na$^+$ channel	SCN5A	I_{Na}	$Na_V 1.5$	3p21	LQTS 3	AD	Mexiletine, flecainide, ranolazine	3p21	Brugada syndrome 1	AD	
									Sick sinus syndrome 1	AD/AR	
	GPD1L	?I_{Na}						3p24	Brugada syndrome 2	AD	
	HCN4	I_f[a]		11q23.3				15q24 – q25	Sick sinus syndrome 2	AD	
	SCN4B	I_{Na}	$Na_V \beta4$	11q23.3	LQTS 10[4]	AD					
	SCN1B	I_{Na}	$Na_V \beta1$	19q13.1	Brugada syndrome 5 + conduction defects[3]						
	SNAT1	I_{Na}	Alpha-1-syntrophin protein	20q11.2	LQTS 12	AD					
K$^+$ channels/anchoring proteins	KCNQ1	I_{Ks}	KvLQT1	11p15	SQTS 2	AD		11p15	LQTS 1	AD	Beta blocker
								11p15	J-LN syndrome 1	AR	
	KCNH2	I_{Kr}	hERG	7q35	SQTS 1	AD	Quinidine, disopyramide	7q35	LQTS 2	AD	Beta blocker, oral K$^+$
	ANK2	Multiple	Ankyrin B					4q25	LQTS 4	AD	
	KCNE1	I_{Ks}	mink					21q22	LQTS 5	AD	
								21q22	J-LN syndrome 2	AR	
	KCNE2	I_{Kr}	MiRP1					21q22	LQTS 6	AD	
	KCNE3	I_{to}	MiRP2	11q13-q14	Brugada syndrome 6	?AD					
	KCNJ2	I_{K1}	IK1	17q23.1-24.2	SQTS 3	AD		17q23	LQTS 7	AD	Flecainide
		I_{Ks}	A-Kinase–anchoring protein	7q21-q22				AKAP-9	LQTS 11	AD	
	KCNJ5	$I_{K,Ach}$	Kir3.4					11q24	Long QT 13	AD	
Calcium channels/anchoring proteins	RYR2 (? Not anchoring to K channel)	I_{Ca}	Ryanodine receptor	1q42-43	CPVT 1	AD	Beta blocker, verapamil, flecainide[5]				
	CASQ2	I_{Ca}	Calsequestrin	1p13-21	CPVT 2	AR	Beta blocker, verapamil				
	CACNA1C	I_{Ca}	$Ca_V1.2$	12p13.3				12p13.3	Short QT syndrome 4 (Brugada syndrome 3)	AD	Quinidine

(Continued)

TABLE 13.2 Gene Mutations Associated With Inherited Cardiac Arrhythmia Syndromes—cont'd

Channel Dysfunction[2,3]	Gene Mutation	Protein/Aliases	Ion Current	GAIN-OF-FUNCTION MUTATION[2]				LOSS-OF-FUNCTION MUTATION[2]			
				Gene Locus	Clinical Syndrome	Inheritance	Drugs to Reduce Risk of VT/VF	Locus	Clinical Syndrome	Inheritance	Drugs to Reduce Risk of VT/VF
	CACNB2b	$Ca_v\beta_{2b}$	I_{Ca}					10q12.33	Short QT syndrome 5 (Brugada syndrome 4)	AD	
	$Ca_v1.2$	Ca_v 1.2 (β_{2b} subunit)	I_{Ca}	6q8A	Timothy syndrome (LQT8)	AD	Verapamil, ranolazine				
	Ca_v3	Caveolin (β_{2b} subunit)	I_{Ca}	3p25	LQTS 9[6]	AD					
	CALM1	Calmodulin 1	IcaL	14q24-q31	Long QT syndrome 14	Sporadic					
	CALM2	Calmodulin 2	IcaL	2p21	Long QT syndrome 15	Sporadic					
	CALM1	Calmodulin 3	IcaL	19q13	Long QT syndrome 16	Sporadic					
?								19q13	Progressive familial heart block II	AD	
?								1q32.2-32.3	Progressive familial heart block II	AD	

AD, Autosomal dominant; AR, autosomal recessive; CPVT, catecholaminergic polymorphic ventricular tachycardia; GPD1L, glycerol-3-phosphate dehydrogenase 1–like gene (?ion channel modulator); J-LN, Jervell and Lange-Nielsen syndrome; LQTS, long QT syndrome; SQTS, short QT syndrome; VF, ventricular fibrillation; VT, ventricular tachycardia.

[a]Not a pure Na current.

Adapted with permission from Giudicessi JR, Wilde AAM, Ackerman MJ. The genetic architecture of long QT syndrome: a critical reappraisal. *Trends Cardiovasc Med.* 2018;28(7):453-464.

TABLE 13.3 Diagnostic Criteria for Long QT Syndrome[8]

Criteria			Points
Electrocardiogram findings[a]	QTc interval[b]	>480 ms	3
		460–479 ms	2
		<460 ms	1
	Torsades de pointes		2
	T wave alternans		1
	Notched T wave in three leads		1
	Low heart rate for age[c]		0.5
Clinical history	Syncope[d]		1
	Congenital deafness		0.5
Family history	A. Family history of definite LQTS		1
	B. Unexplained SCD at younger than 30 years of age among immediate family members[e]		0.5

LQTS, Long QT syndrome; *SCD,* sudden cardiac death.

[a]In the absence of medications or disorders known to affect these electrocardiographic features.

[b]QTc calculated by Bazett formula, where QTc = QT/$\sqrt{R\text{-}R}$.

[c]Resting heart rate below the second percentile for age.

[d]Mutually exclusive.

[e]The same family member cannot be counted in both A and B.

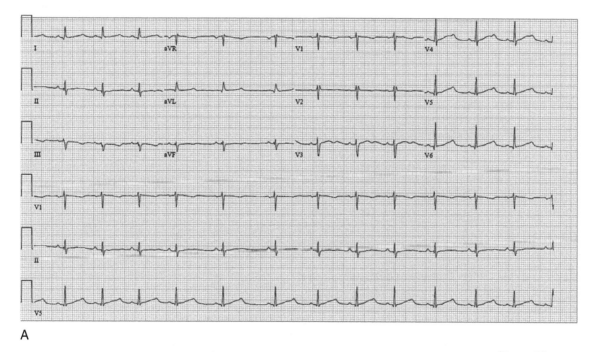

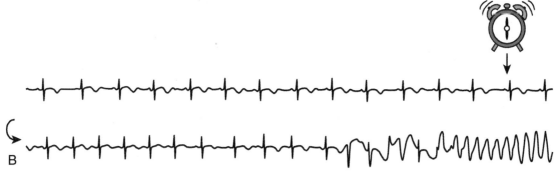

Fig. 13.6 Long QT syndrome 2 (LQTS2) with torsades de pointes provoked by swimming and auditory stimuli. (A) Electrocardiogram of an 11-year-old boy with LQTS2 and family history of sudden death who had appropriate implantable cardioverter-defibrillator shock for ventricular tachycardia during swimming. Electrocardiogram shows QT/QTc intervals of 472/531 ms. T wave is broad, low amplitude, and notched, as typically seen in LQTS2. (B) Auditory stimulus in long QT syndrome: sudden loud sound from alarm clock during early morning shortens R-R interval from 1060 to 680 ms and triggers torsades de pointes in a patient with LQTS2.[9] (Reproduced with permission from Morita H, Wu J, Zipes DP. The QT syndromes: long and short. *Lancet.* 2008;372:750–756.)

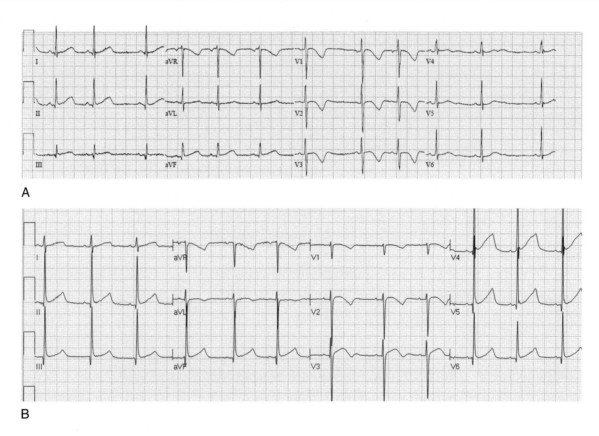

Fig. 13.7 Long QT syndrome 2 (LQTS2). (A and B) Electrocardiograms of two brothers with symptomatic genetically proven LQTS2. Both patients and one of the other unaffected siblings have a seizure disorder. Incidence of seizure disorder is 39% in LQTS, whereas LQTS1 and LQTS3 are not associated with significant risk of seizure disorder.

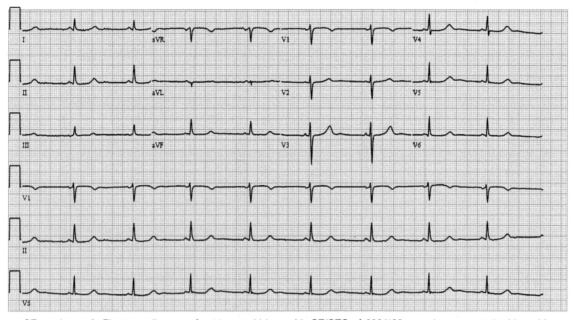

Fig. 13.8 Long QT syndrome 3. Electrocardiogram of a 14-year-old boy with QT/QTC of 633/483 ms who presented with sudden cardiac death. The long JT segment electrocardiogram is consistent with long QT syndrome 3.

Long QT Syndrome 8 (Timothy Syndrome)

LQTS8 (Figs. 13.17–13.19) is a syndactyly associated repolarization disorder caused by missense mutation in $Ca_V1.2$, resulting in a gain of function of the L-type Ca^+ current. It is a multisystem disorder (several cardiac and extracardiac abnormalities). Fetal bradycardia or bradycardia soon after birth is often the initial manifestation of the disease. ECG usually shows markedly prolonged QT interval (> 550 ms) and 2:1 AV block owing to a long ventricular refractory period (Fig. 13.17).[2]

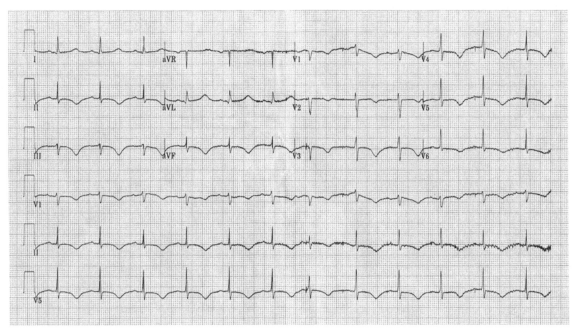

Fig. 13.9 Long QT syndrome 3. Electrocardiogram of a 37-year-old woman with long QT syndrome 3 who developed ventricular tachycardia and ventricular fibrillation storm with cocaine and methadone use. The QT/QTc are 600/667 ms. VT storm was treated successfully with flecainide therapy.

T wave alternans on 12-lead ECG is seen in 62% of patients. VT/VF occurs in approximately 80% of patients (Figs. 13.18 and 13.19). The mortality rate is 58%, with a mean age at death of 2.5 years in these patients. ECGs of LQTS9 (Fig. 13.20) and LQTS12 (Fig. 13.21) with nonischemic dilated cardiomyopathy are also shown.

Long QT Syndrome and Other Associated Cardiac Abnormalities

LQTS can be associated with other cardiac abnormalities, such as Brugada syndrome, hypertrophic cardiomyopathy (Fig. 13.22), and ventricular preexcitation (Fig. 13.23).

Acquired Long QT Syndrome

Acquired LQTS is more commonly associated with electrolyte imbalance (hypokalemia, hypomagnesemia) or the use of QT-prolonging drugs. The risk for developing TdP in the presence of hypokalemia, hypomagnesemia, or both is greatest in patients taking antiarrhythmic drugs. Intracranial (subarachnoid and intraparenchymal) hemorrhage and ischemic stroke can be associated with significant ST-T changes and prolonged QT interval. TdP in stroke is often associated with concomitant hypokalemia. Fragmentation of QRS in acquired LQTS is a predictor of arrhythmic event (Fig. 13.24).[3]

Electrolyte Imbalance

Hypokalemia. Hypokalemia produces changes in the ECG that are not necessarily correlated with the serum potassium level. ECG manifestations of hypokalemia include flattened or inverted T waves, a U wave (more prominent in the lateral precordial leads V4-V6), ST depression, and a prolonged QT interval. Prominent U waves can occur at the end of the T wave with minimum T-U wave fusion (Fig. 13.25). The P wave can become larger and wider, and the P-R interval can prolong slightly (Fig. 13.26). In severe hypokalemia, QRS duration can increase, ST segment can become markedly depressed, and T waves can become inverted. Hypokalemia alone or with concomitant QT-prolonging drug therapy can cause TdP (Fig. 13.27).

Hypocalcemia. Hypocalcemia causes prolongation of the QT interval. This is caused by lengthening of the JT (interval from the end of J wave to initiation of T wave) segment as a result of a delay in the onset of membrane repolarization, whereas the T wave (which correlates with the time for repolarization) onset and duration remain unaltered. QT prolongation is more commonly present with hypokalemia (Fig. 13.28) or hyperkalemia (Fig. 13.29).

Hypomagnesemia. The diagnosis of hypomagnesemia can be made by finding a plasma magnesium concentration of less than 0.7 mmol/L. Because most magnesium is intracellular, a body deficit can be present with a normal plasma concentration. In addition to hypomagnesemia, up to 40% of cases will also have hypocalcemia, and in up to 60% of cases hypokalemia will also be present.

Drug Induced

Drug-induced LQTS is mostly a result of blocking the I_{Kr} current mediated by the potassium channel encoded by the *hERG* gene. Common drugs are class I and III antiarrhythmic agents. Certain antipsychotic medications (chlorpromazine, haloperidol), a few antihistamines (terfenadine, astemizole), a few antibiotics (azithromycin, clarithromycin, levofloxacin, erythromycin), protease inhibitors used for human immunodeficiency virus disease, gastrointestinal drugs (cisapride, domperidone), and opiate agonists (methadone) also cause QT prolongation. A useful website lists QT prolonging drugs: https://www.crediblemeds.org.

Antiarrhythmic Drug-Induced Long QT Syndrome. Class IA and class III drugs are K^+ channel blockers, and therefore prolong the ventricular repolarization, causing lengthening of the QT interval and increasing the vulnerability to TdP. With quinidine use, the incidence of drug-induced TdP is 0.6% to 1.5%, and most cases occur within 48 hours of initiating drug therapy (Fig. 13.30). Concomitant hypokalemia and excessive bradycardia increase the risk of TdP in these patients.

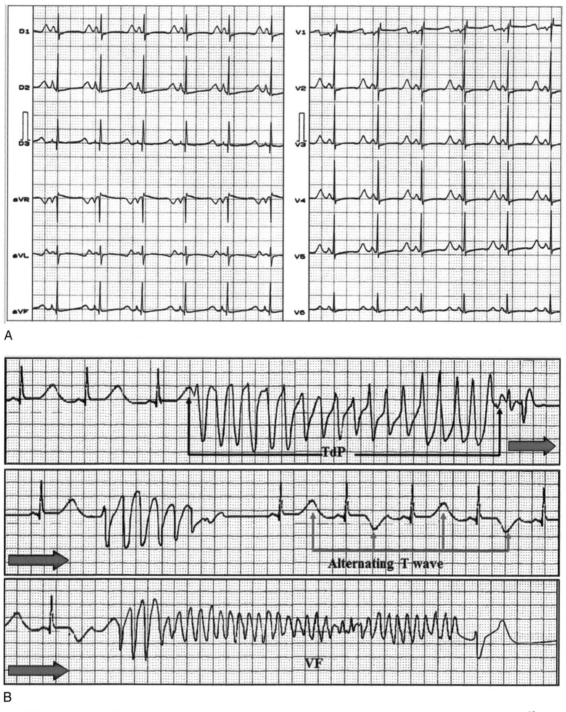

Fig. 13.10 Long QT syndrome 3 (LQTS3). Rhythm strip of a patient of LQTS3 demonstrates the typical prolonged JT segment.[10] Horizontal arrows show continuation of the electrocardiogram (ECG) rhythm strip. (A) ECG of newborn baby with LQTS3. Clear ST segment prolongation and delayed appearance of T wave. (B) ECG shows QTc of 670 ms and short runs of torsades de pointes (*TdP*) after macro wave T alternans. T-wave alternans is a diagnostic feature of the LQT and reflects an enhanced electrical instability during repolarization. (From Perez-Riera AR, Barbosa-Barros R, Daminello Raimundo R, da Costa de Rezende Barbosa MP, Esposito Sorpreso IC, de Abreu LC. The congenital long QT syndrome type 3: an update. *Indian Pacing Electrophysiol J.* 2018;18:25–35.) *VF*, Ventricular fibrillation. Arrows signify that the rhythm is in continuation.

The incidence of TdP is approximately 2% with sotalol (Fig. 13.31), 0.9% to 3.5% with dofetilide (Fig. 13.32), 2% to 3% with ibutilide, and less than 1% with amiodarone (Fig. 13.33) therapy. Beta blockers, calcium blockers, and class IC drugs, as well as class III antiarrhythmic drugs, can cause sinus and AV node dysfunction. Methadone can cause QT prolongation and TdP (Fig. 13.34). Of note, grapefruit juice consumption can also cause QT prolongation.[4]

CEREBROVASCULAR ACCIDENTS

ECG manifestation of cerebrovascular accidents includes transient ST-T changes in lateral leads. The typical findings are flat or slightly negative T waves, horizontal or downsloping ST segments, and sometimes a small ST depression (Fig. 13.35). A transient prolonged QT interval and transient U waves appear in few patients. ECG signs do correlate

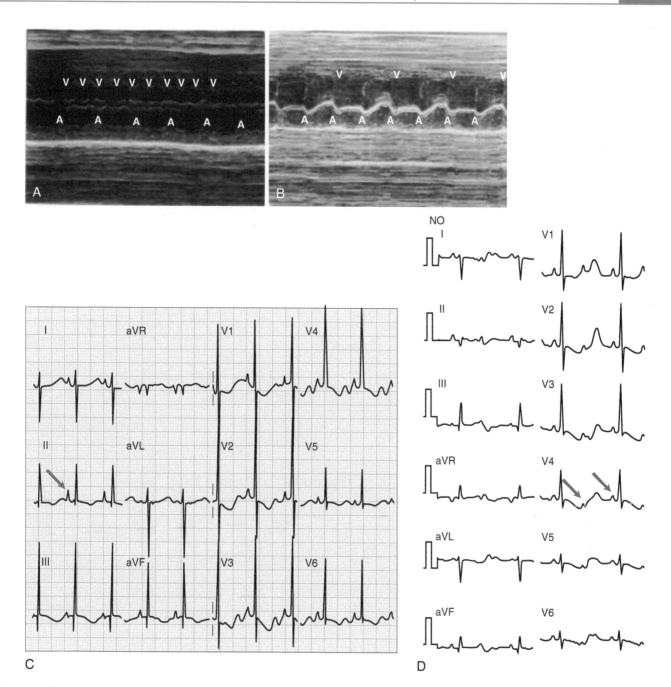

Fig. 13.11 Electrocardiogram and echocardiography of a fetus with long QT syndrome 3 phenotype at gestational week 26 with frequent 2:1 atrioventricular block and nonsustained ventricular tachycardia (VT).[11] Patient had compound effects of hERG pore region mutation and SCN5A N-terminus variant. It is associated with spontaneous or lidocaine-induced VT. (A) M-mode fetal echocardiogram with simultaneous recording of the left ventricle (V) and left atrium (A). VT was diagnosed from the rapid ventricular rate with dissociated ventriculoatrial conduction. (B) Tachycardia stopped after lidocaine was discontinued, and the rhythm showed an atrial rate of 130/min that conducted to the ventricle in a 2:1 fashion. (C) Electrocardiogram recorded soon after birth. Paper speed 25 mm/s; 1 mV = 10 mm. P waves are shown by *red arrows*. The corrected QT interval at a sinus rate of 104/min was 600 ms, and the T wave was broad. (D) On the same day, when the sinus rate accelerated to 140/min, 2:1 block developed as a result of an extremely prolonged QT interval. Arrows show P waves.

with the location of the vascular lesion seen on computed tomography or the clinical outcome.

SHORT QT SYNDROME

Short QT syndrome (SQTS) is associated with gain of function of cardiac K^+ channels as a result of the mutation of genes *KCNH2* (SQTS1), *KCNQ1* (SQTS2), and *KCNJ2* (SQTS3) and loss-of-function mutations in L-type

Ca^{2+} channel genes *CACNA1C* (SQTS4), *CACNB2b* (SQTS5), *CACNB2AD1* (SQTS6), and SCN5A (SQTS7). SQTS4 and SQTS5 share some ECG features of Brugada syndrome with ST elevation in leads V1-V3. Both changes shorten ventricular repolarization. SQTS is associated with risk of VT/VF and SCD, as well as atrial fibrillation. In addition to a short QTc (<370 ms), the following ECG findings are required to make the diagnosis of inherited SQTS:
1. ST segment is universally absent; the QRS complex connects directly to the T wave (Figs. 13.36 and 13.37).

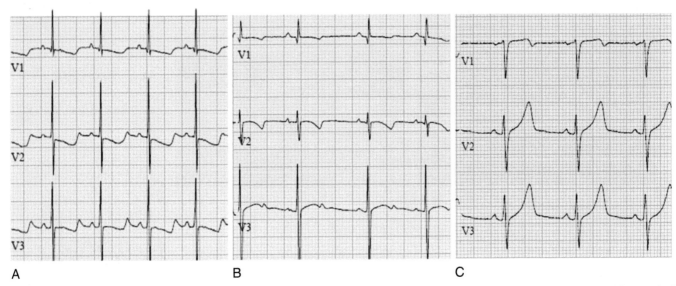

Fig. 13.12 Different T wave morphologies in long QT syndrome 1. (A–C) Electrocardiograms (ECGs) of the affected members with genetically proven long QT syndrome 1. (A and B) are the ECGs of two sisters, and (C) is the ECG of the mother (patient in Fig. 13.5B), which shows biphasic, notched, and tall T waves, respectively.

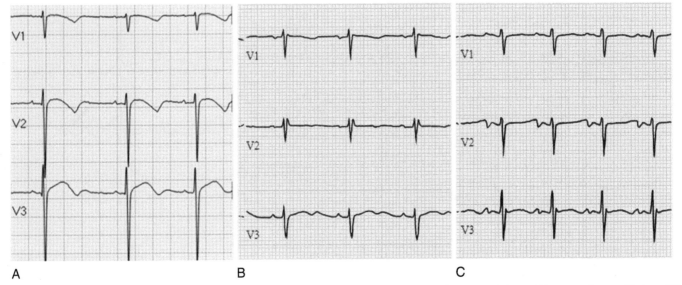

Fig. 13.13 Different T wave morphologies in long QT syndrome 2. (A–C) are the electrocardiograms of three different patients with long QT syndrome 2.

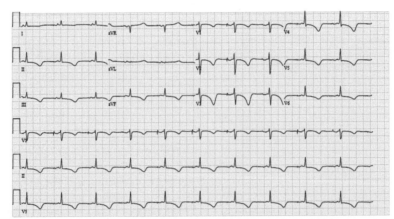

Fig. 13.14 Long QT syndrome 5. Electrocardiogram of a 43-year-old woman shows a prolonged QT/QTc of 536/536 ms and family history of sudden death (one sister and one daughter). Patient received a dual-chamber pacemaker for bradycardia.

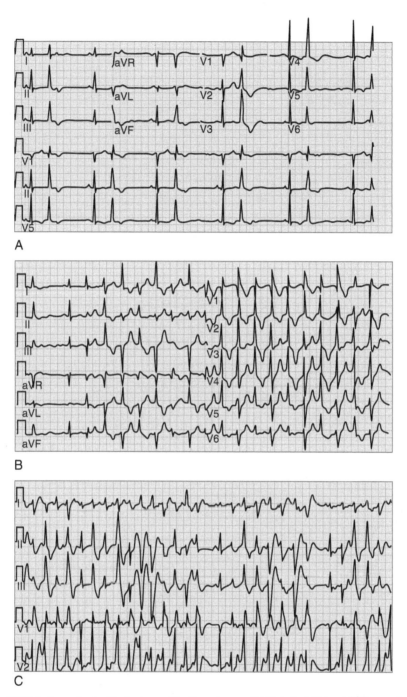

Fig. 13.15 Electrocardiograms (ECGs) of a patient with Andersen-Tawil syndrome. (A) Standard 12-lead ECG recorded at rest demonstrating sinus rhythm and ventricular bigeminy with a right bundle branch block morphology. (B) Standard 12-lead ECG recorded at rest demonstrating bidirectional ventricular tachycardia. These arrhythmias were asymptomatic. (C) Six-lead ECG recorded during exercise stress testing. Note the short bouts of polymorphic ventricular tachycardia.[12] (Reproduced with permission from Schoonderwoerd BA, Wiesfeld AC, Wilde AA, et al. A family with Andersen-Tawil syndrome and dilated cardiomyopathy. *Heart Rhythm.* 2006;3(11):1346–1350.)

2. T waves are tall, peaked, and narrow based, particularly in the precordial leads. These T waves resemble those seen in hyperkalemia.
3. The U wave is often prominent and separated from the T wave by an isoelectric T-U segment.
4. There is minimal rate dependency of the QT interval with changing heart rates. The QT interval fails to prolong even at slow rates.

5. Relatively prolonged $T_{peak}-T_{end}$ interval compared with patients with incidental short QTc for other causes (81 ± 21 ms vs. 67 ± 13 ms, $P < 0.001$) suggestive of augmented transmural dispersion of refractoriness.[5]

Causes of acquired SQTS include hyperkalemia; hypercalcemia (Fig. 13.38); acidosis; hyperthermia; tachycardia; alterations in the

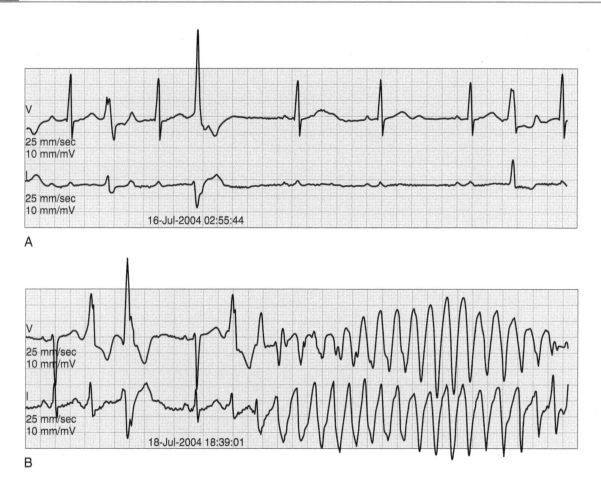

Fig. 13.16 Telemetry tracings. (A) Rare presence of three consecutive sinus beats. Note the prolonged terminal T wave downslope and the prolonged QTU interval with prominent U wave. (B) Torsades de pointes. During this episode, the patient experienced dizziness. Potassium level was 4.0 mmol/L.[12] (Reproduced with permission from Schoonderwoerd BA, Wiesfeld AC, Wilde AA, et al. A family with Andersen-Tawil syndrome and dilated cardiomyopathy. *Heart Rhythm*. 2006;3(11):1346−1350.)

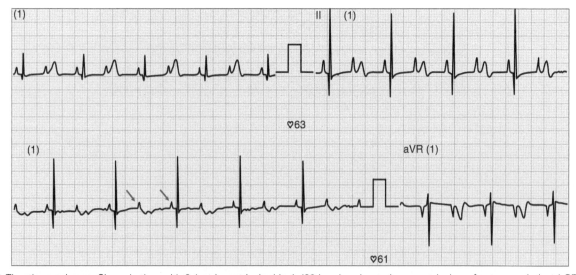

Fig. 13.17 Timothy syndrome. Sinus rhythm with 2:1 atrioventricular block (60 bpm) owing to long ventricular refractory period and QT interval of 570 ms.[14,15] P waves are shown by *red arrows*. (Reproduced with permission from Lo-A-Njoe SM, Wilde AA, van Erven L, Blom NA. Syndactyly and long QT syndrome (CaV1.2 missense mutation G406R) is associated with hypertrophic cardiomyopathy. *Heart Rhythm*. 2005;2 (12):1365−1368.)

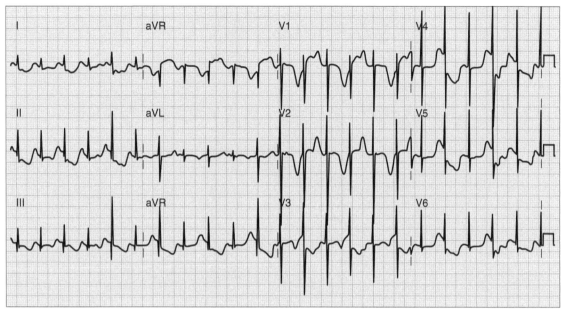

Fig. 13.18 Electrocardiogram of another patient with Timothy syndrome showing QT/QTc of 420/650 ms and T wave alternans. Alternate T waves (inverted) extend until the initiation of the next QRS complexes in lead V2.[15] (Reproduced with permission from Lo-A-Njoe SM, Wilde AA, van Erven L, Blom NA. Syndactyly and long QT syndrome (CaV1.2 missense mutation G406R) is associated with hypertrophic cardiomyopathy. *Heart Rhythm.* 2005;2(12):1365–1368.)

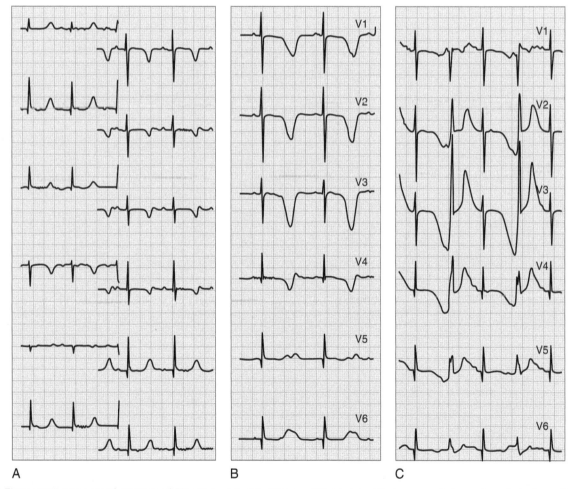

Fig. 13.19 Electrocardiogram manifestations of Timothy syndrome. (A) Long QT syndrome 3–type morphology of repolarization with straight ST segment and small T waves. (B) Giant negative T waves on precordial leads with notches. (C) Macroscopic T wave alternans with extremely prolonged ventricular repolarization, causing intraventricular conduction delay on a beat-to-beat basis. (Zipes DP, Jalife J. *Cardiac Electrophysiology: From Cell to Bedside.* 7th ed. Philadelphia, PA: Saunders; 2017.)

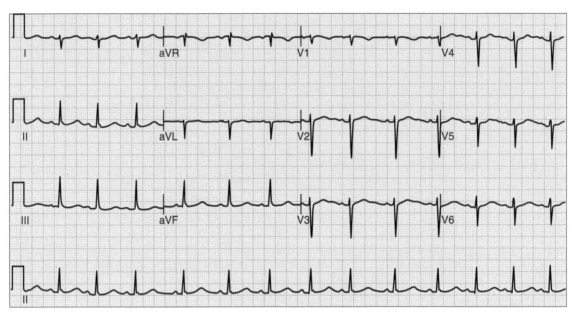

Fig. 13.20 Electrocardiogram of a patient with long QT syndrome 9.[16] (Reproduced with permission from Vatta M, Ackerman MJ, Ye B, et al. Mutant caveolin-3 induces persistent late sodium current and is associated with long-QT syndrome. *Circulation.* 2006;114(20):2104–2112.)

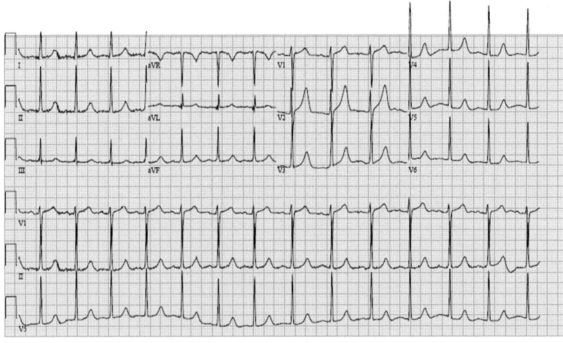

Fig. 13.21 This 12-lead electrocardiogram of a 22-year-old man who presented with syncope shows QT/QTc interval of 420/493 ms. Patient also has nonischemic cardiomyopathy. The genetic study revealed long QT syndrome 12 (owing to the mutation of SNTA1 that encodes Syntrophin α).

autonomic tone; and drugs such as digoxin, mexiletine, testosterone, sympathomimetics, and rufinamide (anticonvulsant). Therefore an SQTS diagnosis is made on the basis of clinical, electrographic, and genetic findings (Table 13.4).

BRUGADA SYNDROME

Brugada syndrome is characterized by ST segment elevation in the right precordial leads (V1-V3); incomplete or complete right bundle branch block, with susceptibility to polymorphic VT; and SCD, occurring mostly at rest or during sleep. It predominantly affects men and is inherited as an autosomal-dominant trait with variable and probably age-dependent expression, with a mean age at onset of 40 years. Only 15% to 30% of families with Brugada syndrome have been found to have mutant *SCN5A* genes. Other sodium and calcium channel mutations with Brugada syndrome include *SCN1B*, *CACNA1C*, *CACNB2*, and *GDP1L* mutation of the glycerol-3-phosphate dehydrogenase 1–like protein. Brugada syndrome is estimated to be responsible for

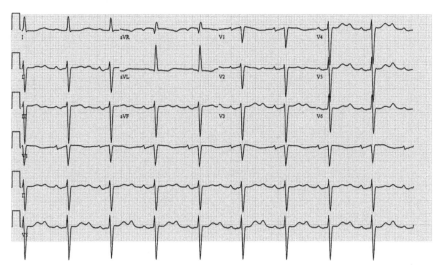

Fig. 13.22 Long QT syndrome with prominent U waves in a patient with hypertrophic cardiomyopathy. Patient presented with syncope and torsades de pointes and was found to have concentric left ventricular hypertrophy with left ventricular outflow tract obstruction.

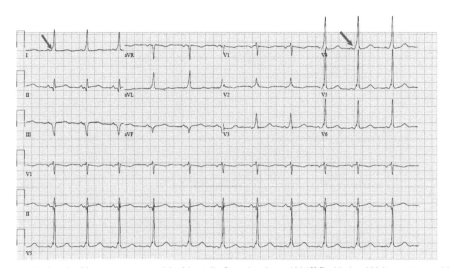

Fig. 13.23 A 45-year-old man admitted with acute gout and incidentally found to have Wolff-Parkinson-White pattern with QT/QTc of 512/552 ms. Delta waves are shown by *red arrows*. He was not taking any QT interval prolonging drugs. The patient developed torsades de pointes during hospitalization and resuscitated successfully with direct current cardioversion.

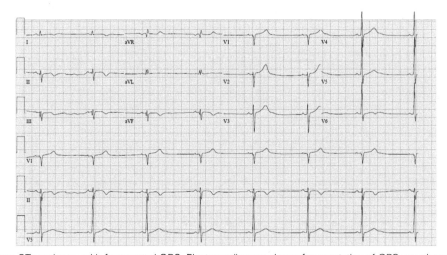

Fig. 13.24 Patient with long QT syndrome with fragmented QRS. Electrocardiogram shows fragmentation of QRS complexes in leads aVL, III, and aVF. Fragmented QRS in acquired long QT syndrome is associated with a high risk of torsades de pointes. This patient presented with sudden cardiac arrest.

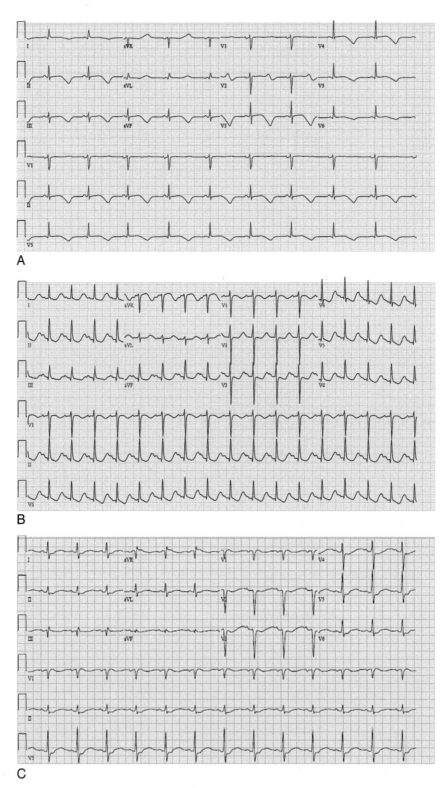

Fig. 13.25 (A) Electrocardiogram of a patient with hypokalemia (K+ 2.8 mMol/L) with QTc/QT interval of 662/645 ms. Patient suffered from torsades de pointes (not shown). (B) A 45-year-old patient with extensive adenocarcinoma who developed long QT syndrome in the setting of K+1.9 and Mg+1.7. Note that QT is difficult to measure because it extends over the next P wave. (C) A 58-year-old man presented with torsades de pointes (not shown) owing to severe hypokalemia associated with diuretic use. The QT/QTC interval is 494/556 ms.

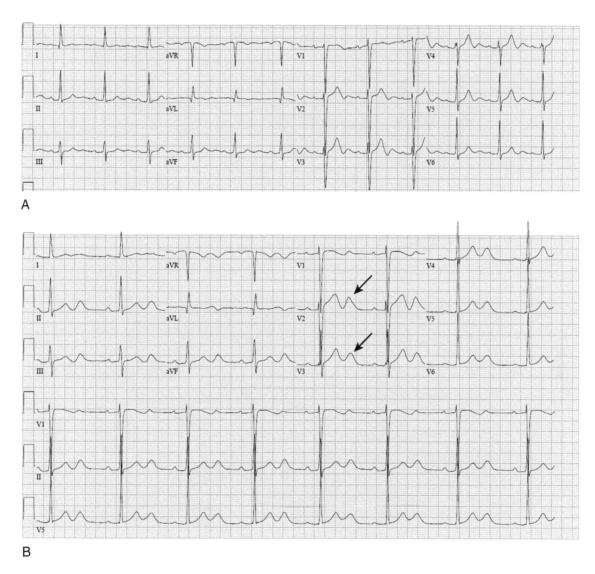

Fig. 13.26 Hypokalemia (2.6 meq/L) with prominent U waves (*arrows*) in an 80-year-old man. (A) Initial electrocardiogram, which worsened with diuretic use. (B) QT/QTc intervals are 457/400 ms, whereas the QTU interval is 760 ms.

4% of all SCD and up to 20% of SCD in patients with structurally normal hearts.[6] The prevalence of Brugada pattern in ECGs recorded from adults is between 0.05% and 0.6%. This ECG pattern cannot be distinguished between asymptomatic and symptomatic patients. Three ECG repolarization patterns in the right precordial leads are recognized (Table 13.5). Type 0 Brugada syndrome is characterized by J wave amplitude or ST segment elevation of 2 mm (0.2 mV) or greater at its peak followed by absent or shallow negative T wave (<1 mm), with little or no isoelectric separation. Type 1 Brugada syndrome pattern includes an ST segment elevation of at least 2 mm, with a "coved" morphology associated with incomplete or complete bundle branch block by a negative T wave. Brugada syndrome is definitively diagnosed when a type 1 ST segment elevation is observed in more than one right precordial lead (V1-V3) in the presence or absence of a sodium channel–blocking agent and in conjunction with one of the following: documented VF, polymorphic VT, a family history of SCD at younger than 45 years of age, coved-type ECGs in family members, inducibility of VT with programmed electrical stimulation, syncope, or nocturnal agonal respiration (Fig. 13.39). Other ECG manifestations of Brugada syndrome include prolonged QT, AV block (prolonged H-V interval),

and atrial arrhythmias (including atrial fibrillation). The incidence of atrial fibrillation in Brugada syndrome is 20%. The ECG manifestations of the Brugada syndrome may vary from day to day or hour to hour and, when concealed, can be unmasked primarily by sodium channel blockers (Fig. 13.40) and with vagal maneuvers. The ECG pattern varies from day to day in the same patient and can be completely normal at times. Shifting ECG types are associated with increased risk of a cardiac event.[18] Myriad physiologic and environmental factors have been shown to play a role in the clinical expression of patients with Brugada syndrome. Vagotonic agents and sympatholytic drugs also enhance the typical ST pattern in Brugada syndrome (Figs. 13.41 and 13.42). VT/VF may be provoked by fever, large meals, cocaine use, excessive alcohol consumption, fever, and overdose of tricyclic antidepressants. Patients with a spontaneous type 1 ECG have a shorter time to first arrhythmic event (VT/VF) than patients in whom the type 1 ECG is shown only during drug challenge. It is important to note that VT in Brugada syndrome is infrequently suppressed by catecholamine administration (e.g., isoproterenol) and enhanced by vagomimetic maneuvers. Long-term quinidine therapy is useful to suppress arrhythmic events in Brugada syndrome. Spontaneous type I Brugada pattern,

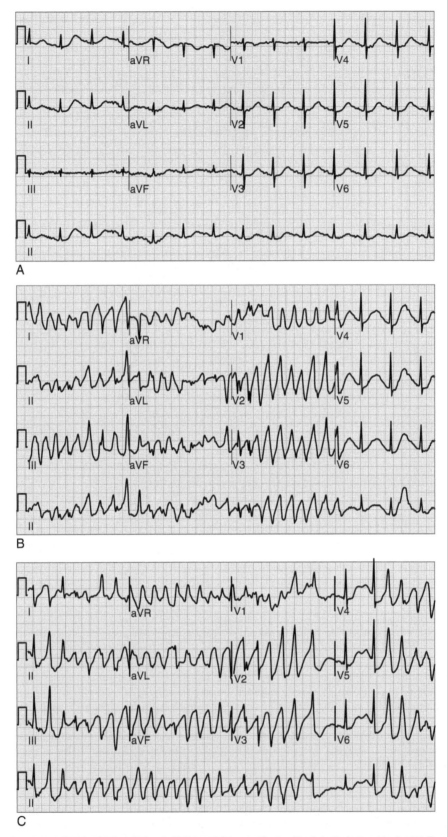

Fig. 13.27 Torsades de pointes associated with hypokalemia (2.5 meq/L) in a patient with diabetic ketoacidosis. (A) Baseline QT/QTc intervals are 560/666 ms. (B and C) Electrocardiograms depict short runs of rapid torsades de pointes. The arrhythmia responded to rapid correction of electrolytes and acidosis.

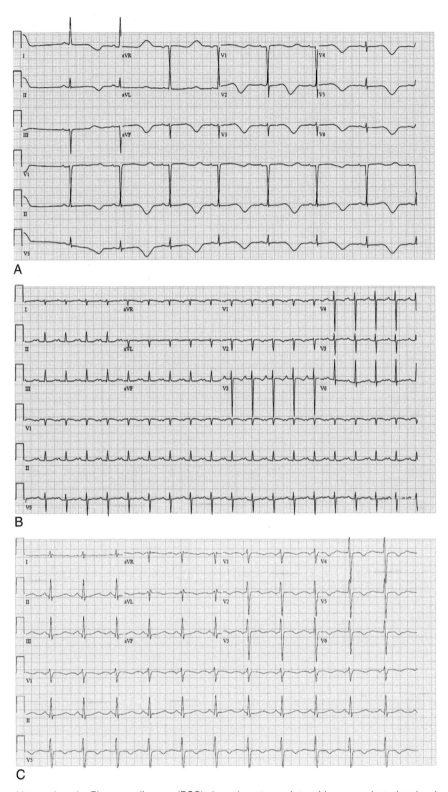

Fig. 13.28 Hypokalemia and hypocalcemia. Electrocardiogram (ECG) signs do not correlate with serum electrolyte levels. (A) ECG of a male patient with renal failure on hemodialysis with K+ level of 3.0 mMol/L and Ca+ level of 7.9 mMol/L. QT/QTc intervals are 730/648 ms. After correction of electrolyte imbalance, the QTc interval was normalized. (B) ECG of a patient with K+ level of 3.0 mMol/L and Ca+ level of 7.9 mmol/L. QT/QTc intervals are 446/614 ms. (C) ECG of a patient with combined hypokalemia (K+ 2.2 mEq/L) and hypocalcemia (Ca+ 7.4 mEq/L).

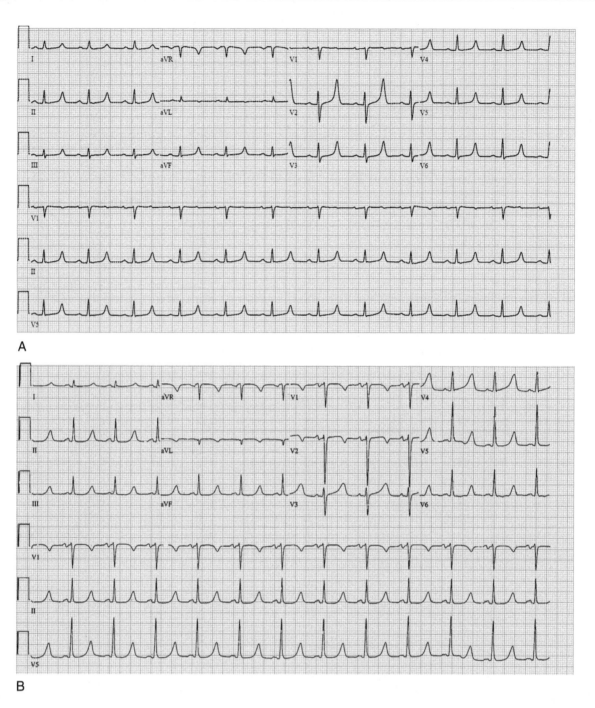

Fig. 13.29 Long QT interval as a result of combined hypocalcemia and hyperkalemia (more commonly seen in patients with chronic renal failure). There is prolongation of JT segment with prominent T waves in the precordial leads. (A) Electrocardiogram was obtained during hypocalcemia (Ca^+ 3.3 mEq/L) and hyperkalemia (K^+ 5.9 mEq/L). QT/QTC intervals are 344/516 ms. (B) Electrocardiogram shows prolonged QT interval during hypocalcemia (Ca^+ 7 mEq/L) and hyperkalemia (K^+ 6.9 mEq/L). QT/QTC intervals are 480/534 ms.

deep S wave in lead I, prominent R wave in lead aVR, and fragmented QRS in the ECG represent markers of high risk in Brugada syndrome.

Brugada pattern of ECG can also be encountered in atypical right bundle branch block, early repolarization, left ventricular hypertrophy, acute pericarditis, acute myocardial ischemia, coronary artery disease (Fig. 13.43), pulmonary embolism, Prinzmetal angina, dissecting aortic aneurysm, various central and autonomic nervous system abnormalities, Duchenne muscular dystrophy, hyperkalemia (Fig. 13.44), hypercalcemia, arrhythmogenic right ventricular dysplasia/cardiomyopathy, pectus excavatum, hypothermia, cocaine use, tricyclic antidepressant overdose, and mechanical compression

of the right ventricular outflow tract, such as occurs in mediastinal tumor. Brugada-like pattern of ECG can occasionally appear for a brief period or for a period of several hours after direct current cardioversion.

CATECHOLAMINERGIC POLYMORPHIC VENTRICULAR TACHYCARDIA

Catecholaminergic polymorphic VT (CPVT) is a highly malignant form of arrhythmogenic disorder characterized by exercise- or emotion-induced

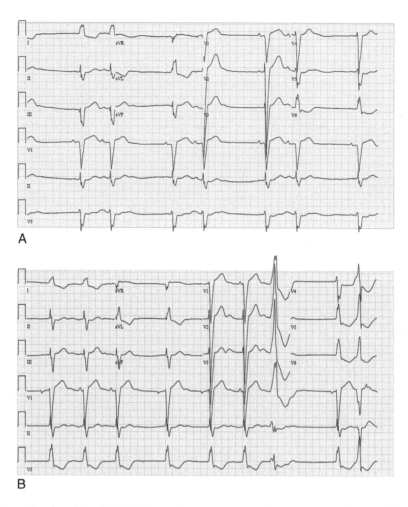

Fig. 13.30 Quinidine-induced torsades de pointes (TdP). Patient with coronary artery disease was receiving quinidine for the management of atrial fibrillation. (A) Baseline electrocardiogram revealed sinus rhythm with possible type I second-degree sinoatrial block, left bundle branch block, and left axis deviation. QT/QTC intervals are 588/508 ms. (B) Sinus and nonsinus atrial rhythm with frequent premature ventricular complexes were noted on the electrocardiogram and telemonitoring before the rhythms in (C). QT/QTC intervals are 535/506 ms. (C) Patient developed self-terminating TdP during sleep. The TdP lasted for 2.5 minutes.

polymorphic VT in patients with structurally normal hearts. CPVT is associated with mutations of cardiac ryanodine receptor *(RyR2)* and cardiac calsequestrin *(CASQ2)*, inherited as autosomal dominant and recessive patterns, respectively. The resting ECG is often unremarkable, although sinus bradycardia and prominent U waves can be observed in some patients. Typically, initially frequent monomorphic or polymorphic PVCs are noted during exercise stress test or Holter monitoring (during exercise). With continued exercise, bidirectional VT and polymorphic VT, as well as supraventricular arrhythmias (in nearly three-fourths of patients), are noted. Ventricular arrhythmias during exercise stress testing appear quite constantly at heart rates of 110 to 130 bpm. The bidirectional VT is the distinguishing arrhythmia of CPVT, which is characterized by alternating QRS axis with a rotation of 180 degrees on a beat-to-beat basis in the frontal plane (Fig. 13.44). Baher and colleagues[8] studied a two-dimensional anatomic model of the rabbit ventricles with a simplified His-Purkinje system, in which different sites in the His-Purkinje system had different heart rate thresholds for delayed after depolarization—induced bigeminy. When the heart rate exceeded the threshold for bigeminy at the first site in the His-Purkinje system, ventricular bigeminy developed, causing the heart rate to accelerate and exceed the threshold for bigeminy at the second site. Thus the triggered beat from the first site induced a triggered beat from the second site. The triggered beat from the second site next reciprocated by

inducing a triggered beat from the first site, and so forth. Bigeminy from two sites produced bidirectional VT, and that from three or more sites produced polymorphic VT.

Bidirectional VT occurs in only 35% of patients, and the remaining patients have polymorphic VT or VF (Figs. 13.45–13.47). When the exercise stops, arrhythmias gradually disappear. The presence of a prominent U wave is a frequent finding, although it cannot be considered to be a diagnostic indicator of CPVT. U wave alternans (beat-to-beat variability) in the recovery phase of exercise can be seen when VT is induced. Bidirectional VT is also encountered in other diseases (Table 13.6). CPVT (emotion- or exercise-induced VT) phenotypes can occur in other conditions as well (Box 13.1)

IDIOPATHIC VENTRICULAR FIBRILLATION

Idiopathic VF accounts for up to 8% of victims of SCD. Recently, early repolarization abnormality (defined as an elevation of the QRS-ST junction of at least 0.1 mV from baseline in the inferior or lateral lead and manifested as QRS slurring or notching) has been reported to be present in 31% patients with idiopathic VF compared with only 5% in the general population $(P < 0.001)$[19] (Fig. 13.51). Otherwise, the ECG typically shows no depolarization abnormalities (sinus rhythm with normal P-R interval and QRS interval)

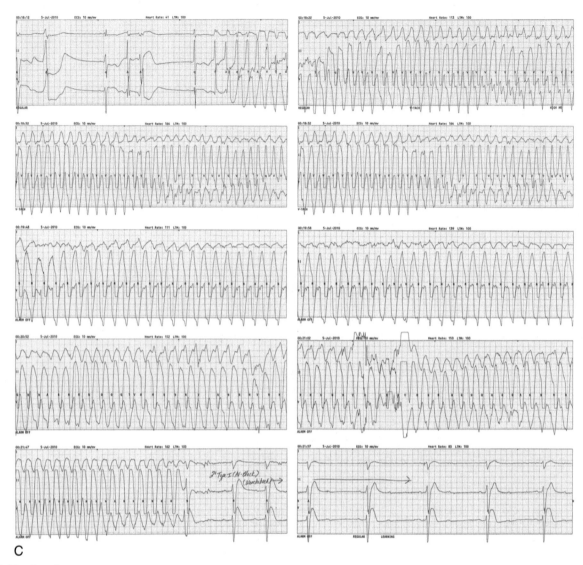

C

Fig. 13.30 (Continued).

or major repolarization abnormalities (no ST-T changes or prolongation of QT interval). The VF typically is initiated by a single monomorphic PVC. Purkinje network is shown to be the trigger PVC that initiates VF. Ablation targeting specific Purkinje potentials that precede the culprit PVC cures or reduces the recurrence of VF. The PVCs can originate in any ventricle. In a study of 38 patients with idiopathic VF, the mean coupling interval was 291 ± 39 ms.[17] The coupling interval of the PVC was longer when originating from the right ventricular outflow tract compared with the left ventricular Purkinje system (355 ± 23 ms vs. 276 ± 22 ms, $P < 0.001$). Similarly, monomorphic PVCs originating from the His-Purkinje network can cause VT/VF in patients with coronary artery disease (Fig. 13.52).

SHORT-COUPLED TORSADES DE POINTES

Short-coupled variant of TdP was described by Leenhardt and associates[18] in 14 patients with SCD or family history of SCD. It is defined by the presence of short coupling interval ($<245 \pm 28$ ms) of PVCs that initiate polymorphic VT.[18] The definition of TdP may not be correct because these patients have a normal QT interval; it probably could be included in the idiopathic VF group. The VT/VF episodes are partially suppressed by verapamil, but verapamil does not prevent SCD (Fig. 13.53).

Early repolarization abnormality: Early repolarization is generally a benign ECG finding with a rare risk of VF and SCD.[20] The diagnosis criteria for early repolarization are following:

1. The presence of J-point elevation ≥ 1 mm in ≥ 2 at the end QRS notch (J wave) or slur on the downslope of a prominent R wave with and without ST-segment elevation in contiguous inferior and/or lateral leads of a standard 12-lead ECG in a patient resuscitated from otherwise unexplained VF/polymorphic VT;
2. The peak of the notch or J wave (J_p) ≥ 0.1 mV in ≥ 2 contiguous leads of the 12-lead ECG, excluding leads V_1-V_3; and
3. QRS duration (measured in leads in which a notch or slur is absent) less than 120 ms.
   (Figs. 13.54 and 13.55)
   Pause-Dependent Torsades De Pointes

Bradycardia-dependent TdP is rarely encountered in patients with or without structural heart disease. Commonly, it occurs in the presence of advanced AV block or marked bradycardia associated with "R" on "T" phenomenon and initiation of TdP (Fig. 13.56). This phenomenon can also occur during asynchronous temporary ventricular pacing (Fig. 13.57). Increasing ventricular rate with pacing or catecholaminergic medications usually cures the arrhythmia.

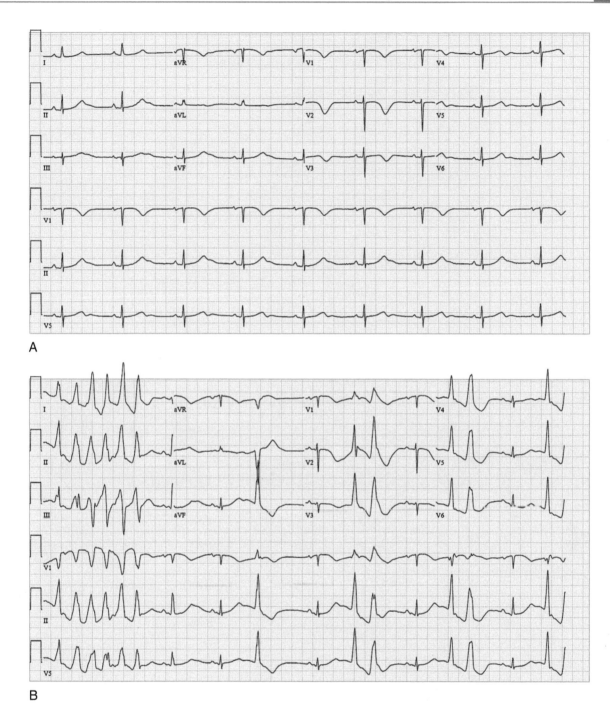

A

B

Fig. 13.31 Sotalol therapy–induced torsades de pointes. (A) Electrocardiogram reveals pronged QT interval after initiation of sotalol therapy. The patient later developed short runs of torsades de pointes, premature ventricular complexes, and ventricular couplets (B). The arrhythmia responded to intravenous magnesium and discontinuation of sotalol therapy.

ASYNCHRONOUS PACING-INDUCED POLYMORPHIC VENTRICULAR TACHYCARDIA

The R-on-T phenomenon predisposes to malignant ventricular arrhythmias. Typically, a PVC occurring at the critical time during the T wave of the preceding beat precipitates VT and VF. This phenomenon can occur with asynchronous ventricular pacemakers, and even with synchronous pacemakers if there is loss of sensing of the intrinsic rhythm (Fig. 13.57).

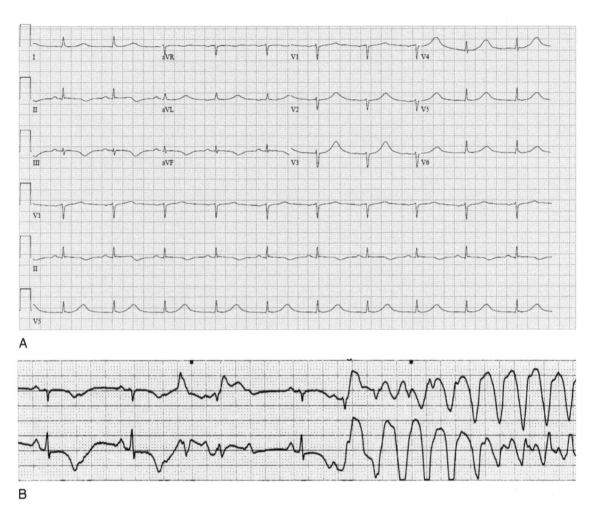

A

B

Fig. 13.32 Dofetilide-induced long QT prolongation. (A) Patient suffered ventricular fibrillation and cardiac arrest during acute inferior wall myocardial infarction. He was treated with amiodarone after the cardiac arrest. The QT/QTc interval is 566/569 ms. The risk of torsades de pointes is less than 1% with amiodarone even with marked prolonged QT interval. (B) After receiving dofetilide (500 mcg twice daily, for 3 months) the patient developed torsades de pointes, which required external direct-current shock.

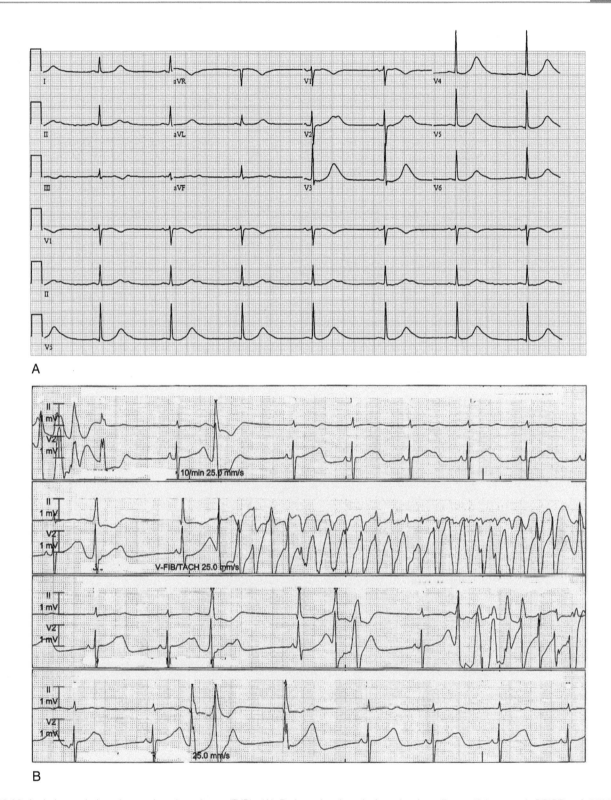

Fig. 13.33 Amiodarone-induced torsades de pointes (TdP). (A) Patient developed sinus bradycardia at 43 bpm and QT/QTc of 672/568 ms. (B) Rhythm strip shows frequent premature ventricular complexes (*PVCs*), ventricular couplets, and two episodes of TdP. Both episodes of TdP are initiated by short-long-short cycles.

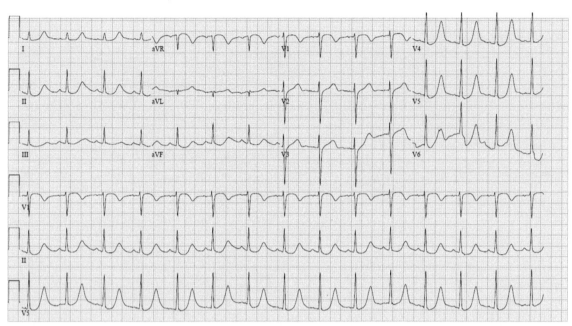

Fig. 13.34 Methadone-induced long QT syndrome (QT/QTc = 400/511 ms). Patient developed torsades de pointes (not shown) while receiving methadone therapy.

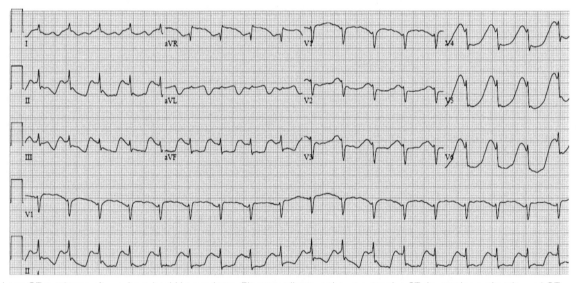

Fig. 13.35 Long QT syndrome after subarachnoid hemorrhage. Electrocardiogram shows extensive ST depression and prolonged QT.

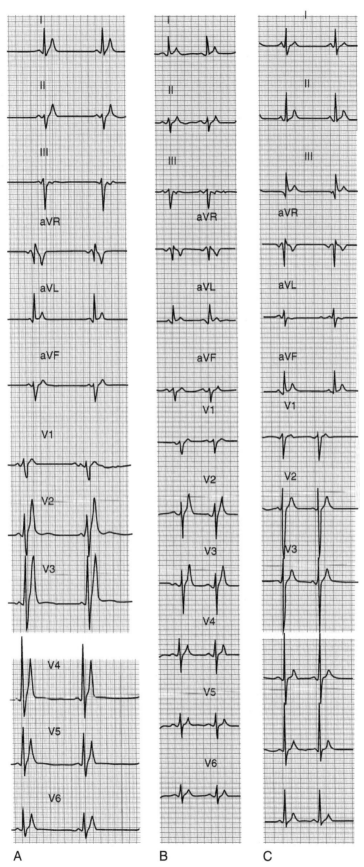

Fig. 13.36 Short QT syndrome. This 12-lead electrocardiogram of a patient in sinus rhythm shows a heart rate of 52 bpm, left axis deviation, and QTc of 280 ms. Paper speed: 25 mm per second. (Gaita F, Giustetto C, Bianchi F, et al. Short QT syndrome: a familial cause of sudden death. *Circulation*. 2003;108:965–970.)

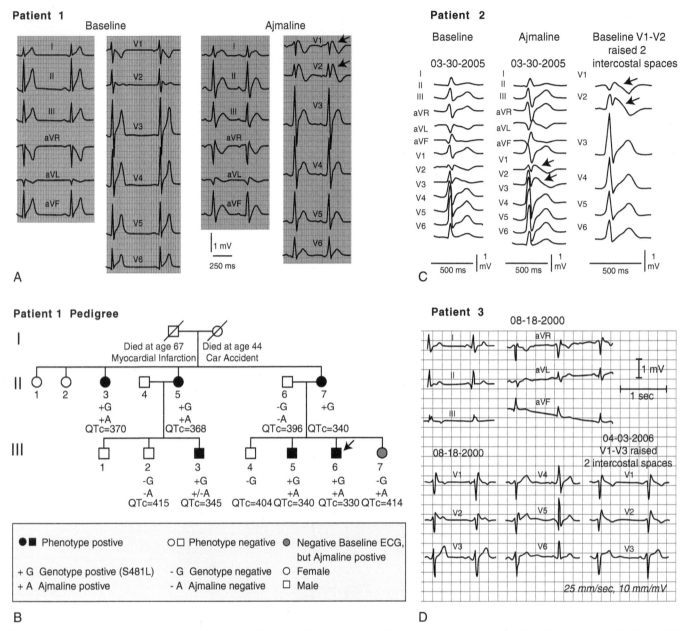

Fig. 13.37 Twelve-lead electrocardiogram of patient with short QT syndrome 4 before and after ajmaline administration recorded with V1 and V2 displaced superiorly two intercostal spaces, which shows Brugada pattern of ST-T changes in leads V1-V2. Arrows show pronounced ST-T changes during ajmaline administration. (Reproduced with permission from Antzelevitch C, Pollevick GD, Cordeiro JM, et al. Loss-of-function mutations in the cardiac calcium channel underlie a new clinical entity characterized by ST-segment elevation, short QT intervals, and sudden cardiac death. *Circulation.* 2007;115(4):442–449.)

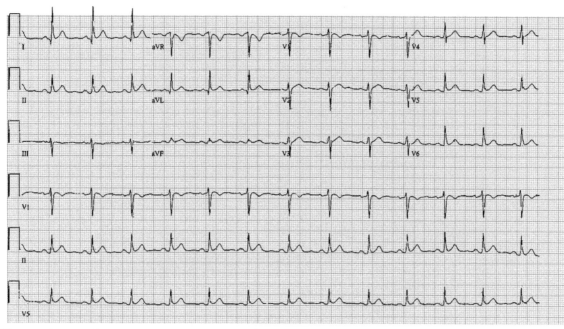

Fig. 13.38 Electrocardiogram of a patient with hypercalcemia (Ca^+ level: 11.6 mEq/L) shows loss of the JT segment resulting in short QT interval owing to shortening of myocardial repolarization. QT/QTc intervals are 320/368 ms.

TABLE 13.4   Short QT Syndrome Diagnostic Criteria[17]

Parameters	Points
QT$_C$ (ms)	
<370	1
<350	2
<330	3
J point-T$_{peak}$ interval <120 ms	1
Clinical history[a]	
History of sudden cardiac arrest	2
Documented polymorphic ventricular tachycardia/ventricular fibrillation	2
Unexplained syncope	1
Atrial fibrillation	1
Family history[a]	
First- or second-degree relative with high probability of SQTS	2
First- or second-degree relative with autopsy-negative sudden cardiac death	1
Sudden infant death syndrome	1
Genotype[a]	
Genotype positive	2
Mutation of undetermined significance in a culprit gene	1

SQTS, Short QT syndrome.

[a]A minimum of 1 point must be obtained in the electrocardiographic section to obtain additional points. High-probability SQTS: ≥ 4 points, intermediate-probability SQTS: 3 points, low-probability SQTS: ≤ 2 points. Electrocardiogram: must be recorded in the absence of modifiers known to shorten the QT. J point-T$_{peak}$ interval must be measured in the precordial lead with the greatest T wave amplitude. Clinical history: events must occur in the absence of an identifiable etiology, including structural heart disease. Points can be received for only one of cardiac arrest, documented polymorphic ventricular tachycardia, or unexplained syncope. Family history: points can be received only once in this section.

TABLE 13.5   Electrocardiogram Types of Brugada Syndrome[18]

ECG Pattern	ST Segments in Leads V-V3	ST Segment Configuration	ECG
Type 0	J wave amplitude or ST segment elevation ≧2 mm (0.2 mV) at its peak followed by absent or shallow negative T wave (<1 mm), with little or no isoelectric separation	Coved	
Type 1	J wave amplitude or ST segment elevation ≧2 mm (0.2 mV) at its peak followed by a negative T wave, with little or no isoelectric separation	Coved	
Type 2	High take-off ST segment elevation, but the J wave amplitude (≧2 mm) gives rise to a gradually descending ST segment elevation (remaining ≧1 mm above the baseline), followed by a positive or biphasic T wave that results in a saddle-back configuration	Saddle back	
Type 3	J wave amplitude ≧2 but right precordial ST-segment elevation <1 mm	Saddle back or coved or both	

ECG, Electrocardiogram.

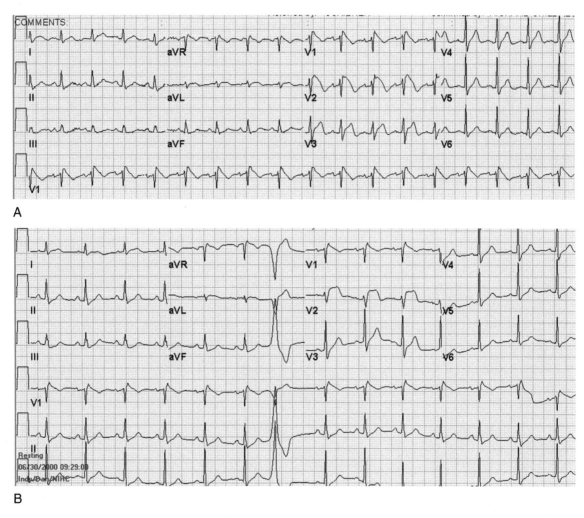

Fig. 13.39 Electrocardiogram of a patient who suffered sudden cardiac arrest as a result of Brugada syndrome. (A) Electrocardiogram shows 2-mm J point elevation and coved-type ST-T changes in leads V1-V2. (B) Single premature ventricular complex is originating from the right ventricular outflow tract. Most ventricular tachycardias are initiated by similar premature ventricular complexes from the right ventricular outflow tract.

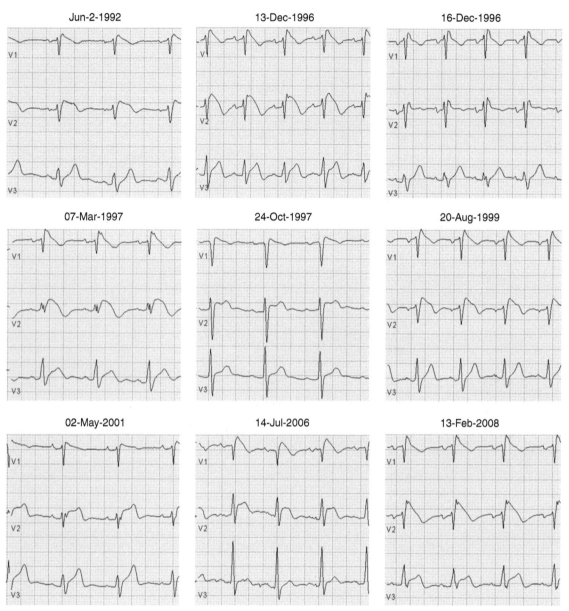

Fig. 13.40 Serial electrocardiograms (ECGs) of the patient in Fig. 13.39 with Brugada syndrome who suffered ventricular fibrillation (VF) and cardiac arrest. ECG shows waxing and waning ST-T changes over the period of 18 years. The initial ECG is from 1992. The patient suffered VF in 1996 and received an implantable cardioverter-defibrillator (ICD). He had an appropriate ICD shock for polymorphic ventricular tachycardia/VF in 2001. He has not suffered any ICD shock since his last follow-up in February 2010.

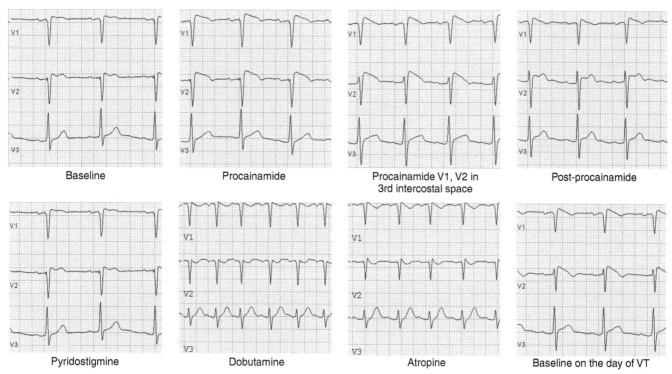

Baseline   Procainamide   Procainamide V1, V2 in   Post-procainamide
                                        3rd intercostal space

Pyridostigmine   Dobutamine   Atropine   Baseline on the day of VT

Fig. 13.41 Electrocardiograms of a patient with type 1 Brugada pattern that resolved spontaneously. Later serial drug testing demonstrated ST-T changes from type 3 to typical type 1 (coved) ST elevation greater than 2 mm in lead V1 and V2 after infusion of procainamide, whereas ST changes became minimal after infusion of dobutamine and atropine. *VT,* Ventricular tachycardia.

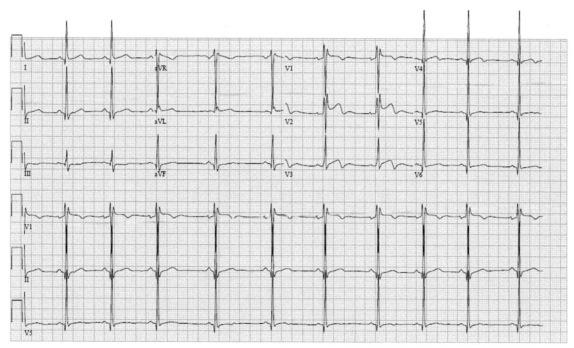

Fig. 13.42 Saddle-back pattern of ST-T wave in lead V2 in a patient with Brugada syndrome.

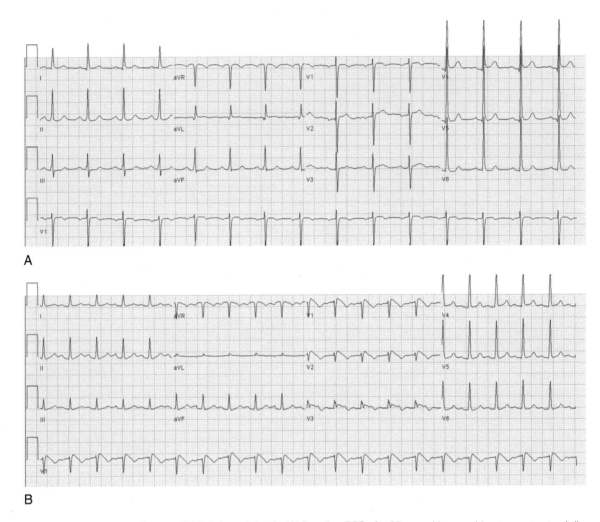

Fig. 13.43 Brugada pattern electrocardiogram (ECG) in hyperkalemia. (A) Baseline ECG of a 62-year-old man without any structural disease with K+ level of 4.1 mEq/L. (B) Patient developed Brugada-pattern ECG during hyperkalemia (K+ level: 6.5 mEq/L) and acidosis secondary to sepsis and renal failure.

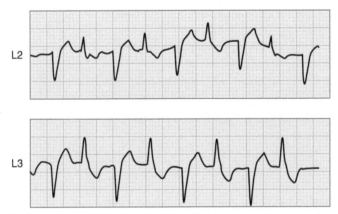

Fig. 13.44 Rhythm strip showing bidirectional ventricular tachycardia in an 11-year-old patient with catecholaminergic polymorphic ventricular tachycardia.

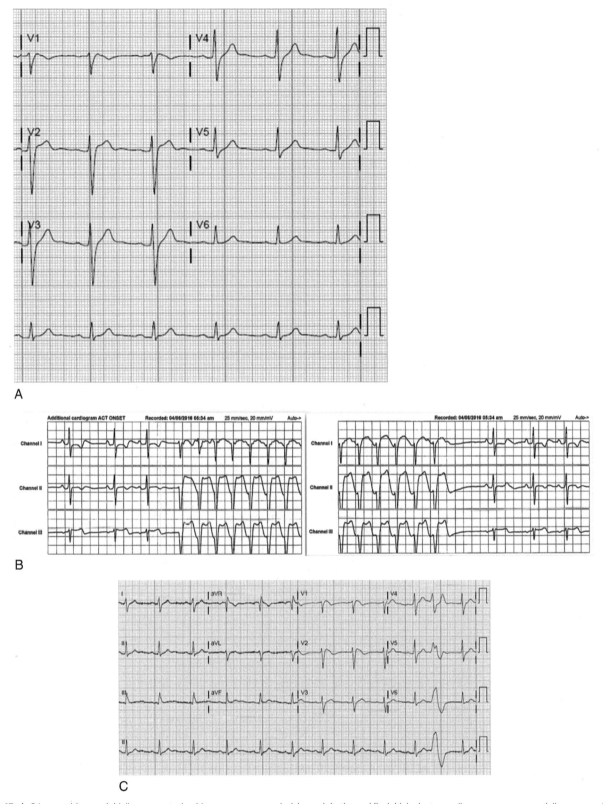

Fig. 13.45 A 24-year-old man initially presented with syncope preceded by palpitations. His initial electrocardiogram was essentially unremarkable (A), and the Holter showed nonsustained ventricular tachycardia (B). Careful review of his prior electrocardiograms subsequently showed type I Brugada pattern (C). Therefore he received a subcutaneous implantable cardioverter-defibrillator. However, within 1 month, he received multiple appropriate implantable cardioverter-defibrillator shocks for ventricular fibrillation storm. Some of these shocks failed as well. (D) He was unresponsive to amiodarone and lidocaine. Subsequently, the arrhythmia responded to intravenous isoproterenol. He underwent electrophysiology (EP) study (E) with electroanatomic mapping of epicardium and endocardium (F). It revealed epicardial areas of slow conduction/scar (*blue and green dots*) in the basal right ventricle and right ventricular outflow tract with inducible ventricular tachycardia/ventricular fibrillation, which was successfully ablated (*maroon dots*). *Red areas* represent scar zones, *purple areas* are healthy myocardium, and the *green areas* represent scar border zones. The ECG after ablation shows normalization of ST-T changes in leads V1 to V3 (G). The patient has been arrhythmia free for the past 3 years. *Abld,* Ablation distal; *Ablp,* ablation proximal; *CS,* coronary sinus; *HisP,* his proximal; *HisM,* His middle; *HisD,* His distal; *LAD,* left anterior descending artery; *LV,* left ventricle; *RCA,* right coronary artery; *RV,* right ventricle; *RVA,* right ventricular apex; *RVOT,* right ventricular outflow tachycardia.

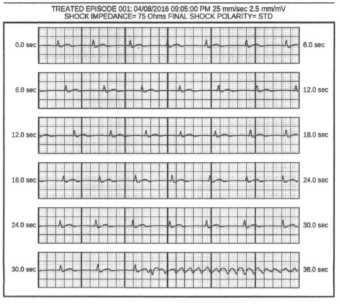

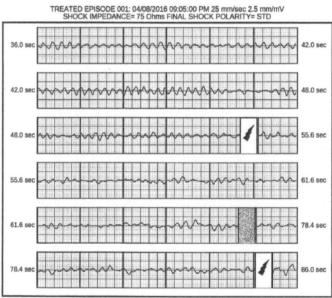

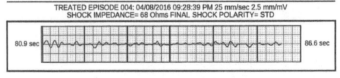

D

Fig. 13.45 (Continued).

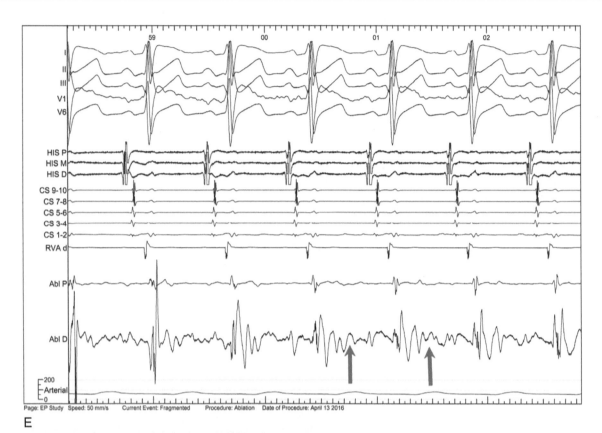

E

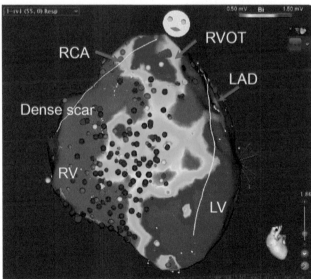

Purple dots: sites of ablation
Blue dots: sites of late potentials
Green dots: sites of delayed activation

F

Fig. 13.45 (Continued).

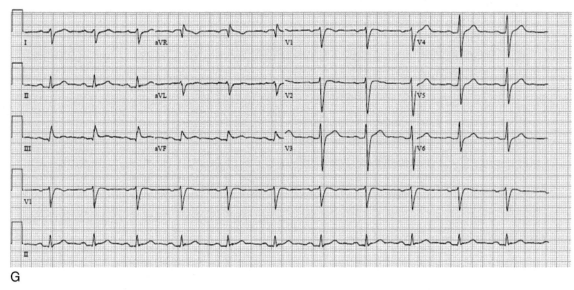

G

Fig. 13.45 (Continued).

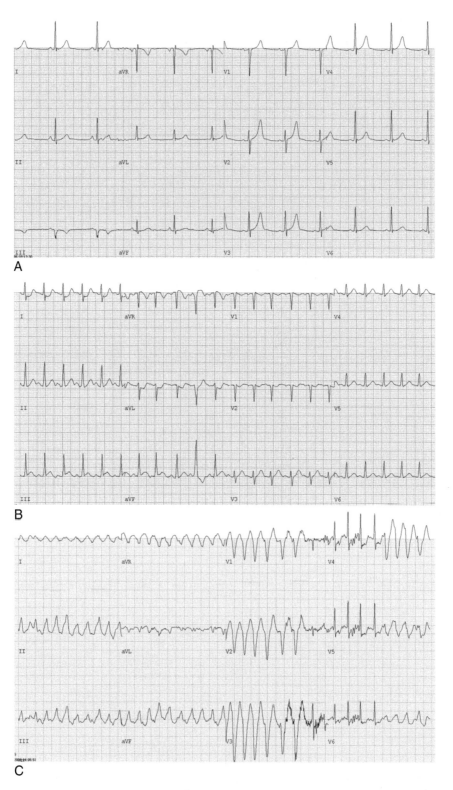

Fig. 13.46 Electrocardiogram of a 64-year-old man who presented with syncope (A). The exercise test revealed rapid polymorphic ventricular tachycardia (B–D), which subsided on rest (E). He was found to have catecholaminergic polymorphic ventricular tachycardia.

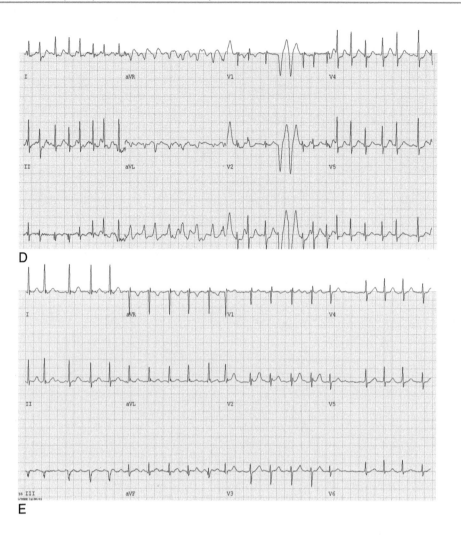

Fig. 13.46 (Continued).

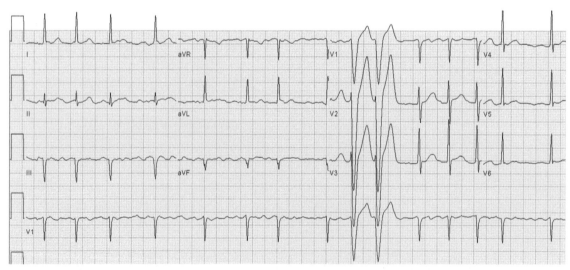

Fig. 13.47 The patient in Fig. 13.46 developed bradycardia and ultimately developed paroxysmal atrial fibrillation. Atrial arrhythmias, such as atrial tachycardia and atrial fibrillation, are common in patients with catecholaminergic polymorphic ventricular tachycardia.

TABLE 13.6   Catecholaminergic Polymorphic Ventricular Tachycardia

Variant	Chromosomal Locus	Gene	Inheritance	Phenotype
CPVT1	1q42-43	*RYR2*	AD	CPVT, IVF
CPVT2	1p23-21	*CASQ2*	AR	CPVT
CPVT3	7p14-22	Unknown	AR	CPVT, QT interval prolongation
CPVT4	14q32.11	CALM1	AD	CPVT
CPVT5	6q22.31	Triadin	AR	CPVT, long QT syndrome
CPVT-Related Phenotypes				
LQTS4	4q25-26	*ANK2*	AD	IVF, QT prolongation (atypical), stress-induced bidirectional VT
ATS	17q23.1-q24.2	*KCNJ2*	AD	U waves, bidirectional VT, periodic paralysis, facial dysmorphisms
CPVT/DCM	1q42-43	*RYR2*	AD	Stress-induced VT, sinus node dysfunction, dilated cardiomyopathy

AD, Autosomal dominant; *AR*, autosomal recessive; *ATS*, Andersen-Tawil syndrome; *CALM1*, calmodulin1; *CPVT*, catecholaminergic polymorphic ventricular tachycardia; *DCM*, dilated cardiomyopathy; *IVF*, idiopathic ventricular fibrillation; *VT*, ventricular tachycardia.
Adapted with permission from Sumitomo N. Current topics in catecholamingergic polymorphic ventricular tachycardia. J Arrhythm. 2016 Oct; 32(5): 344–351.

BOX 13.1   Causes of bidirectional ventricular tachycardia

CPVT	(Figs. 13.45–13.47)
LQTS4	(Fig. 13.48)
Andersen-Tawil syndrome	(Fig. 13.48)
Acute coronary ischemia	(Fig. 13.49)
Digoxin toxicity	(Fig. 13.50)

CPVT, Catecholaminergic polymorphic ventricular tachycardia; *LQTS4*, long QT syndrome 4.

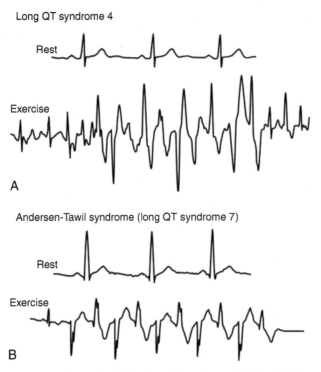

Fig. 13.48 Exercise-induced bidirectional ventricular tachycardia (VT) in long QT syndrome (LQTS). (A) Electrocardiogram recorded during exercise stress testing in a patient with LQTS 4 (*ANK2* mutation) reveals bidirectional VT. (B) Resting electrocardiogram in a patient with LQTS 7 (*KCNJ2* mutation) also shows bidirectional VT.

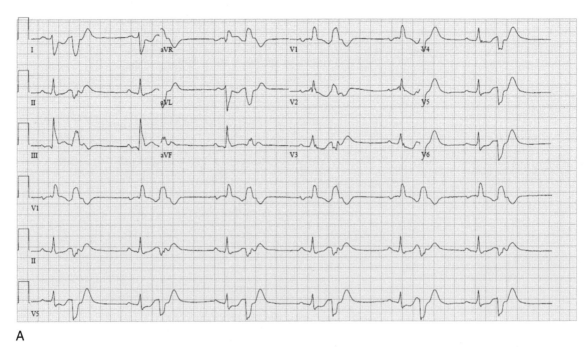

Fig. 13.49 Bidirectional ventricular tachycardia (VT) in the presence of coronary artery disease. Bidirectional VT can occur infrequently in coronary artery diseases, such as acute coronary ischemia. (A) Baseline electrocardiogram shows frequent premature ventricular complexes in a bigeminal pattern. (B) Nonsustained bidirectional VT.

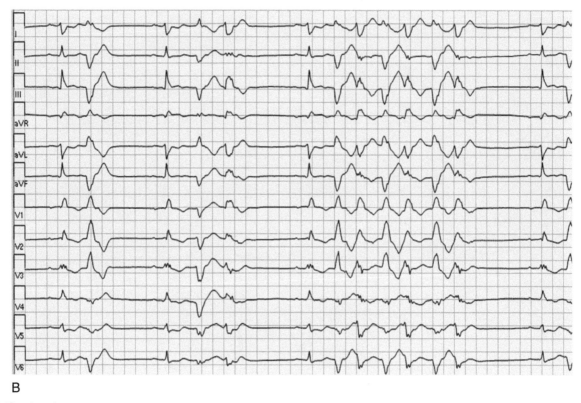

B

Fig. 13.49 (Continued).

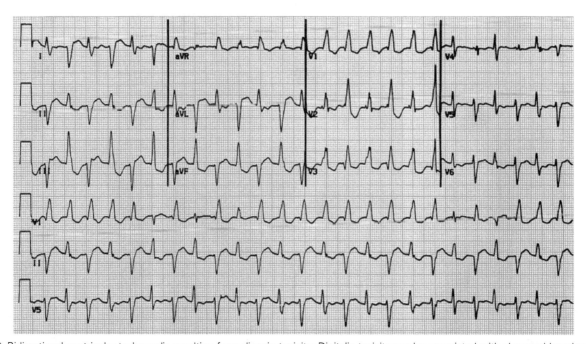

Fig. 13.50 Bidirectional ventricular tachycardia resulting from digoxin toxicity. Digitalis toxicity can be associated with abnormal impulse formation in the bundle branches and Purkinje tissue. This tachycardia has a relatively narrow QRS complex (120–140 ms) and a right bundle branch block morphology QRS. Bidirectional ventricular tachycardia results when foci alternate between the anterior and the posterior fascicles of the left bundle branch, causing the frontal plane axis to alternate.

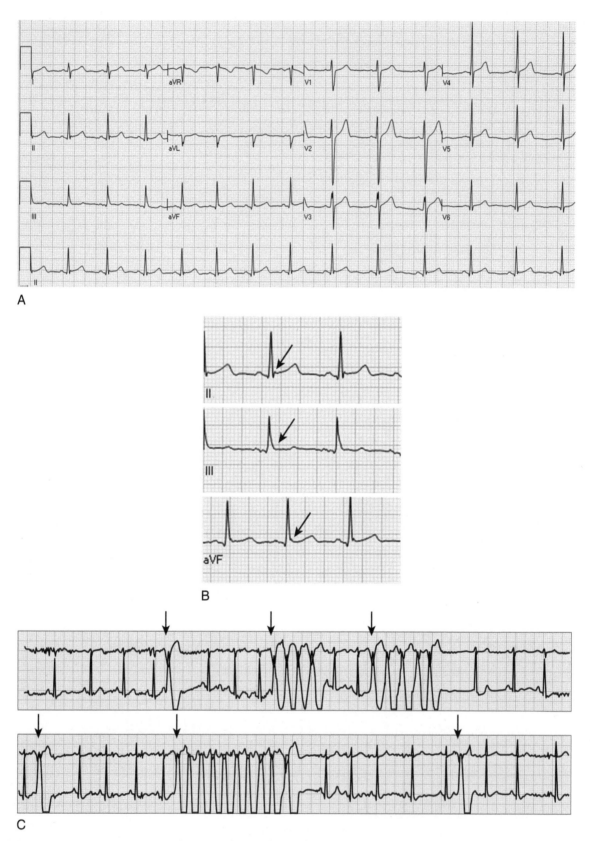

Fig. 13.51 Idiopathic ventricular tachycardia. (A) Electrocardiogram of a 17-year-old male patient without any structural heart disease shows J point elevation in the inferior leads (*arrows* in B). (C) Rhythm strip shows a single monomorphic premature ventricular complex (shown by *arrows*) that initiates nonsustained rapid polymorphic ventricular tachycardia.

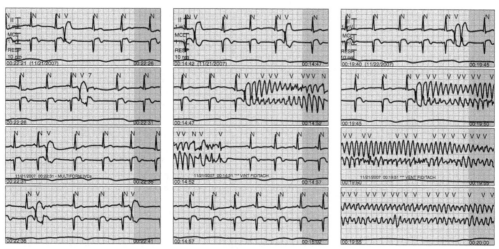

Fig. 13.52 Frequent single monomorphic premature ventricular complexes trigger polymorphic ventricular tachycardia and ventricular fibrillation in a patient with ischemic cardiomyopathy. Catheter ablation of the premature ventricular complexes focus on eliminated episodes of ventricular tachycardia/ventricular fibrillation.

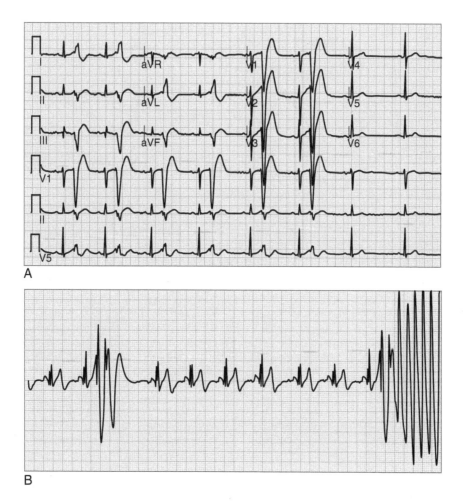

Fig. 13.53 Short-coupled torsades de pointes in a 45-year-old man. (A) Electrocardiogram shows sinus rhythm with very short coupled premature ventricular complexes originating from the right ventricle, probably close to the apex. The patient received multiple implantable cardioverter-defibrillator shocks when verapamil therapy was discontinued (B).

Classic Definition of Early Repolarization:ST Elevation

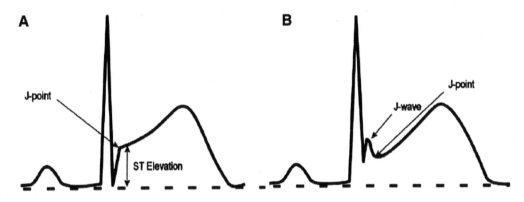

A

J-point

ST Elevation

Classic Early Repolarization Without a J-wave

B

J-point

J-wave

Classic Early Repolarization With a J-wave

New Definitions of Early Repolarization

C

New J-point

Terminal QRS Slurring

Slurred QRS Downstroke without STE

D

J-wave / New J-point

J-wave or the new "J-point Elevation" without STE

A

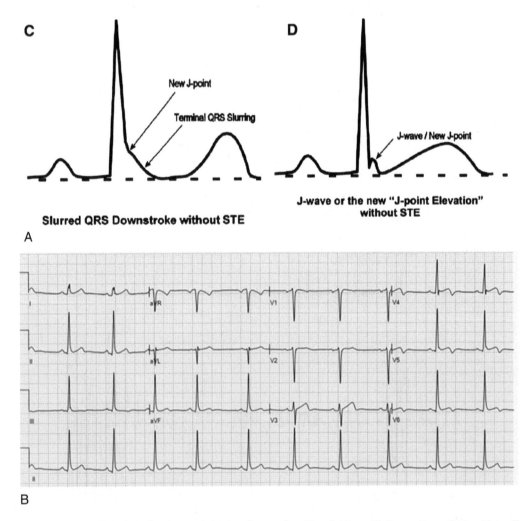

B

Fig. 13.54 (A) Shows different morphologies of early repolarization abnormality. (Part A Marco V. Perez, Karen Friday, Victor Froelicher, Semantic Confusion: The Case of Early Repolarization and the J Point, *The American Journal of Medicine*, 125 (9), 2012, 843–844.) (B) J point elevation in lateral leads with low amplitude T waves suggest high-risk early repolarization abnormality. (C) Significant J point elevation (6 mm) in lateral precordial leads in a patient presenting with polymorphic ventricular tachycardia. *STE*, ST segment elevation.

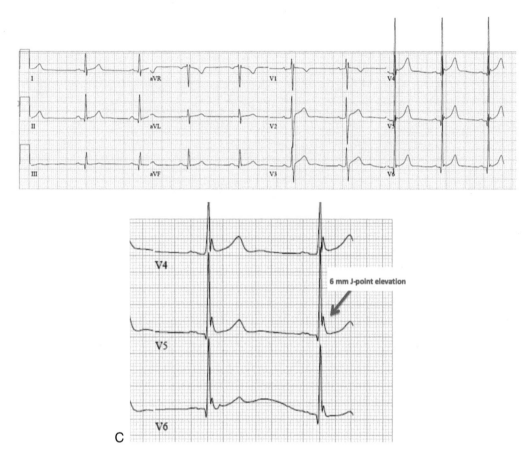

Fig. 13.54 (Continued).

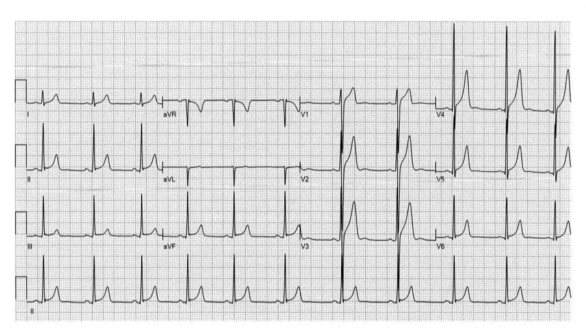

Fig. 13.55 Short QT syndrome with early repolarization abnormality. The electrocardiogram shows short QT (QTc 360 ms) and early repolarization in inferior leads.

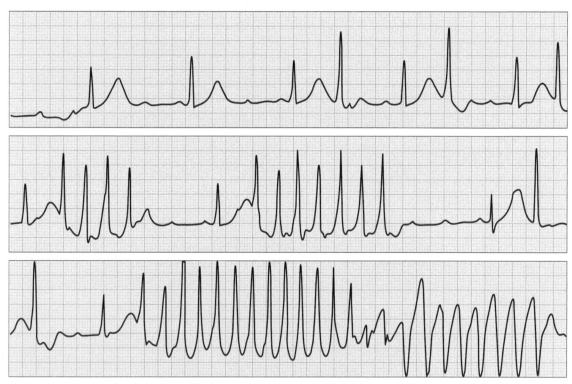

Fig. 13.56 Pause-dependent torsades de pointes. Rhythm strip reveals advanced atrioventricular block and short runs of torsades de pointes related to bradycardia.

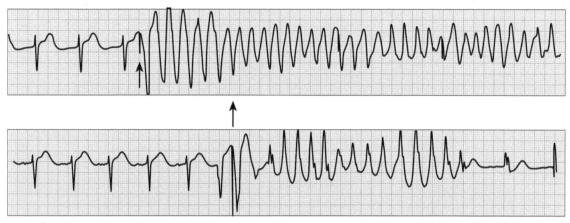

Fig. 13.57 R-on-T phenomenon. Patient received epicardial temporary pacing during cardiac surgery. Asynchronous pacing with intermittent loss of sensing resulted in pacing-induced (*arrows*) nonsustained and sustained polymorphic ventricular tachycardia and ventricular fibrillation due to R-on-T phenomenon. The sustained ventricular tachycardia/ventricular fibrillation required external defibrillation. The *arrow* indicates pacing stimulus.

REFERENCES

1. Singh M, Morin DP, Link MS. Sudden cardiac death in long QT syndrome (LQTS), Brugada syndrome, and catecholaminergic polymorphic ventricular tachycardia (CPVT). *Prog Cardiovasc Dis.* 2019;62:227–234.
2. Walsh MA, Turner C, Timothy KW, et al. A multicentre study of patients with Timothy syndrome. *Europace.* 2018;20:377–385.
3. El-Sherif N, Turitto G, Boutjdir M. Acquired long QT syndrome and electrophysiology of torsade de pointes. *Arrhythm Electrophysiol Rev.* 2019;8:122–130.
4. Chorin E, Hochstadt A, Granot Y, et al. Grapefruit juice prolongs the QT interval of healthy volunteers and patients with long QT syndrome. *Heart Rhythm.* 2019;16:1141–1148.
5. Campuzano O, Sarquella-Brugada G, Cesar S, Arbelo E, Brugada J, Brugada R. Recent advances in short QT syndrome. *Front Cardiovasc Med.* 2018;5:149.
6. Coppola G, Corrado E, Curnis A, et al. Update on Brugada syndrome 2019. *Curr Probl Cardiol.* 2019;100454.
7. Al-Khatib SM, Stevenson WG, Ackerman MJ, et al. 2017 AHA/ACC/HRS guideline for management of patients with ventricular arrhythmias and the prevention of sudden cardiac death: executive summary: a report of the American College of Cardiology/American Heart Association Task Force on Clinical Practice Guidelines and the Heart Rhythm Society. *Heart Rhythm.* 2018;(15)e190–e252.
8. Baher AA, Uy M, Xie F, Garfinkel A, Qu Z, Weiss JN. Bidirectional ventricular tachycardia: ping pong in the His-Purkinje system. *Heart Rhythm.* 2011;8:599–605.

9. Morita H, Wu J, Zipes DP. The QT syndromes: long and short. *Lancet.* 2008;372:750−763.

10. Perez-Riera AR, Barbosa-Barros R, Daminello Raimundo R, da Costa de Rezende Barbosa MP, Esposito Sorpreso IC, de Abreu LC. The congenital long QT syndrome type 3: an update. *Indian Pacing Electrophysiol J.* 2018;18:25−35.

11. Lin MT, Wu MH, Chang CC, et al. In utero onset of long QT syndrome with atrioventricular block and spontaneous or lidocaine-induced ventricular tachycardia: compound effects of hERG pore region mutation and SCN5A N-terminus variant. *Heart Rhythm.* 2008;5:1567−1574.

12. Schoonderwoerd BA, Wiesfeld AC, Wilde AA, et al. A family with Andersen-Tawil syndrome and dilated cardiomyopathy. *Heart Rhythm.* 2006;3:1346−1350.

13. Totomoch-Serra A, Marquez MF, Cervantes-Barragan DE. Clinical heterogeneity in Andersen-Tawil syndrome. *Neuromuscul Disord.* 2017;27:1074−1075.

14. Sherman J, Tester DJ, Ackerman MJ. Targeted mutational analysis of ankyrin-B in 541 consecutive, unrelated patients referred for long QT syndrome genetic testing and 200 healthy subjects. *Heart Rhythm.* 2005;2:1218−1223.

15. Lo ANSM, Wilde AA, van Erven L, Blom NA. Syndactyly and long QT syndrome (CaV1.2 missense mutation G406R) is associated with hypertrophic cardiomyopathy. *Heart Rhythm.* 2005;2:1365−1368.

16. Vatta M, Ackerman MJ, Ye B, et al. Mutant caveolin-3 induces persistent late sodium current and is associated with long-QT syndrome. *Circulation.* 2006;114:2104−2112.

17. Knecht S, Sacher F, Wright M, et al. Long-term follow-up of idiopathic ventricular fibrillation ablation: a multicenter study. *J Am Coll Cardiol.* 2009;54:522−528.

18. Leenhardt A, Glaser E, Burguera M, Nurnberg M, Maison-Blanche P, Coumel P. Short-coupled variant of torsade de pointes. A new electrocardiographic entity in the spectrum of idiopathic ventricular tachyarrhythmias. *Circulation.* 1994;89:206−215.

19. Haissaguerre M, Derval N, Sacher F, et al. Sudden cardiac arrest associated with early repolarization. *N Engl J Med.* 2008;358:2016−2023.

20. Bourier F, Denis A, Cheniti G, et al. Early repolarization syndrome: diagnostic and therapeutic approach. *Front Cardiovasc Med.* 2018;5:169.

Page numbers followed by *f* indicate figures; *t*, tables; *b*, boxes.

0-9, and Symbols

2:1 atrioventricular block, 62−63, 72*b*, 73*f*, 75*f*, 91*f*

A

Accelerated junctional rhythm, 99

Acceleration (tachycardia) dependent blocks or delays, 4, 18*f*

Accessory pathway(s), concealed, 151, 152*f*
  in atrial flutter or atrial tachycardia, 161, 167*f*
  atypical, 172, 173*f*
  bilateral conduction in, 152*f*
  bundle branch block effect on, 161, 164*f*
  common and less common. *See also* Wolff-Parkinson-White syndrome, 153*f*
  in congenital anomalies, 172, 172*f*
  and enhanced atrioventricular nodal conduction, 172, 176*f*
  intermittent preexcitation in, and risk of ventricular fibrillation, 165, 167*f*
  latent, 160*f*, 161
  localization of, 151
    anteroseptal, 151, 158*f*
    left lateral or anterolateral, 151, 160*f*
    posterior or posteroseptal, 151, 159*f*
    posterior, in coronary sinus or middle cardiac vein, 151, 159*f*
    right lateral or anterolateral, 151, 155*f*, 158*f*
  multiple, 165−171, 170*f*
  in preexcitation variants, 172
  in Wolff-Parkinson-White syndrome, 152*f*, 172

Adenosine-sensitive atrial tachycardia, 210*f*

Adenosine-sensitive idiopathic ventricular tachycardia, 329, 330*f*
  malignant, 332*f*

Adrenergic drug infusion, junctional rhythm in, 99, 116*f*

Advanced atrioventricular block, 62−63, 74*f*
  with atrial tachycardia, 75*f*
  in inferior wall infarction, 77*f*
  with intact ventriculoatrial conduction, 75*f*

Alternating left and right bundle branch blocks, 64−65, 88*f*

Andersen-Tawil syndrome, 412−417, 423*f*
  genetics of, 411

Antiarrhythmic drugs, long QT syndromes induced by, 419−420, 434*f*

Antibiotics, long QT syndromes induced by, 419−420

Antidromic reciprocating tachycardia, 151, 153*f*, 172
  atriofascicular pathway associated with, 172, 174*f*
  latent accessory pathway in, 163*f*
  multiple accessory pathways in, 165
  reentrant pathway in, 153*f*, 172

Antihistamines, long QT syndromes induced by, 419−420

Antipsychotic drugs, long QT syndromes induced by, 419−420, 438*f*

Arrhythmia syndromes, inherited, and associated gene mutation(s), 415*t*

Arrhythmogenic right ventricular dysplasia/cardiomyopathy, ventricular tachycardia in, 371−373, 403*t*, 406*f*

Ashman phenomenon, 4, 16*f*
  atrial fibrillation with, QRS morphology, 286*f*
  atrial tachycardia associated with, 190*f*

Asynchronous pacing, polymorphic ventricular tachycardia induced by, 435, 460*f*

Atrial arrhythmia
  second-degree atrioventricular block type 2 with, 72*f*
  in Wolff-Parkinson-White syndrome, and risk for sudden cardiac death, 161−164, 165*f*

Atrial conduction abnormalities, P waves in, 1, 3*f*

Atrial fibrillation, 273
  with aberrancy and premature ventricular contractions, differentiation of, 273, 294*t*
  atypical, 284*f*
  autonomic mediation of, 273, 293*f*
  with controlled ventricular rate, 274*f*
  focal, originating in right superior pulmonary vein, 273, 278*f*
  with intermittent right bundle branch block aberrancy, 285*f*
  leading to tachycardia-induced tachycardia, 273, 292*f*
  paroxysmal, 273, 279*f*
  QRS morphology during, 273
    with aberrancy, 283*f*
    with Ashman phenomenon, 286*f*
    after catheter ablation, 284*f*
    with left atrial flutter, 284*f*
    with left bundle branch block aberrancy, 287*f*, 289*f*
    normalized, 290*f*
    with rapid ventricular rate, 282*f*
    with right bundle branch block aberrancy, 285*f*, 289*f*
    in wide complex tachycardia, 280*f*, 288*f*
  with rapid ventricular rate, 274*f*, 282*f*
  with regular ventricular rate, 273, 275*f*
    regular narrow complex rhythm in, 278*f*
  with slow ventricular rate, 275*f*
  and Wolff-Parkinson-White syndrome, 273, 291*f*

Atrial flutter, 179
  and atrial tachycardia, classification of, 180*t*
  concealed accessory pathways in, 161, 167*f*
  effect of drug therapy on, 179
  left, 284*f*
  QRS alternans in, 11−13, 26*f*
  with variable AV response, wide complex tachycardia in, 326*f*

Atrial hypertrophy, right and left, P waves in, 1, 3*t*

Atrial tachycardia, 179
  adenosine-sensitive, 210*f*
  anatomic distribution of focal, 181*f*
  and atrial flutter

  classification of, 180*t*
  in patient with history of atrial fibrillation, 216*f*
  automatic, 187*f*, 213*f*
  concealed accessory pathways in, 161, 167*f*
  drug therapy and effects on, 179
  electrophysiologic studies of, 179
  focal, 179, 186*f*
    at coronary aortic cusp, 184*f*, 191
    at coronary sinus, 183−191
      close to septum, 203*f*
      P wave morphology in, 182*f*
    at crista, 183
      high, 193*f*, 196*f*
      low, 198*f*
      mid, 197*f*
      P wave morphology in, 182*f*, 185*f*
    mitral annular, 192−193
    tricuspid annular, 183
      inferior, close to septum, 202*f*
      low lateral, 200*f*
      P wave morphology in, 182*f*
  and inappropriate sinus tachycardia, 183
  left, 182*f*, 191−194
    at inferolateral mitral annulus, 210*f*
    with left superior pulmonary vein focus, 187*f*
    at midseptal region, 211*f*
    P wave morphology in, from several sites, 185*f*
    in patient with history of atrial fibrillation, 215*f*, 217*f*
    with posterosuperior focus near right superior pulmonary vein, 212*f*
    at superomedial mitral annulus, 214*f*
  left bundle branch block aberrancy in. *See also* Wide complex tachycardia, 19*f*
    QRS morphology, 2, 10*f*, 26*f*
  localization of, 179−181
  macroreentrant, 218*f*
  multifocal, 221*f*
  noncoronary cusp origins of, 184*f*, 191, 208*f*
  P and QRS relationship during, 179
  P wave morphology in locating, 179, 180*f*
  paraseptal, with left bundle branch block aberrancy, 195*f*
  paroxysmal rapid, with wide and narrow QRS complexes, 190*f*
  pulmonary vein origin of, 194, 218*f*, 220*t*
    left superior, 187*f*, 213*f*, 217*f*
    right inferior, 215*f*
    right superior, 185*f*, 216*f*
  rapid, 212*f*
    resulting in left atrial thrombus, 191*f*
    with wide and narrow QRS complexes, 190*f*
  right, 182−183
    with focal and reentrant morphologies, 206*f*
    high focus in, 189*f*
    lateral focus in, 183, 189*f*, 190*f*, 199*f*
    low lateral focus in, 199*f*
    posterior, close to septum, 205*f*

Atrial tachycardia (*Continued*)
  with septal focus, 195*f*
  right bundle branch block aberrancy in, 18*f*, 190*f*
  second-degree atrioventricular block type 1 in, 68*f*
  septal and midline origins of, 183–191, 195*f*, 204*f*, 207*f*, 209*f*
    P wave morphology in, 182*f*
  sinus node reentrant, 183, 187*f*
  with wide and narrow QRS complexes, 191*f*
  wide complex tachycardia presenting as, 193*f*
Atriofascicular pathway, 172, 173*f*
Atriohisian accessory pathway, 174*f*
Atrioventricular block(s), 61, 62*t*, 64*f*
  2:1, 62–63, 72*b*
  advanced, 62–63
  alternating left and right bundle branch blocks, 64–65
  atrioventricular dissociation in, 66–71
  congenital, 64
  exercise-induced and paroxysmal, 66
  first-degree, 61
  pathophysiology of, 61
  right bundle branch block with alternate fascicular block, 64–65
  second-degree type 1, 61
    atypical, 61
  second-degree type 2, 62
  third-degree (complete), 63–64
  ventriculophasic sinus arrhythmia in, 71
Atrioventricular dissociation, 66–71
  four causes of, 66–71, 91*f*
  in sinus bradycardia, peaked T waves, 92*f*
  type 1, 92*f*
  type 2, 93*f*
    with idioventricular rhythm, 77*f*
  type 2 intermittent, 95*f*
  with wide complex tachycardia, diagnostic of ventricular tachycardia, 316*f*
Atrioventricular nodal reentrant tachycardia, 125, 126*f*
  anterograde and retrograde echo beats in, 129*f*
  atrial fibrillation initiated by, 273, 292*f*
  cycle length alternans in, 128–129, 143*f*
  cycle length prolongation with aberrancy in, 128
  cycle length variation during supraventricular tachycardia, 128, 142*f*
  differentiation of, from atrioventricular reentrant tachycardia, 151, 160*f*, 177*f*
  dual atrioventricular nodal physiology of, concealments and blocks, 127*f*
  effect of PVC during short R-P' tachycardia with refractory His bundle, 128, 142*f*
  left-sided AV nodal inputs in, 130–132, 146*f*
  with lower and upper common pathway block, 132–135, 147*f*
  mode of onset, heart rate variation, and SVT termination mode, 126–128, 135*f*
  P wave morphology and axis in, 128, 139*f*
  P wave position within R-R interval in, 125–126, 131*f*
    atypical AVNRT, 125, 133*f*
    slow-slow or slow-intermediate AVNRT, 126, 134*f*
    typical AVNRT, 125, 131*f*
  QRS alternans in, 130, 146*f*

QRS morphology during supraventricular tachycardia in, 130, 144*f*
  slow pathway modification in, 99, 122*f*
  tachycardia cycle length oscillations in, 128
  tachycardia rate in, 125
Atrioventricular node
  concealed conduction at. *See also* Atrioventricular reentrant tachycardia, 17, 33*f*
  enhanced conduction at, P-R interval and P-R segment in. *See also* Enhanced atrioventricular nodal conduction, 1, 7*f*
  gap phenomenon at, 14, 30*f*
Atrioventricular reentrant tachycardia, 151
  accessory pathways in, 151, 152*f*
    in atrial flutter or atrial tachycardia, 161, 167*f*
    atypical, 172, 173*f*
    bilateral, 152*f*
    bundle branch block effect on, 161, 164*f*
    in congenital anomalies, 172, 172*f*
    and enhanced atrioventricular nodal conduction, 172, 176*f*
    latent, 160*f*, 161
    localization of, 151, 155*f*
    multiple, 165–171, 170*f*
    in preexcitation variants, 172
    ventricular preexcitation and risk of ventricular fibrillation, 165, 167*f*
    in Wolff-Parkinson-White syndrome. *See also* Wolff-Parkinson-White syndrome, 152*f*, 172
  antidromic. *See also* Antidromic reciprocating tachycardia, 151, 154*f*
  differentiation of, from atrioventricular nodal reentrant tachycardia, 151, 160*f*, 177*f*
  forms of, 151
  orthodromic. *See also* Orthodromic reciprocating tachycardia, 151, 154*f*
  in Wolff-Parkinson-White syndrome, 151, 152*f*
Atypical accessory pathway(s), 172, 173*f*
Automatic atrial tachycardia, 187*f*

B
Bidirectional ventricular tachycardia, 362*t*, 432–433, 446*f*
  causes of, 453*b*, 454*f*
  exercise-induced, in long QT syndrome, 454*f*
Bifascicular block, 2, 16*t*
Bilateral bundle branch block, 2
Bilateral conduction, in accessory pathways, 152*f*
Brugada algorithm (differentiation of ventricular tachycardia from supraventricular tachycardia), 301*f*
Brugada pattern ECG, 432
  in hyperkalemia, 446*f*
  J wave in, 4, 22*f*
Brugada syndrome, 426–432, 442*t*, 443*f*
  genetics and types of, 426–432, 442*t*
Bundle branch block(s), 2–4, 14*t*
  alternating left and right, 64–65, 88*f*
  bilateral, 2
  effect of
    on accessory pathways, 161, 164*f*
    in orthodromic reciprocating tachycardia, 161, 164*f*
  junctional rhythm in presence of, 99, 101*f*
  left, 15*f*

pattern and wave morphologies in structural heart disease ventricular tachycardia, 361, 366*f*
  right, 13*f*
Bundle branch reentrant ventricular tachycardia, 369–370
  resting ECG in, 361
  types of, 361, 394*t*, 397*f*

C
Calcium ion transport dysfunction, and associated genetic mutations, 415*t*
Cardiac arrhythmia syndromes, inherited, and associated gene mutation(s), 415*t*
Cardiac conduction disease, 61
Carotid sinus hypersensitivity, sinus node dysfunction in, 38*t*, 55*f*
Catecholaminergic polymorphic ventricular tachycardia, 432–433, 452*f*
  bidirectional ventricular tachycardia in, 432–433, 446*f*
Cerebrovascular accidents, long QT syndrome in, 420–421, 438*f*
Chronotropic incompetence, 37, 38*t*, 54*f*
Circus movement tachycardia, 151
Concealed conduction. *See also* Accessory pathway(s), concealed, 14–17
  at atrioventricular node, 17, 33*f*
  at His-Purkinje level, 17, 34*f*
Congenital anomalies, accessory pathways in, 172, 172*f*
Congenital atrioventricular block, 64, 85*f*
Congenital heart repair, late ventricular tachycardia in, 373–375, 408*f*
Congenital junctional tachycardia, 99, 118*f*
Congenital long QT syndrome, 411, 413*f*
  and associated gene mutation(s), 415*t*
  with deafness (Jervell and Lange-Neilsen syndrome), 413*f*
  gene specific ECG patterns in, 411, 417*f*
  LQTS9 and LQTS12 in, 418–419, 426*f*
  LQTS7 (Andersen-Tawil syndrome) in, 412–417, 423*f*
  LQTS1 through LQTS5 in, 411–420, 414*f*
  LQTS8 (Timothy syndrome) in, 418–419, 424*f*
  presentation of, 411, 413*f*
  sudden death after physical exertion or emotional stress in, 411, 422*f*
  variant T wave morphologies in, 411, 422*f*
Coronary artery disease, 9–11
  J wave in, 4
  monomorphic ventricular tachycardia in, 361, 368–369, 391*f*
  polymorphic ventricular tachycardia in, 369, 393*f*

D
Deceleration (bradycardia)-dependent blocks or delays, 4, 20*f*
Deceleration-dependent aberrancy, 289*f*
Delta wave, 151, 152*f*
  in localization of accessory pathways, 151, 155*f*
  in Wolff-Parkinson-White syndrome, 152*f*
Dextrocardia, 9
  P waves in, 1, 4*f*
Digitalis toxicity, junctional rhythm in, 99, 115*f*

E

Early repolarization, J wave in, 4, 20*f*
Ebstein anomaly, 165–171, 172*f*
Electrocardiography, 1
 of atrial fibrillation, 273
 of atrial flutter, 223
 of atrial tachycardias, 179
 of atrioventricular conduction abnormalities,
  61
 of atrioventricular nodal reentrant tachycardia
  (AVNRT), 125
 of bundle branch blocks and fascicular blocks,
  2, 14*t*
 of concealed accessory pathways, Wolff-
  Parkinson-White syndrome, and variants,
  151
 of concealed conduction, 14–17
 in coronary artery disease, 9–11
 in electrolyte imbalance, 13–14
 of fascicular blocks, 4
 gap phenomenon in, 14
 of generalized low voltage, 9
 of idiopathic ventricular tachycardia, 329
 J point and J wave in, 4
 of junctional tachycardia, 99
 of multifascicular blocks, 2–4, 16*t*
 normal 12-lead, 1, 2*f*, 2*t*, 14
 P waves in, 1
 of parasystole, 14
 of polymorphic ventricular tachycardia and
  ventricular fibrillation, 411
 P-R interval and P-R segment in, 1
 Q waves in, 2
 QRS alternans and T wave alternans in, 11–13
 QRS complexes in, 1–2
 Q-T interval in, 5–8
 right sided precordial lead placement, 9
 of sinus node dysfunction, 37
 ST and T waves in, 4–5
 of supernormal conduction, 36
 U wave in, 4
 of unexpected facilitation of conduction,
  17–35
 in ventricular hypertrophy, 8, 23*b*, 23*t*
 of ventricular tachycardia in normal heart, 329
 of ventricular tachycardia in structural heart
  disease, 361
 of wide complex tachycardia, 297
Electrolyte imbalance, 13–14, 21*f*
 long QT syndromes associated with, 419–420
  hypocalcemia, 419, 431*f*
  hypokalemia, 419, 428*f*
  hypomagnesemia, 419
Enhanced atrioventricular nodal conduction
 P-R interval and P-R segment in, 1, 7*f*
 and putative Lown-Ganong-Levine syndrome,
  172, 176*f*
Epicardial ventricular tachycardia, in nonischemic
 cardiomyopathy, 371, 402*f*
Epsilon waves, 371–373, 408*f*
Exercise-induced heart block, 66, 91*f*

F

Fascicular block(s), 2–4, 14*t*
Fascicular ventricular tachycardia
 and papillary muscle ventricular tachycardia,
  differentiation of, 329, 360*t*
 verapamil-sensitive idiopathic, 340, 359*f*

 wide complex tachycardia in, 304*f*
First-degree atrioventricular block, 61, 64*f*
 junctional rhythm manifesting as, 99, 110*f*
Flutter waves, 223
Fragmented QRS complexes, 2
 representing anteroseptal and inferoposterior
  scar, 12*f*
 representing inferior myocardial scar, 11*f*
Fragmented right bundle branch block, 12*f*
Frequent atrial premature complexes, 1, 6*f*
Frequent single monomorphic premature
  ventricular complexes, 433–434, 457*f*
Fusion complexes, 367*f*

G

Gap phenomenon, 14, 30*f*
 at atrioventricular node, 14, 30*f*
Generalized low voltage, 9

H

His bundle tachycardia, 99
His-Purkinje bundles, concealed conduction at.
  See also Accessory pathway(s), concealed,
  17, 34*f*
Hypercalcemia, 14, 29*f*
 short QT syndrome in patient with, 423–426,
  441*f*
Hyperkalemia, 14, 27*f*
 Brugada pattern ECG in patient with, 446*f*
 sinus junctional escape rhythm associated with,
  41*f*
Hypertrophic cardiomyopathy, inherited, multiple
  accessory pathways in, 172, 173*f*
Hypocalcemia, 14, 28*f*
 long QT syndrome associated with, 419, 431*f*
Hypokalemia, 14, 27*f*
 long QT syndromes associated with, 419, 428*f*
Hypomagnesemia, long QT syndrome associated
  with, 419
Hypothermia, J wave in, 4, 21*f*

I

Idiopathic ventricular tachycardia, 329–340
 adenosine-sensitive, 329, 330*f*
 electrocardiography and sites of origin in,
  329–340, 333*t*
  aortic cusp, 334, 353*f*
  epicardial, 334
   coronary sinus and cardiac veins, 340, 356*f*
   crux, 340, 358*f*
   left ventricular outflow tract, 334–340
   right ventricular, 340
  left ventricular, 330, 345*f*
  left ventricular outflow tract, 330–331
   aortomitral continuity, 348*f*
   lateral, 347*f*
   septal, 346*f*
  mitral annular, 331–334, 350*f*
  papillary muscles, 334, 351*f*
  parahisian ventricular, 330, 331*f*
  pulmonary artery, 329–330, 341*f*
  right lateral ventricular, 330, 344*f*
  right septal ventricular, 330, 342*f*
  right ventricular outflow tract, 329, 334*f*
   anterior, 335*f*
   lateral, 340*f*
   posterior, 337*f*

  septal, 336*f*
  tricuspid annular, 330
  verapamil-sensitive, 340, 359*f*
Idioventricular rhythm, junctional rhythm
  presenting as, 99, 101*f*
Inappropriate sinus tachycardia, 183
 syndrome of, 58, 58*f*
Intraventricular conduction delays
 junctional rhythm in presence of, 99, 101*f*
 QRS complexes in, 2–4, 10*f*
Isorhythmic atrioventricular dissociation
 P-R interval and P-R segment in, 1, 9*f*
 in same junctional and sinus rate, 99, 105*f*

J

J point, 4
J wave, 4
 in Brugada pattern, 22*f*
 in early repolarization, 20*f*
 in hypothermia, 21*f*
 in methadone overdose and severe acidosis, 21*f*
Jervell and Lange-Neilsen syndrome, 413*f*
 ECG during syncopal episode, 414*f*
 genetics of, 411
Junctional ectopic tachycardia, 99
Junctional rhythm, 99, 101*f*
 in adrenergic drug infusion, 99, 116*f*
 in digitalis toxicity, 99, 115*f*
 and junctional tachycardia with different
  ventriculoatrial intervals (with P wave
  positions), 99, 104*f*
 manifesting as first-degree or type 2 second-
  degree AV block, 99, 110*f*
 in myocardial ischemia, 99, 114*f*
 in presence of bundle branch block or
  intraventricular conduction delays, 101*f*
 presenting as idioventricular rhythm, 99, 101*f*
 with retrograde atrial echo, 99, 120*f*
 and same sinus rate, isorhythmic AV
  dissociation in, 105*f*, 109*f*
 in septal ventricular tachycardia, 99, 116*f*
 in slow pathway modification of
  atrioventricular nodal reentrant
  tachycardia, 99, 122*f*
Junctional tachycardia, 99
 in complex congenital heart disease, 99, 118*f*
 junctional rhythm and, with different
  ventriculoatrial intervals (with P wave
  positions), 99, 104*f*
 paroxysmal, after aortic valve surgery, 99, 119*f*
 presenting as wide complex tachycardia, 327*f*

L

Latent accessory pathway(s), 160*f*, 161
Left atrium (LA), 260*f*
Left bundle branch block, 2, 14*t*, 15*f*, 20*f*
 rate related, 4, 19*f*
 sinus rhythm with, 16*f*
Left ventricular assist devices, ventricular
  tachycardia in patients with, 376, 410*f*
Lev-Lenègre disease, 61
LGL syndrome, 172
Long QT syndrome(s), 411–420
 acquired (electrolyte imbalance, antiarrhythmic
  drugs). *See also* Antiarrhythmic drugs,
  long QT syndromes induced by,
  419–420

Long QT syndrome(s) (*Continued*)
  fragmented QRS in, 419, 427*f*
  in cerebrovascular accidents, 420–421, 438*f*
  congenital or inherited, 411, 413*f*
    and associated gene mutation(s), 415*t*
    with deafness (Jervell and Lange-Neilsen syndrome), 413*f*
    gene specific ECG patterns in, 411, 417*f*
    LQTS9 and LQTS12 in, 418–419, 426*f*
    LQTS7 (Andersen-Tawil syndrome) in, 412–417, 423*f*
    LQTS1 through LQTS5 in, 411–420, 414*f*
    LQTS8 (Timothy syndrome) in, 418–419, 424*f*
    presentation of, 411, 413*f*
    sudden death after physical exertion or emotional stress in, 411, 422*f*
    variant T wave morphologies in, 411, 422*f*
  diagnostic criteria of, 411, 417*t*
  exercise-induced bidirectional ventricular tachycardia in, 454*f*
  in hypertrophic cardiomyopathy, 419, 427*f*
  in ventricular preexcitation, 419, 427*f*

M
Mahaim fibers, 172
Manifest accessory pathways, 151, 152*f*
Maze surgery, for atrial fibrillation, post surgery P waves, 1, 7*f*
Mobitz type 2 atrioventricular block, 62
Monomorphic ventricular tachycardia, in coronary artery disease, 361, 362*t*, 368–369
  differentiation of focal and reentrant, 368–369, 391*f*
Multifascicular blocks, 2–4, 16*t*
  acceleration (tachycardia) dependent, 4
  Ashman phenomenon, 4, 16*f*
  deceleration (bradycardia) dependent, 4
Multifocal atrial tachycardia, 179
Myocardial infarction
  anterior wall, ventricular fibrillation in, 24*f*
  inferior wall
    complete heart block in, 24*f*
    second-degree atrioventricular block type 1 associated with, 69*f*
    wide complex tachycardia in, 327*f*
  non-ST elevation, 24*f*
  remote, ventricular fibrillation in, 25*f*
Myocardial ischemia, junctional rhythm in, 99, 114*f*
Myocardial scar, 9–11

N
Nonischemic cardiomyopathy
  epicardial ventricular tachycardia in, 371, 402*f*
  ventricular tachycardia in, 370–371, 375*f*
Nonparoxysmal junctional tachycardia, in digoxin toxicity, 277*f*
Nonsustained ventricular tachycardia, 362*t*

O
Orthodromic reciprocating tachycardia
  bundle branch block and cycle length in, 161, 164*f*
  concealed accessory pathways in, 151, 153*f*, 172–177

  in anterolateral mitral annulus, 161*f*
  in left side, 151, 160*f*
  reentrant pathway in, 153*f*
  short R-P', 161, 164*f*
  differentiation of, 172–177
Osborn wave, 4, 21*f*

P
P wave(s), 1
  in atrial conduction abnormalities, 3*f*
  in atrioventricular nodal reentrant tachycardia morphology and axis, 128, 139*f*
    position within R-R interval, 125–126, 131*f*
      atypical AVNRT, 125, 133*f*
      slow-slow or slow-intermediate AVNRT, 126, 134*f*
      typical AVNRT, 125, 131*f*
  in dextrocardia, 4*f*
  after maze procedure for atrial fibrillation, 7*f*
  normal, 1, 3*f*
  in paroxysmal atrial fibrillation, 1, 6*f*
  in wandering atrial pacemaker, 5*f*
Parasystole, 14
  intermittent ventricular, 31*f*
  intermittent, with exit block, 32*f*
  ventricular, 32*f*
Paroxysmal atrial fibrillation, P waves in, 1, 6*f*
Paroxysmal atrioventricular block, 66, 91*f*
Permanent junctional reciprocating tachycardia, 177, 177*f*
Polymorphic ventricular tachycardia, 362*t*, 369, 411, 412*f*
  asynchronous pacing-induced, 435
  Brugada syndrome in, 426–432
  catecholaminergic, 432–433
  idiopathic ventricular fibrillation in, 433–434
  long QT syndrome and torsades de pointes in. *See also* Long QT syndrome(s), 411–420
  pause-dependent torsades de pointes in, 435
  short QT syndromes in, 421–426
  short-coupled torsades de pointes in, 434
Postural orthostatic tachycardia syndrome, sinus tachycardia in, 56*f*, 58
Potassium ion channel dysfunction, and associated genetic mutations, 415*t*
P-R segment and P-R interval, 1, 2*f*
  in atrioventricular reentrant tachycardias, 151, 152*f*
  in enhanced AV nodal conduction, 7*f*
  in isorhythmic atrioventricular dissociation, 9*f*
  in ventricular preexcitation, 8*f*
Precordial lead placement, right sided, 9
Preexcitation syndrome, 151
  accessory pathways in, 152*f*
  reentrant pathway in, 153*f*
Preexcitation variants, atypical accessory pathways in, 172, 173*f*
Preexcitation, intermittent, and risk of ventricular fibrillation, 165, 167*f*
Premature ventricular complexes, 362*t*
  frequent single monomorphic, 433–434, 457*f*
Putative Lown-Ganong-Levine syndrome, 172, 176*f*

Q
Q waves, 2
QRS alternans, 11–13, 26*f*

  in atrial flutter, 26*f*
  in atrioventricular nodal reentrant tachycardia, 130, 146*f*
QRS complex(es), 1–2
  in atrial fibrillation, 273, 280*f*
  in atrioventricular reentrant tachycardias, 151, 152*f*
  in bundle branch blocks and fascicular blocks, 2, 14*t*
  conduction delay in, analytic value of, 300*f*
  in coronary artery disease, 9–11
  in differentiation of ventricular tachycardia and supraventricular tachycardia. *See also* Wide complex tachycardia, 297
  in fascicular blocks, 4
  fragmented, 2
  in generalized low voltage, 9
  in idiopathic ventricular tachycardia, 329–340, 333*t*
  in intraventricular conduction abnormalities, 2
  in multifascicular blocks, 2–4, 16*t*
  normal, 1–2, 2*f*
  and P wave relationships during atrial tachycardias, 179
  in paroxysmal rapid atrial tachycardias, 190*f*
  Q wave and duration in, 2
  in QRS alternans, 11–13
  Q-T interval of, 5–8
  in rapid atrial tachycardias, 191*f*
  ST segment in, 4–5
  in supraventricular tachycardia in AVNRT, 130, 144*f*
  in ventricular hypertrophy, 8, 23*b*, 23*t*
  in ventricular tachycardia in structural heart disease, 362–368
QRS morphology, 9
QT dispersion, 5–8
Q-T interval, 5–8, 22*f*

R
Rapid automatic tachycardia, 99
Rapid JT, 99
Retrograde atrial echo, junctional rhythm with, 99, 120*f*
Right bundle branch block, 2, 13*f*, 14*t*
  with alternating fascicular block, 64–65, 88*f*
  rate-related, 4, 18*f*, 20*f*
Right-sided precordial lead placement, 9
Right ventricular infarction, 9
Romano-Ward syndrome, genetics of, 411

S
Second-degree atrioventricular block type 1, 61, 65*f*
  associated with acute inferior myocardial infarction, 69*f*
  in atrial tachycardia, 68*f*
  atypical, 61, 65*f*, 69*f*
    concealed discharge from His bundle in, 66*f*
    long AV node Wenckebach (10:9) pattern, 69*f*
  with sinus bradycardia, 68*f*
  with variable AV conduction (4:3 to 6:5), 67*f*
Second-degree atrioventricular block type 2, 62, 71*f*
  with atrial arrhythmia, 72*f*
  junctional rhythm manifesting as, 99, 110*f*

Septal ventricular tachycardia, junctional rhythm in, 99, 116f
Severe His-Purkinje disease, 64, 88f
Short QT syndrome, 421–426
    diagnosis of, 421–423, 439f, 441t
Short R-P tachycardia versus long R-P tachycardia, 126b
Sinoatrial exit block, 37, 38t
    second-degree type 1, 50f
    second-degree type 2, 52f
Sinus arrhythmia, 37
    in child with long QT syndrome, 42f
    in normal respiration or vagal stimulation with drugs, 42f
    and normal respiratory variation of P wave in inferior leads, 43f
    in patient with dextrocardia, 43f
    with P-R prolongation during sinus slowing, 43f
Sinus atrial tachycardia, 187f
Sinus bradycardia, 38t
    atrioventricular dissociation in, peaked T waves, 92f
    with intermittent junctional rhythm after maze procedure, 40f
    marked, and junctional rhythm emergence, 37, 39f
    marked, with ST elevation in coronary artery occlusion, 41f
    after mitral valve replacement, 40f
    with prolonged QTc, in amiodarone therapy, 41f
    second-degree atrioventricular block type 1 with, 68f
    in well-trained athletes, 37, 38f
Sinus junctional escape rhythm, associated with hyperkalemia, 41f
Sinus node dysfunction, 37, 38t
    in carotid sinus hypersensitivity, 38t
    in chronotropic incompetence, 37
    in sinoatrial exit block, 37
    in sinus arrhythmia, 37
    in sinus bradycardia and junctional escape rhythms, 37
    in sinus tachycardia, 38–57
    in tachycardia-bradycardia syndrome, 38t
    in ventriculophasic sinus arrhythmia, 37
Sinus node reentrant tachycardia, 38–57, 183, 187f
    in patient with nonischemic cardiomyopathy, 55f
    in patient with normal heart, 55f
    in postural orthostatic tachycardia syndrome, 56f
Sinus pause, or sinus arrest, 38t, 47f
    in presentation of seizure disorder, 48f
    simultaneous EEG and ECG in seizure disorder, 49f
Sinus rhythm, 135–148
Sodium ion channel dysfunction, and associated genetic mutations, 415t
ST segment, 4–5
ST segment elevation, 4, 23b
ST-T waves, 4–5
    in atrioventricular reentrant tachycardias, 151, 152f
    nonspecific changes in, 5
Supernormal conduction, 36, 36f

Supraventricular tachycardia
    common QRS morphologies in, 299f
    multiple accessory pathways in. See also Atrioventricular reentrant tachycardia, 125, 126b, 151
    and ventricular tachycardia, differentiation of, 298t, 301f
Sustained ventricular tachycardia, 361, 362t
Syndrome of inappropriate sinus tachycardia, 58, 58f

T
T wave alternans, 11–13
Tachycardia-bradycardia syndrome, 38t, 53f
Tachycardia-induced tachycardia, atrial fibrillation leading to, 273, 292f
Third-degree (complete) atrioventricular block, 63–64, 76f
    after atrioventricular nodal–blocking therapy, 85f
    in calcium blocker therapy, 84f
    in His-Purkinje system, 79f
    paroxysmal, in severe His-Purkinje disease, 80f
    retrograde P waves in, 85f
    in sarcoidosis, 83f
    in severe conduction disease or drug toxicity, 82f
    in sinus rhythm with pauses up to 17 seconds, 81f
    in vagal maneuver, 80f
    3:1 with prolonged P-R interval, left bundle branch block, left axis deviation, 79f
Timothy syndrome, 418–419, 424f
    genetics of, 411
Torsades de pointes, 362t, 411–420
    associated with hypokalemia in patient with diabetic ketoacidosis, 430f
    induced by antiarrhythmic drugs, 419–420, 434f, 437f
    nonsustained and sustained, 413f
    pause-dependent, 435, 460f
    short-coupled, 434, 457f
Trifascicular block, 2, 16t

U
U wave, 4
Unexpected facilitation of conduction, 17–35

V
Vagal stimulation, J wave in, 4
Ventricular aberrancy, 2–4
Ventricular arrhythmias, 361, 362t
Ventricular fibrillation. See also Polymorphic ventricular tachycardia, 362t, 369, 411
    disorders causing, in structurally normal heart, 412t
    idiopathic, 412f, 433–434, 456f
    intermittent preexcitation and risk of, 165, 167f
Ventricular flutter, 362t
Ventricular hypertrophy, left and right, QRS complexes in, 8, 23b, 23t
Ventricular preexcitation
    long QT syndrome associated with, 419, 427f
    P-R interval and P-R segment in, 1, 8f
    and risk of ventricular fibrillation in atrial flutter or fibrillation, 165, 167f
Ventricular tachycardia
    in arrhythmogenic right ventricular dysplasia/cardiomyopathy, 371–373, 403t, 406f

bidirectional, 432–433, 446f
bundle branch reentrant, 369–370
    resting ECG in, 361
    types of, 361, 394t, 397f
common QRS morphologies in. See also Wide complex tachycardia, 299f
epicardial, in nonischemic cardiomyopathy, 371, 402f
idiopathic, 329–340
    adenosine sensitive, 329, 330f
    electrocardiography and sites of origin. See also Idiopathic ventricular tachycardia, 329–340, 333t
    verapamil-sensitive, 340, 359f
late, after repair of congenital heart disease, 373–375, 408f
monomorphic, in coronary artery disease, 361, 368–369, 391f
in nonischemic cardiomyopathy, 370–371, 375f
in patients with left ventricular assist devices, 376, 410f
septal, junctional rhythm in, 99, 116f
of structural heart disease, 361, 362t
    algorithmic analysis of, 361, 366f
    electrocardiographic analysis of, 361–368, 363t
    electrocardiography and sites of origin. See also Ventricular tachycardia of structural heart disease, electrocardiography and sites of origin, 361, 363f
and supraventricular tachycardia, differentiation of, 298t, 301f
and ventricular fibrillation
    in coronary artery disease, 369, 393f
    in structurally normal heart, 412t
Ventricular tachycardia of structural heart disease, electrocardiography and sites of origin, 361, 363f
    epicardial with right bundle branch block
        left superior axis, inferobasal left ventricle, 388f
        right inferior axis, basal anterior left ventricle, 389f
    with left bundle branch block, inferior axis, anterior left ventricle, 371f
    with left bundle branch block, left superior axis
        apical left ventricle, near septum, 368f
        inferior left ventricle, mid-septum, 377f
        at mitral annulus, close to septum, 368f
        posterior left ventricle, near mitral annulus, 379f
        right ventricular origin, near mid-septum, 372f
    with left bundle branch block, right axis deviation, apical left ventricle, near septum, 369f
    with left bundle branch block, right inferior axis
        anterior septum, 381f
        mid-anterior septum, 371f
        at mitral isthmus, 372f
    with narrow QRS
        inferior apex of left ventricle, 390f
        septal ventricular tachycardia, 367f
    with right bundle branch block, inferior axis, anterolateral base of left ventricle, 373f
    with right bundle branch block, left superior axis, inferior left ventricle at mid-septum, 378f

Ventricular tachycardia of structural heart disease, electrocardiography and sites of origin (*Continued*)
  inferolateral left ventricle, 375*f*
  inferoposterior left ventricle, near mitral annulus, 380*f*
  inferoseptal, near mitral valve, 374*f*
  with right bundle branch block, right inferior axis, variations in same patient, 387*f*
  with right bundle branch block, right superior axis, mid-inferior left ventricle, 383*f*, 385*f*
  with right bundle branch block, superior axis, inferior septum, 370*f*
Ventriculophasic sinus arrhythmia, in advanced atrioventricular block, 37, 44*f*, 71, 97*f*

W
Wandering atrial pacemaker, 221*f*
  P waves representing, 5*f*
Wenckebach block. *See* Second-degree atrioventricular block type 1
When Brugada syndrome, 9
Wide complex tachycardia, 280*f*, 297
  with acceleration-dependent right bundle branch block and left posterior fascicular block, 311*f*

in acute inferior myocardial infarction, 327*f*
in atrial flutter with variable AV response, 326*f*
atrial tachycardia presenting as, 193*f*
with atrioventricular dissociation, in ventricular tachycardia, 316*f*
and differentiation of ventricular tachycardia from supraventricular tachycardia, 298*t*
irregular, in sudden cardiac death, 328*f*
junctional tachycardia presenting as, 327*f*
with left bundle branch block pattern
  in atrial tachycardia in low right atrial wall, 312*f*
  in atrial tachycardia in right lateral wall, 313*f*
  in sinus tachycardia during exacerbation of heart failure, 314*f*
with positive and negative concordances, in ventricular tachycardia, 317*f*
QRS conduction delay and QRS analysis of, 300*f*
with right bundle branch block pattern
  in atrial fibrillation with variation in cycle length, 324*f*
  in atrial flutter with right axis deviation, 323*f*
  in atrial flutter with variable AV response, 322*f*

in atrial tachycardia with variable atrioventricular block, 310*f*
in atrial tachycardia with ventricular aberrancy, 309*f*
diagnostic for ventricular tachycardia, 307*f*
in fascicular ventricular tachycardia, 304*f*
in reentrant ventricular tachycardia, 308*f*
in supraventricular tachycardia, 303*f*
with sinus capture and fusion beats, 316*f*
with slurred upstroke, in ventricular tachycardia originating in inferior left ventricle, 325*f*
in ventricular tachycardia, 315*f*, 321*f*
  in patient with myocardial infarction history, 193*f*
  with retrograde ventriculoatrial conduction, 320*f*
Wolff-Parkinson-White syndrome, 151, 172
  accessory pathways in, 152*f*, 172, 172*f*
  atrial fibrillation in, 273, 291*f*
  latent accessory pathway in, 161, 163*f*
  pattern, 151
  supraventricular tachycardias associated with, 153*f*
  ventricular fibrillation and sudden cardiac death in, 161–164, 165*f*